ICONOCLAST

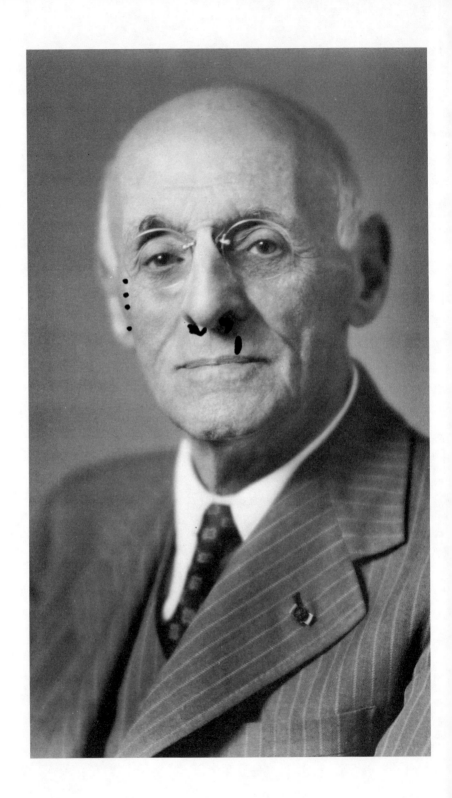

Thomas Neville Bonner

Iconoclast

ABRAHAM FLEXNER AND A LIFE IN LEARNING

The Johns Hopkins University Press
Baltimore and London

Frontispiece: *Abraham Flexner. Courtesy Rockefeller Archive Center.*

© 2002 The Johns Hopkins University Press
All rights reserved. Published 2002
Printed in the United States of America on acid-free paper
9 8 7 6 5 4 3 2 1

The Johns Hopkins University Press
2715 North Charles Street
Baltimore, Maryland 21218-4363
www.press.jhu.edu

Library of Congress Cataloging-in-Publication Data
Bonner, Thomas Neville.
Iconoclast: Abraham Flexner and a life in learning / Thomas Neville Bonner
   p.   cm.
Includes bibliographical references (p.   ) and index.
ISBN 0-8018-7124-7 (hardcover: alk. paper)
1. Flexner, Abraham, 1866–1959.
2. Educators—United States—Biography.
I. Title.
LB875.F583 B66 2002
370′.92—dc21

                                        2002003252

A catalog record for this book is
available from the British Library.

Members of a noble profession

V. James Morgan
Vice-Principal, Monroe High School
Rochester, NY, 1940–41

and

Perley C. Perkins
Professor and Debate Coach
Middlebury College, 1941–42

who helped to bend the twig

Contents

Introduction ix

1 "Our Children Will Justify Us" 1

2 A University Like No Other 20

3 Mr. Flexner's School 32

4 Breaking Free 48

5 A Legend Is Born 69

6 Master of the Survey 91

7 A Secure Berth—at Last 114

8 At the Pinnacle 144

9 A Fall from Olympus 175

10 Phoenix Rising 213

11 A Last Hurrah 236

12 Final Battles 264

13 "I Burn That I May Be of Use" 290

Notes 311

A Note on Sources 353

The Published Writings of Abraham Flexner 359

Acknowledgments 361

Index 363

Illustrations appear following p. 174.

Introduction

In 1939, the year I passed my sixteenth birthday, Abraham Flexner departed from the national scene. I could not have foreseen how closely my life would be connected with his. Flexner was stepping down after nine eventful years as the founding director of the Institute for Advanced Study in Princeton, New Jersey. Millions knew him as the man who brought Einstein to America.

For thirty years Abraham Flexner had stood in the limelight as reformer and critic of the way Americans learn, from elementary school through postgraduate study. No one raised so many questions that have persisted into our own time. Many of them directly affected my life and work.

How are children best taught? What should they learn, and when should they learn it? Should all children be taught the same thing? Do only those planning on college need to know foreign languages or history or science or mathematics? What standard should be set for the graduate? What is the teacher's role? How should teachers be taught? How important is class size? Why do Americans spend more time in school than others, with no better results?

He asked other questions.

What of the American college? Is it a place to get a broadly liberal education, or does it represent an unnecessary postponement of serious study? And the American university? Is it a uniquely democratic opening of higher education or an undigested potpourri of academic and vocational study? How is professional study, especially for doctors, best structured to produce a scientifically trained and practical yet humane practitioner? What institutional arrangements stimulate the most rapid advances in research?

These questions affected, and still affect, millions of Americans. Sixty years later, they are the subject of acrimonious debate.

Although I did not know it, I grew up in an atmosphere much influenced by Flexner. His questions applied very personally to me. In the public schools of Rochester, New York, educators were strongly affected by the stream of influences coming from the experimental Lincoln School in New York City. The school, founded in 1917, was built on Flexner's ideas and supported at his behest by the philanthropy of John D. Rockefeller. Many of the principles behind the school were derived from the private school Flexner had opened in Louisville in 1892, four years before John Dewey launched his Laboratory School at the University of Chicago.

Flexner taught that students learn best through activities of mind and body rather than traditional "bookish" learning and daily recitations. Rote teaching and memorization should give way to more imaginative teaching; the teacher was extremely important; Latin and other traditional studies are of little value in the twentieth century; science should be taught by experimenting and by observing objects in nature; every student profits from such real-world skills as shopwork and dressmaking; children learn best in small groups and at their own pace, never in lockstep. The schooling Flexner proposed was highly individualized and aimed at better training of the mind—it was not "soft" or "lacking in vigor." It was important, and it was expensive.

In my own schooling, I remember the pride I felt when both teacher and principal praised an apron I made in an elementary grade. I recall with pleasure the "activity projects" that took us out of routine, and the frequent trips to museums and local industries. A memorable course in "sex hygiene" (in 1936!) was taught by the basketball coach, a man we all admired. I enrolled in a course in woodworking in high school and earned my only failing grade. "Current events" was a staple of every class in "social studies." I learned to read a newspaper. To learn at a faster rate, I was "skipped" over two half-grades in elementary school and found myself in the company of older, more assured classmates.

In the seventh grade, I was summoned with my mother to the office of the school psychologist, herself influenced by the Lincoln School, who explained that I was being taken out of the classroom altogether and placed in an "experimental" group that encouraged children to proceed at their own pace. We would work in the library and seek help only when needed. Two weeks later, I pleaded tearfully to return to the comfort of a structured curriculum and classroom.

I was not prepared for so radical a learning environment. Mine was a home without books, my parents had not finished elementary school, and for seven long years we were recipients of federal "relief" from the nation's first national welfare program. No one in my neighborhood, parent or child, had ever gone to college. I never carried books to and from school (I relied on study halls), so as not to betray any interest in schoolwork. Like most of my contemporaries, I did not question the largely academic education I was given, though I had no expectation of ever going to college. I took for granted that schooling would provide the mental skills and knowledge needed to live the fullest life open to me. There were no separate "tracks" for those bound for different stations in life.

On graduation from high school a year after Flexner's retirement, I went to work, as expected, in a neighborhood grocery store. I spent nearly two years at menial jobs and made a largely fruitless attempt to begin a college education. I enrolled briefly as a day student at the local university with the help of a full scholarship, made possible by the intervention, long after my graduation from high school, of the school's vice-principal (to whom, along with another educational Samaritan, this book is dedicated). Each day, as I went to class, I took the long bus ride to the end of the line at the University of Rochester medical school, and from there I walked to the university's main campus.

The school of medicine in Rochester owed its very existence to a deal struck by Flexner with the local Kodak camera king, George Eastman. In the 1920s Flexner had persuaded Eastman to join in the launching of an entirely new school of medicine with full-time appointments in the clinical sciences. At its head was George H. Whipple, who had won a Nobel Prize for his work on pernicious anemia. Whipple was still dean when I arrived in 1942. Years later, I would listen to a recorded memoir in which he credited Flexner with his decision to come to Rochester.

America owes to Flexner, more than any other person, the rapid implementation of the full-time medical school, allied to a teaching hospital, and integrated into a university. It was he who defined what a medical school should and should not be. His 1910 report on medical education remains, even after ninety years, a remarkably well-known study.

The questions he raised about medical education still reverberate. How are scientific principles best joined to clinical problem solving and broadly liberal knowledge in a doctor's education? How long and by what steps should a student prepare to practice medicine? What part of training should be spent in learning about disease prevention and health promotion, what part about treating illness? Should the boundary between preclinical courses (anatomy, physiology) and clinical study (medicine, surgery) be relatively firm, or can learning proceed simultaneously in both fields? How much free election of studies should be encouraged? How is new scientific knowledge best incorporated into the medical curriculum? Should clinical teachers devote all, most, or part of their time to teaching and research? Is there an essential place in the curriculum for humanistic studies, communication skills, and the history of medicine?

In the twenty-first century, a writer in a study by the Association of American Medical Colleges and the Milbank Memorial Fund asks, in words that could have been Flexner's, whether it is possible to maintain a "nurturing learning environment" where teachers have enough time to teach, learners have enough time to learn, and leaders care more about service to patients than cash flow or market share.[1] Flexner's questions remain.

My future, like those of many in my generation, was changed by war. My brief career in college abruptly ended when I began my military service. After three years in the army, I returned home certain that this time I would finish college. The GI bill made possible a belated A.B. and then a Ph.D. degree. The University of Rochester generously granted credit for courses I had left unfinished before my service and for a year of "physical education" while in the army. Like Abraham Flexner, I was awarded my undergraduate degree after having spent barely two years in residence.

In my final year as an undergraduate, I first encountered Abraham Flexner himself, in a book called *The American College*. I learned, strange as it seemed to me then, that he believed the American college to be a largely useless prolongation of high school, a patchwork of random courses without a core of common learning. Such weird and unfamiliar charges, it seemed to me, were hardly to be taken seriously.

I did not know then that as teacher and administrator I would confront the same issues over the next forty years. What *is* the purpose of a liberal arts college? How much "general education" does a student need? Should every student be made to take a "core curriculum" of subjects and, if so, what subjects? Can narrowly trained faculty members serve as effective advisers to students confronted with cafeteria-like choices of subjects? Can academic politics be kept out of the setting of curriculum requirements? As I write these lines, I have before me the words, written just a few weeks ago, of Jacques Barzun, the long-time professor and provost of Columbia University. No one today, he writes, "knows what a college is," and it is "social lunacy" to try to define its meaning.[2]

In my graduate study at Northwestern University, I encountered Abraham Flexner once more. In writing a dissertation on the history of Chicago medicine, I became sharply aware of his famous report of 1910 on medical education. Chicago, with its fourteen medical schools, he had called the "plague spot of the nation."[3] I took issue with Flexner's claims, calling them "exaggerated." I accused him of making hurried inspections. I charged that he had prepared his conclusions a priori.[4] But in the following pages, I tell a different story.

After graduate school I encountered him again and again. New generations of students and readers found value in the questions he raised. In teaching the history of America's schools and colleges, I was struck by how pervasively his ideas had seeped into the ways in which my colleagues, as well as Americans generally, think about learning, from kindergarten to postgraduate study. At times I grew irritated with his relentless attacks on the "contradictory" character of public schools, the "uselessness" of the American college, and the "confusion" of the American university. But the questions he raised were endlessly provocative—and they have never been fully answered.

When I came to write the history of medicine in Kansas, I again found that he had wreaked havoc in that state. Virtually all of the schools in the Kansas City area were, in Flexner's opinion, "utterly wretched." The medical college in Topeka, he said, had a dissecting room indescribably filthy and, aside from "a single, badly hacked cadaver," it was "used as a chicken yard."[5] At one point, I sought his personal counsel (he was then close to 90) about a book I planned on the study of American doctors in Germany. He responded promptly with suggestions of specific books and persons who might be of help, and sent me a copy, now dog-eared, of his 1910 report. I wish now that I had gone to see him. As historian and provost at the University of Cincinnati, I came to know the heritage of President Charles Dabney, who worked with Flexner to create the modern medical center in that city.

Over the years, as president of several colleges and universities, I found myself periodically returning to Flexner's 1930 book criticizing American universities and comparing them with those of England and Germany. I used the book in a course I taught in the German university at Freiburg in the 1980s. More recently, in a study of comparative medical education in Europe and America, I paid tribute to the book Flexner had written on the same subject seventy years before.

I learned of his concern for the education of African Americans and how he helped to keep alive the remaining schools for educating black physicians, at Meharry Medical College in Nashville and Howard University in Washington, D.C. So powerful was his influence that the nation's foremost black scientist called him "the dictator in all matters concerning Negro education."[6]

My own repeated encounters with Abraham Flexner are not special or unique—except to me. Rather, they indicate the depth of his influence on Americans seeking to improve their world and education in particular. They show the remarkable impact, often unrealized, of an extraordinary individual on generations of Americans. "No one of our generation," said Henry James, nephew of the novelist, "has rattled the bones in the academic closet so effectively."[7]

Who was Abraham Flexner? How did he come to play such a multitude of significant roles in American learning? His climb to fame was slow and halting. He was born in Louisville in 1866, the son of hard-pressed immigrants, and was brought up in the Reconstruction South. Nothing in his background distinguished him. He was a Jew in a consciously Christian world. He was imperfectly educated and burdened into middle age by family responsibilities. He was a teacher and schoolmaster for nearly twenty years. Not until the age of forty-four did he burst on the national scene as the scourge of medical education. Only his companionate, often transatlantic, marriage to the Louisville playwright Anne Crawford, whose best-known play dominated Broadway for seven seasons, enabled him to escape the ties that bound him to his childhood home and family. Together, they raised two remarkable daughters who won fame in their own right.

Flexner owed his success not to education or family or chance—the forces that Flexner himself credited with propelling him to such a high position—but to the power of his mind. His intellect and his unmatched instinct for new organizational possibilities enabled him to see new relationships among the separate worlds of education, business, government, professional life, and philanthropy. He was one of a small number of persons, such as the British John Maynard Keynes in economic matters and William Beveridge in unemployment and health policy, and the American Wilbur Cohen in health and social legislation, who moved across intellectual boundaries while working with great organizations. They stimulated new approaches to the great policy questions facing health, science, education, and welfare in the modern age. It was Flexner's genius to create and help implement new models of organization to improve education, train better doctors, and bring science into the hospitals. In this respect, he was a very modern figure who combined "real intellectual power with vision and action in the public sphere."[8]

No one was more successful than he in raising money for educational purposes. Persuasive, charming, at times nearly hypnotic in promoting his ideas, he was unmatched in his skill at wooing owners of great fortunes. He won the confidence of Andrew Carnegie, the John D. Rockefellers, *père* and *fils,* J. P. Morgan, George Eastman, Robert Brookings, Julius Rosenwald, and other benefactors of American learning. As a principal agent of Rockefeller beneficence, he distributed the equivalent of more than a billion dollars in today's currency to medical schools and other educational projects, and helped raise several times that amount in matching funds and fundraising efforts. Never had a representative of learning moved so surefootedly amidst the places of great power and influence. At the peak of his power, his word was virtually law across broad swaths of education and medicine.

Abraham Flexner's encounter with his times is the stuff of heroic legend. He walks these pages not only with the Rockefellers and Carnegies but with such figures as Albert Einstein, John von Neumann, Charles A. Lindbergh, John Dewey, Charles W. Eliot of Harvard, Nicholas Murray Butler of Columbia, the historians Arnold Toynbee and Charles A. Beard, the Egyptologist James H. Breasted, the geneticist Thomas Hunt Morgan, and the pathologist William Henry Welch. The conflict among the mammoth egos of these men creates the backdrop for drama. Flexner was never awed by the formidable figures with whom he shared the stage.

The combative schoolmaster from Louisville quarreled with Einstein, forced Felix Frankfurter from the board of the Institute for Advanced Study, and feuded with the American Medical Association's Arthur Dean Bevan, perhaps the most powerful man in American medicine, threatening to create an organization that would rival the American Medical Association. He humiliated before his own board the iron-willed Frederick T. Gates, right-hand man to John D. Rockefeller. He refused all aid to A. Lawrence Lowell, president of Harvard University, whom he found insufferable for his stubborn insistence on Harvard's privileged place in the educational world. He debated at length the purpose of a university with the eminent historian Charles A. Beard. He turned down, without consulting the invitee, an invitation for Einstein to lunch with President Franklin D. Roosevelt. To him, the renowned president of Columbia University Nicholas Murray Butler was a "Tammany politician" who lacked both ideas and common sense, while John Dewey was an able but indecipherable writer on education who repeated the same ideas for thirty years. Seldom has history produced a figure who so thoroughly enjoyed controversy and intellectual jousting with those around him.

Understandably, his life has caught the attention of historians. But their attention has focused on one or another of his contributions—on medical education, as in the work of Kenneth Ludmerer and Steven Wheatley, or on the Lincoln School, as in the writings of Lawrence Cremin, or on the Institute for Advanced Study. But these achievements have remained separate, unconnected, with little sense of the man behind them. When joined together, they form a story of a man of enormous significance for the twentieth century.

It is indeed a marvel that so rich and colorful a life, so full of contradictions, has found no biographer. The issues with which Abraham Flexner wrestled, readers will find, are as fresh as today's headlines. He confronted and tried to solve major social problems—and his story challenges us to do the same. He did much good in the world. Can the world today hope for a similar figure, someone with the vision and the fortitude, the ideals and the pragmatic skills, to make a difference?

ICONOCLAST

1

"Our Children Will Justify Us"

In the spring of 1940, in the quiet of his New York study, Abraham Flexner reflected on the seventy-four crowded years that lay behind him. He was struck, he said, by the strange turnings that had brought him to this point in life. For nearly forty years, more than half his life, he had grown up, studied, taught school, and run a private academy in Louisville, Kentucky. Then, suddenly, he was catapulted almost overnight from obscurity to national and international fame as a reformer of medical education, though he was not a physician. He went on to become a leading critic of America's colleges, though he had spent only two years in college himself. Finally, he was the founder of the Institute for Advanced Study, in Princeton, though he was never a research scholar.

A wild roller-coaster ride had turned his life upside down, brought him great success, and baffled his efforts to explain it. From inauspicious beginnings, he had gone on to encounter some of the giant figures of twentieth-century life. Nothing puzzled him more, he said, than the great distance that separated him and his remarkable brothers from their obscure origins in an immigrant ghetto in the post–Civil War South. All the children had made a significant mark on their times. All had moved far up the social ladder. In a time of heroic achievement by immigrant families, the Flexners nevertheless stood out. No fewer than five members of the close-knit family were listed in *Who's Who in America*. Remarkably, all of them reached success late in life and with little formal education. How did it happen?

It all began with Flexner's parents. The years did not dim the admiration and respect he felt for them. Never would he understand, he said, the courage and confidence with which they had confronted so unpromising a future. Somehow, they had "faced facts, endured, clung to ideals, and acted fearlessly."[1] Nine children had been born between 1859 and 1873 to Moritz and Esther Flexner, struggling German-Jewish immigrants, in the politically torn border city of Louisville.

They lived in a small Jewish island in a moderately prosperous community convulsed by divisions of loyalty, slavery, and war. They enjoyed only a few years of relatively comfortable living during their first quarter-century in America—years that were marked mainly by privation, struggle, and hopes deferred. All the children would survive to adulthood, itself unusual in that day. The life they led together in Louisville, the crippling adversities they suffered, and the contracted futures they faced left an enduring mark. How were they able to put behind them the limitations of their childhood and achieve so much?

The path to Louisville of Moritz and Esther Flexner, like that of so many of their friends and neighbors, began in the Orthodox Jewish enclaves of German-speaking Europe. Amid the political upheavals and pogroms beginning in the 1840s, the first wave of German Jews had swept westward from all parts of central Europe. Esther Abraham had come from the small town of Roden, a few miles from Saarlouis, in a western German outpost in the Saarland, adjacent to France, while Moritz Flexner was being reared on the opposite side of German-speaking Europe in Bohemia, in the village of Vserby, close to the Bavarian border. Moritz was not alone in following the path to Louisville. Other such acquaintances and soon-to-be-prominent families from Bohemia as the Dembitzes, the Brandeises, and the Taussigs would join him.[2] These early Jewish settlers from German Europe were but a tiny minority of inhabitants in the Ohio River city, having built their first small temple in 1849. By the time of Abraham's birth in 1866, the Jewish community numbered fewer than a thousand persons.[3]

What the Flexner family owed to its Orthodox heritage, according to those who knew them, was a fierce sense of family loyalty, unusual even by Jewish standards, an unshakeable determination to get ahead in a raw, new environment, and an almost mystical faith in the power of learning to shape their children's lives. Although hard-pressed, the Flexners valued a life of learning far more than the humdrum occupations of business and trade in which Moritz was indifferently engaged. In their Jewish heritage lay concepts that left a special mark on young Abraham: learning and doing are related, education lasts a lifetime, and differences among individuals are important in the learning experience.

Moritz and Esther were proud of the teachers and learned men in their ancestry and spoke often to their children of what lay open to them in the new country. Moritz, whose father and grandfather had been teachers and rabbis but who himself held no steady job, had left his Bohemian birthplace at age thirteen because the "nest was crowded" and had gone to live and study with an uncle, also a rabbi, in French Strasbourg. Later, according to family tradition, he was briefly a public school teacher.[4]

Esther's father, too, had once been a teacher. Her education-minded parents sent her to the Hebrew school in Saarlouis rather than to the public schools of her hometown. There she would have a chance at a broader education than at home, including instruction in both French and German, as well as in Hebrew. Years later, she recalled proudly for her children the excitement when a teacher at her school, a Mr. Levy, learning that she owned no book of her own, presented her one with the inscription "From Mr. Levy, for industry and good behavior, I present this book to Esther Abraham." Her schoolmates promptly labeled her "Mr. Levy's sweetheart."[5] So much did the family value learning, their recollections of educational achievements often bordered on myth.

Why Esther and Moritz came to America is not entirely clear. Moritz must have been something of a political activist, for as a result of his involvement in politics, by his own account, he was "forced suddenly to leave Strasbourg."[6] He had lived through the revolutions of 1848 and the years of Louis Napoleon but now found himself forced to flee. No other account of Moritz's abrupt departure for America in 1853 survives. We know that he traveled steerage across the Atlantic and arrived "penniless" in New York.

The ambitious Esther, by contrast, had won a degree of independence and prosperity before she and her sister left for America in 1855. Five years before her departure, she and her older sister Caroline had been sent to Paris to live with her mother's cousin, whose husband owned a dress and millinery shop. There the sisters learned the dressmaking trade and became skilled at their work. Invited by an uncle in Louisville to seek still better opportunities abroad, they hesitated, not wishing to leave their family and friends, and only after an interlude lasting several years did they finally accept. The two sisters, twenty-one and twenty-three years old, forbidden by their parents to go on a more dangerous steamship, traveled second-class on a sailing ship across the Atlantic. The trip, arduous enough at a scheduled three weeks, actually took "nine awful weeks" because of storms and poor sailing conditions and became part of the family's lore.[7]

Moritz's first encounter with America was far from happy. His early years were filled with disappointment and misadventure. When he arrived he was thirty-three years old, knew no English, and lacked the experience or skills required for most jobs. Since he felt himself more French than

German after two decades in Strasbourg, he sought out fellow French immigrants in New York, who helped him get a job with a French wine
dealer. A few weeks of work were enough to make him realize that he was
unfit for clerical duties. He was not able to find a steady job in the months
following, so in 1854 he left New York with five friends, bound for New
Orleans, where it was believed "there were more Frenchmen" and a better living was possible. Upon arriving in the Southern port, he learned
that the city was suffering from a savage epidemic of yellow fever. Within
two weeks, four of his friends were dead and he lay delirious with fever in
the great Charité Hospital. It was not an auspicious beginning.

He could not remember how long he lay near death before he slowly,
very slowly, began to recover. His salvation he attributed to a good
Samaritan he identified only as "a Frenchman." The man nursed Moritz
constantly, never leaving his room and supervising his food and drink.
When at last able to stand with the aid of crutches, he was urged by
his savior to go to Louisville, where friends would help him. The name-
less Frenchman even bought his ticket and gave him a small amount
of money to travel. Traveling by steamship, he arrived in Louisville
hobbling weakly, unable to work, and had to be sheltered and nursed
for months.[8]

When at last able to work, he started a new life, like so many of his
countrymen, as a traveling peddler. On his back he carried an assortment
of wares from house to house, occasionally enjoying the luxury of resting
his bundle on the horse-drawn wagon of a friendly traveler. It was not an
easy life, Esther told their children, but "man can accustom himself to
anything," she said, if necessity demanded it. After many months, he was
able, with a partner in a nearby town, to buy his own horse and wagon
and to begin selling goods wholesale to storekeepers as well as to farmers
and other customers along his route. Abraham would recall his father's
glee in describing the horse, which had a stiff knee, making it necessary
to stop when another vehicle passed on the road, then step aside so that
the awkward horse would not become entangled in the other wagon.[9]

His journeys took him away from home for days at a time, and like
other peddlers he stayed with friends and customers along the way. Genial
and unaggressive, Moritz had a talent for selling, and his stock of stories
and good-humored wit made him popular along the route. Periodically he
returned to Louisville to restock his inventory in the Market Street stores.
There in the close-knit community of merchants and sellers, most of them
German Jews, Morris (as he now called himself) made many friends.

Among those he called on was Esther and Caroline Abraham's uncle, who was taken by the newcomer's personality and growing success.

By the time Esther met Morris, she and her sister were well known in the small Jewish section of Louisville. To old-time residents, the attractive sisters, with their Parisian experience and needlework skills, represented a level of sophistication and charm that was hitherto unknown. The whole city was aware that the sisters had come from Paris "and could do everything." At a New Year's ball, they created a sensation by arriving dressed in the latest Parisian fashions. After a number of months in which Esther took over much of the housekeeping in her uncle's house (aided by the family's house slave), the sisters went to work for the owners of a large dry goods store. There they were put to work finishing "the finest clothes" to be found in Louisville.[10]

Esther had many suitors, but she was attracted by Morris's good humor and easy ways, and encouraged by her uncle's praise of his potential in business. When he proposed, Esther was pleased but asked for time to consider her response. Perhaps she was concerned about what she felt was the social distance between them. Several of the Flexner children remembered her comparing their father's penniless arrival in steerage with her own more dignified journey to America. At any rate, Morris, who was traveling during the time she was deciding his future, decided to hasten a decision by asking a fellow salesman returning to Louisville to make further entreaties. But the treacherous messenger proposed to her himself. "Paradoxically," according to her grandson, "this hastened Morris's suit. In turning the interloper down, Esther made up her own mind."[11]

Morris and Esther became engaged in April 1856 and were married in September. "Of one thing I am sure," Esther told her children, "that Father felt as if he had suddenly become a wealthy man." Their grandson, the historian James Thomas Flexner, has described the couple at the time of their marriage. Morris, about five feet eight inches tall, was "lank with narrowish sloping shoulders." His head appeared long because of a receding hairline and black sideburns. His eyebrows were narrow, his eyes were sunken, his nose jutted out, and his mouth was full. The overall impression was of "a handsome head, both shrewd and innocent." Esther, by contrast, was petite and small-boned. Her face, apple-like in appearance, was short and round, with prominent cheekbones. Her dark hair, always parted in the middle, fell in ringlets behind her shoulders. She looked sober and firm, with her mouth "turned down over a strong chin." But she was, in her grandson's view, "an extremely pretty girl."[12] Esther was twenty-two and Morris thirty-six as they began their life together.

The newlyweds were apart much of the time as Morris followed his peripatetic calling. For days and sometimes weeks at a time Esther was alone while he was on the road. Morris, too, was lonely. When their first child, Jacob, was born the following year, Morris decided to try to settle down in one place and devote more time to his family. His desire to have a home of his own and to keep his children together, Abraham would recall, "never left him as long as he lived."[13] The family now settled in Lawrenceburg, a small town about fifty miles southeast of Louisville, where Morris entered into a partnership with one of Esther's relatives. Lawrenceburg was a center of the bourbon whiskey business, and Morris was now often paid for his goods in kegs of bourbon, a valued means of exchange in the area.

They were deep in the Kentucky bluegrass region, an area strongly sympathetic to the Southern cause in the looming sectional war. Jacob recalled incidents of drinking and street fighting in Lawrenceburg during the war that began in 1861 and especially the burning of his father's barn— Morris was an opponent of slavery—by a group of Morgan's raiders, a band of Confederate cavalrymen bent on destroying the property of Union sympathizers. He recalled vividly the fright he felt as a five-year-old when the family fled westward to Louisville on a spring night in 1862. While in Lawrenceburg, Esther had given birth to two more sons, Henry and Isadore, and was pregnant with a fourth child, Simon, when they left Lawrenceburg.

In Louisville the growing family found refuge with Esther's sister but now faced the threat of a Confederate invasion, led by General Braxton Bragg. Louisville was the supply depot for all the Union armies in the western theater of war. At one point, before Bragg's defeat at nearby Perryville, women and children were ordered to leave the city, but Jacob remembered Esther, with young Isadore in her arms, saying in her crisp German speech, "Ich gehe nicht" (I'm not going). For a period, Morris served in the city's home guard until the danger of attack receded. While the family was living in a small house on East Street, a "shabby" part of town, with the Civil War still raging, Simon and Bernard, the fourth and fifth members of the young family, were born. Other incidents kept the war constantly before the Flexners as Morris, now in his forties, tried once more to establish himself as a businessman in Louisville.[14]

This time he was more successful. Using the proceeds of the business in Lawrenceburg, he entered in 1863 with a new partner into the whole-sale hat business at a good location on Main Street. For the next ten years, until the panic of 1873, his fortunes prospered. After the war's end, his trade expanded across the South. For long periods of time he was again away from home, this time searching for new outlets in Tennessee, Georgia, Texas, and Alabama. These years, the most prosperous of his life, were a time of great loneliness and homesickness, for he was, in Simon's memory, as in Abraham's, "naturally a home-loving, domestic person." Although good-humored and witty around others, he was to his children a serious man who talked little and often gravely. To Simon, the most sensitive of the children, his talk carried "the stamp of thought and authority." While he "seemed to love children," said Simon, he was not "strikingly demonstrative" in the case of his own.[15]

It was the diminutive Esther who was the real force in their lives. Iron-willed yet gentle, patient, determined that her children succeed, she prodded them to learn self-confidence and to grow close to each other, building bonds that would enable them to help one another in later life. Abraham remembered her as "absolute mistress of herself, her family, and every situation which arose." In intelligence, he said, she was not equaled by any of her children. He adored her. Like her husband, she wanted her children to be doctors, lawyers, or teachers, not merchants or salespeople. Abraham said that his parents discouraged the children from entering business because they "saw through the folly of mere money-making as an end." Both parents, he said, dealt with their children in a way that encouraged the children to develop both initiative and intimacy.[16]

Even after Morris's death in 1882—an event that shook the close-knit family—Esther continually reminded her children of their father's steadfast belief: "Our children will justify us." All the children would remember her as the one who did more to shape their lives.

The children would remember their stern father as a disciplinarian when it came to their education. When Abraham complained about a teacher, Morris accompanied him silently to school the next day and told the principal, "I should like you and all his teachers to know that if any question arises between my son and his teachers I shall always regard the teacher as being in the right." Simon was likewise warned of the consequences of flouting the authority of the school. When told of Simon's rebellious behavior in one of his classes, his father took him to the local prison and asked the warden to take Simon on a somber tour through the prisoners' cells.[17]

By the time Abraham was born, on November 13, 1866, the war had ended, the city was slowly returning to normal, and Morris had started his profitable journeys into the defeated South. He was now able to move the family into a three-story brick house on Center Street with an open gutter, outside privies, and a hydrant "offering yellowish muddy water" behind the house. A few years later, the Flexners were in an even larger Sixth Street house, the first Abraham would remember. Here were born the last three of the Flexner children, Washington, Gertrude, and Mary. The family now lived on a wide street that separated the Jewish inhabitants of the city from the middle-class gentile community. The Jews and the gentiles never mingled, Simon reminisced, and the children played separately. "Even if the men had business connections during the day, their families never visited across the street." Years of prosperity enabled the growing family to move into better and larger housing. A number of friends and relatives, including several of Morris's brothers and their families, joined them in Louisville and for brief periods resided at their home.[18]

The world into which Abraham was born still stood in the shadow of war. Ex-confederate Democrats were in control of the state government, and Kentuckians cast their ballots with the solidly Democratic South for decades to come. Outside the large cities, most of the state's people were "unprogressive, hardy, and reckless," he wrote, and "blood feuds of medieval character were common." Wartime tensions spilled over into conflicts about taxation, transportation routes, and especially the treatment of the freed slaves. In Louisville, thousands of fleeing former slaves crowded into ramshackle quarters in what came to be known as Smoketown. Crosses were burned from time to time by local members of the Ku Klux Klan. Only strenuous efforts by the federal Freedmen's Bureau staved off wholesale starvation and disease.[19] Many whites believed that the massive problems caused by the former slaves' presence were the direct result of Northern policies and that the federal government should solve them. By 1866, the city was nearing one hundred thousand inhabitants, with freed blacks accounting for 20 percent of the total.

Prosperity began to return as the city resumed its entrepôt position between North and South as a center for trade in leaf tobacco, cotton, whiskey, and pork. To its wholesaling and distributing role, it added a new "mania for manufacturing," especially of steam engines and boilers. It was still a river town, a meat-packing town, "a wholesale-merchandise town," the grocer and clothier to a very large segment of the Middle West and the upper South. A racetrack for thoroughbred racing was opened in

1875. By 1880, it was being called "one of the four great cities of the West [along with Chicago, St. Louis, and Cincinnati]." Gradually the urban milieu of Louisville, growing steadily as business and population expanded, made for a somewhat more tolerant and less repressive atmosphere than in the rest of the state. In 1870, the city created separate funds for black and white schools, and within four years, more than eighteen hundred black children were enrolled. A high school for blacks was added in 1873, and a night program for black children and adults was begun. In its readiness to establish public schools for the newly freed population and to tolerate an education that went beyond an elementary vocationalism, Louisville, though scarcely progressive, was "a generation ahead" of much of the South and led parts of the North as well. Not until 1905 was a program of manual training introduced into the public schools.[20]

By the time Flexner left Louisville, a dozen public schools were open to blacks, as well as schools for teacher training, law, and medicine. In the 1880s, nearly one hundred black students, a large number by contemporary standards, completed high school. By 1900, the proportion of African-American homeowners in Louisville was higher than that in any other American city. The freedmen were able to vote and were not without influence during Flexner's childhood years. Black businesses, including a newspaper, were beginning to multiply. Kentucky was one of only eight states, three of them in the North, to pass antilynching laws in those years. Flexner's own relatively progressive views about blacks and their educability owed not a little to these formative years.

Socially, the city was stratified into the prewar landed class, the rising merchant and professional groups, a growing army of laborers, and the poor whites and blacks. Racial lines in residential housing were not yet firmly drawn, and many whites, including the Flexners, lived in close proximity to blacks. In 1870, black families could be found on three of every four blocks of the city. Flexner recalled that blacks "were indeed our playmates." Although playgrounds were nonexistent, there was "little to interfere with baseball played in the streets by teams indiscriminately white and black."[21] How close the family actually came to any real social contact with blacks, however, is doubtful. When he later undertook a survey of southern schools for the General Education Board, he admitted that only then did he become acutely aware of the social and educational disadvantages of the blacks he had known.

In the small Jewish community, liberal ideas about politics, race, and religion were common. The city was a center of Reform Judaism, and

prominent Jewish families played a quiet role in civic life. The Adath Israel congregation to which the Flexner family belonged was led by liberal
and scholarly rabbis active in political reform. Rabbi Isaac M. Wise of
Cincinnati, the nation's leading Reform rabbi and a frequent visitor to
Louisville, found the temple a congenial second home. By the time Abraham reached adolescence, Adath Israel had the second largest Reform
congregation in the United States.[22]

The Flexner children attended the temple school and were duly confirmed as members of the congregation. The parents, although faithful in
attending the temple, never gave up the Orthodox practices of their
youth. Simon recalled the surprise he felt on entering his father's bedroom
to find him wearing a leather tape around his head and mumbling sounds
that Simon did not understand. He remembered, too, the two sets of
dishes his mother kept and her Friday night prayers over the white table-
cloth with candlesticks.[23]

But the children were falling away from their parents' faith. Not only
were they indifferent to the ancient customs, they were becoming, in
Bernard's words, "indifferent to Jewish interests." The liberal teachings of
the temple and the distractions of school and city life made their parents'
pious faith seem remote. "They saw us drift away into streams of thought
and feeling that they did not understand," Abraham wrote in his autobiography, but "they interposed no resistance." The theories of Charles Darwin, which had gained ground slowly, were finding acceptance in the liberal Jewish community. For Abraham and his older brothers, Herbert
Spencer and T.H. Huxley took the place of the Bible and the prayer book.
The parents, however, were shrewd enough to realize that their hold upon
their children was stronger when the reins were kept loose. Esther was not
disturbed, Abraham said, when he and Simon married Christian women
and left their childhood faith altogether. Their wives, by his account, became "not daughters-in-law, but daughters."[24]

If the children were sensitive to social slights against Jews, they made
no mention of it. Bernard told an inquiring New York friend in later years
that he had grown up in a small city where "human contacts were close
and associations were largely non-Jewish." Jacob, the only child to spend
his entire life in Louisville, makes no mention of religion in his account
of these years. Simon believed that despite his own occasional experience
with prejudice, it was not important and was best ignored.[25]

Of all the siblings, Abraham became the most impervious to anti-
Semitism. All his life he believed himself to be a completely assimilated

Jew and felt little identification with the self-consciously Jewish associations around him. "I ceased to believe," he told a wartime GI who questioned his loss of faith, "that the Jews were the chosen people in the sense in which the orthodox Jews were chosen people."[26] His own steep rise in American life and that of his brothers strengthened his conviction that anti-Semitism was at most a minor hindrance to those of ability. When he encountered prejudice in others, he dismissed it as ignorance and refused to see any deep malice in the offender.

The Flexner brothers, although they did not know it, were members of a rising generation of secular Jews who would make a special mark on American intellectual life. Like Adolph Ochs of the *New York Times,* the anthropologist Franz Boas, the biologist Jacques Loeb, and many others, they sought to demonstrate "through their energy, industry, and rectitude" that they could make their way in a strongly Christian culture. By shedding the habits and religious practices of their parents, by embracing the public schools, by becoming as much like their Protestant countrymen as possible, they set out on the road to respectability and fame. "Live quietly, happily, unostentatiously," advised Ochs. "Don't be too smart. Don't know too much." If anti-Semitism threatened, it was best to ignore it and not fight back. When Loeb was blackballed by the Century Club in New York, Abraham Flexner criticized a member who charged that Loeb's rejection stemmed from anti-Semitism. "The fool," wrote Flexner of that member, "has thus humiliated Loeb in the face of the town." As they gained success, especially in New York, where three of the Flexner brothers came to live, these secular Jews played an important part in breaking down the Protestant cast of American public culture.[27]

Abraham and his brothers' tranquil childhood years were rudely shattered by the failure of their father's business in the financial panic of 1873. Like many of the Jewish merchants along Main and Market Streets, Morris had allowed his customers to buy on extended credit, and now the severe shortage of money caused many to default on their payments. Without adequate capital, the business he ran with his partner was one of the first to fall before the financial hurricane. Only the generosity of his brother-in-law, Caroline's husband, enabled him to survive by financing a small hat outlet. But the new venture failed to prosper and the store was moved farther down Market Street into ever poorer neighborhoods. Morris's status gradually fell to that of a poorly paid clerk. His pride badly damaged, he more and more saw himself as a failure and began to drink heavily.

Morris's collapse runs like a red line across the Flexner family history. "It broke his spirit," said Bernard, "and a complete change came over family life." Moving into smaller and more crowded quarters in ever poorer surroundings, the children were sharply aware of the change in their fortune. Different neighborhoods meant different schools as well as different playmates. For the older children, it meant leaving school and putting aside plans for the future. The eldest son, Jacob, now sixteen, who in family tradition was to be a doctor, expected his father to send him to medical school and then on to Paris, where Morris had friends. One of the saddest days of his life, Jacob remembered, was a Christmas on which he took a walk with his father. As they walked along icy streets, his father suddenly stopped and confessed that he was a ruined man. It would not be possible for Jacob to continue his schooling, and he would be expected to help his father in supporting the younger brothers and sisters. Since Jacob's hopes were set on medicine, his father told him, his only chance was to work as an apprentice in a drugstore. The next brothers in age, Henry and Isadore, fifteen and thirteen years old, likewise relinquished their hopes and plans for school and dutifully went to work. Soon they were joined by the still younger Simon and Bernard.[28]

Childhood illnesses threatened the Flexner children, as they did many children at the time. Although Simon would become one of America's most influential medical scientists, he disliked school, had behavioral problems, and never completed elementary school. At age sixteen, he contracted a nearly fatal case of typhoid fever that kept him home and away from work for several months. In the case of Bernard, a future leading attorney in New York, a severe attack of what was called "chloriditis" left him nearly blind and kept him out of the workplace for a year or more. The youngest brother, Washington, later America's leading legal printer, also came close to death with a severe case of diphtheria that kept him at home for a period during these dark years.

Only seven years old when his father lost his business, Abraham was exempt from the requirement to work, but his father's failure nevertheless left a deep mark on him. "One should never forget the enormous volume of pain and illness in this world," he wrote his own daughter many years later, "especially for the poor. I saw Grandpa Flexner struggle against a combination of poverty and other afflictions that changed our entire family." Only his mother's heroic efforts to hold the family together, he believed, had concealed the horror from the children. As he sat at his mother's death bed in 1905, he told his wife, her whole life had "tossed through" his mind. While she had the strength to endure and combat poverty, she "never compromised her self-respect by reason of it." Her ideals of home, cleanliness, and dignity and her hold on the future of her children were "unshakeable." Born into the simplest of circumstances, she had come to love books and to achieve a kind of "moral greatness" that had impressed all her children.[29] Abraham's own sympathy for the efforts of women, including his wife and daughters, to seek education and opportunities outside the home and to be independent was, as he made clear, strongly influenced by the gratitude and respect he felt for his mother.

Life in the Flexner household reflected the changed circumstances of their lives. The older boys worked long hours in menial jobs while the younger children remained at home or at school. Yet their mother refused to let them sell papers—"tho' the pennies would have helped"—because she thought it demeaning. In a small house on Fifth Street, the upstairs rooms served as a dormitory for the seven boys. Crowded into a small number of beds, the younger ones engaged in pillow fights and other play. Jacob wondered how his mother survived this "team of wild boys," for these were very "black days" for her.

The small earnings of the boys, when added to the father's declining income, enabled them to pay off some bills and buy the necessities for a large family. Esther made the family clothes and helped her husband by sewing shirts and other garments for his store, even as she managed the household income and kept the house in spotless condition. As the children grew, their earnings increased and a communal plan of living was begun. As each child reached maturity and left home, that child's place was taken by one of the younger boys or girls.[30] In time Abraham would take his place among the wage earners and eventually become the mainstay of the entire family.

As Morris declined in health, Jacob often dominated the conversation at the family dinner table. He was intelligent, self-assured, and often voluble, and he brought news of politics, books, and town happenings to the rest of the family. He was the first to turn his back on his parents' orthodoxy. He absorbed conversations among doctors at the drugstore and read the new works of Darwin and Huxley. His intellectual impact on the older children, especially Abraham, was greater than that of their parents.

In Simon's recollection, Jacob would lead the family in discussions of books he had read. From the head of the table, Jacob "pounced on any of the younger children who disagreed with him, easily routing them all, except, as time passed . . . Abraham [who] was as voluble as Jacob, thought more or less on similar lines, and was equally argumentative." An exasperated Isadore once threw a fork at Jacob, and Simon never forgot the sight of the fork quivering in the wall.

The shy and sensitive Simon was overwhelmed by the vigor and mental aggressiveness of his older brother. He would remain ambivalent about his debt to him. Although Jacob introduced him to the world of books and ideas and gave him the opportunity to work as an apprentice in the drugstore that started his remarkable career, he never forgot his brother's harshness to him. Jacob once destroyed a collection of Simon's children's magazines that Jacob regarded as "trash," and sixty-three years later Simon told his son, "I have never forgiven Jake."[31]

Abraham's experience was different. Of all the children, he romanticized most his childhood years. He alone had escaped the penalty paid by his older brothers for his father's failure. Still very young in 1873, he continued his education and became the first in the family to finish high school and go on to college. Precociously bright, personable, fun-loving, sensitive, prone to disputation, he became the favorite of his parents and older brothers. Like Jacob, Abraham loved to read and to declare his conclusions to his admiring family. Simon remembered him as "an infant prodigy" and said that he was "extraordinarily persuasive." His earliest pictures show a disarmingly sweet-faced, innocent boy, wide-eyed, dark-haired, with a serious, almost melancholy expression, looking far into the distance. The family accounts mention no behavioral problems. His early self-confidence and assured manner set him off from his peers. He was the closest of all the family to Jacob, to Simon, and to his younger sisters and brother.

In Abraham's memory, the dark days of his father's ruin were overshadowed by his own success in school, the warmth of his family's love, and the opportunities for play and enjoyment. The reader should not infer, he wrote in his autobiography, that a poor boy growing up in the 1870s and 1880s led a dreary or unhappy life. He remembered other neighborhood children no better off than he with whom he played in backyards or "on uncongested and ill-paved streets." In the background was always the Ohio River, where the adventurous swam and fished or skated in the winter. Books could be found in the two privately financed libraries where he spent as much time as he could. The family owned a series of Dickens's works, a complete edition of Keats, as well as the plays of Shakespeare and the Bible. This reflected Esther's influence. On his thirteenth birthday Abraham was given a complete Plutarch, which he devoured. Soon he was reading Hawthorne and Thoreau and had begun a lifelong habit of reading literature, history, biography, and the ancient classics.[32] Although the parents spoke German at home, he early developed a keen sense for the idioms and grammar of the English language.

By age fifteen, he was working part-time in the Louisville Library, one of the two lending libraries in the city. His time for play came to an end, as he worked from two-thirty each afternoon until ten in the evening. His pay was sixteen dollars a month, an amount, he proudly recalled, "that told effectually in relieving the family budget." The two years he spent at the library, he maintained, were important in his intellectual growth. He had time to not only read some of the ten thousand books in the collection but to listen silently to leading townspeople's discussions about topics in current newspapers and opinion magazines. Here he acquired a lifelong devotion to the *Nation* magazine; its editor, E.A. Godkin, became his youthful hero. Among those who frequented the library were the eminent lawyer Louis N. Dembitz (the uncle of Louis D. Brandeis), the learned rabbi Adolph G. Moses, the Semple sisters, Patty and Ellen, the latter a future distinguished geographer at the University of Chicago, the blind poet Morrison Heady, and the Baptist theologian John A. Broadus. "Thus, from my fifteenth year," he reminisced, "I was continuously in contact with mature persons who were infinitely my superiors." Always he would learn from personal observation and close attention to those around him.

A lively interest in politics sprang from observing these meetings and discussions at the library. He hung about the polls on Election Day, followed political news in the newspapers, and could recall years later the names of local candidates in elections long forgotten by others. He remembered vividly the national tensions of the Hayes-Tilden election, the shock of the assassination of President Garfield, and the first election of Grover Cleveland, Abraham's favorite president. Throughout his life, Abraham admired President Cleveland's honesty and straightforwardness.[33]

Abraham's views on government were those of a sensitive young man growing up in the Reconstruction South. A Democrat and a laissez-faire individualist, he admired sincerity and efficiency in public leaders, distrusted wealth, hated corruption, and feared strong government. He was optimistic that personal effort and private charity would remedy the nation's industrial ills long after such efforts proved unable to deal with the nation's want and suffering. He believed that the best way for the less advantaged to get ahead was, following his own family's example, through education and hard work. Before he left Louisville, he became a cautious follower of Theodore Roosevelt and the progressives in urging that big business be disciplined and some degree of balance restored between capital and those it affected. But he was always part of the mainstream in his belief in personal responsibility and limited government.

Abraham found his studies easy and enjoyable. He gained self-confidence as he outdistanced his classmates and won the praise of his teachers and parents. "Such was the schooling of that day," he recalled; life at school was "almost as free from intellectual strain, effort or interest" as "the long Southern afternoons and evenings." He played down his own achievement in what became a lifelong habit by pronouncing the teachers "elderly and untrained" and the schoolrooms barren of books, photographs, or scientific equipment. Nor could his schooling compare, he said, with that of his own children, with its emphasis on ideas and music and drama. But in attending school at all he was far in advance of the majority of school-age children in his state: fewer than two of five children in Kentucky at that time were educated in any school at all.[34]

His high school, too, he later denigrated. This was unfair. Fewer than 5 percent of adolescents were in school nationally in the 1880s, and public high schools in the South were almost nonexistent. Public high schools, it was said, were the "people's colleges," preparing students for life as well as college. Course offerings varied widely from school to school, from Greek and Latin to elementary mathematics, American history, drawing, and manual training.

By Flexner's own admission, the high school he attended included teachers whose scholarship would stand out in any age. One of his teachers, Ashley B. Hurt, principal of the school and later a professor at Tulane University, cultivated Flexner's interest in Greek, which later became his major focus in college. For English, he had the well-trained R.H. Carothers, who encouraged his efforts at writing and inspired him to read Spenser, Marlowe, Byron, and the classical English authors. He was taught physiology by C. Leo Mees, a future president of Rose Polytechnic Institute, and chemistry by Harlow W. Eaton, a Leipzig Ph.D. whom he described as a "master of his field." He attended weekly lectures on scientific subjects at the local polytechnic institute, winning a prize, and on Saturday evenings took a prominent part in the school's debating society, of which he was president. Few schools of that day exceeded Louisville Male High School in breadth of curriculum, and few teachers were as well prepared. The small number of students received as good an education as was available in the United States. The school, in fact, was highly selective, requiring an entrance examination, and had previously been known as the "academic department" of the city-run University of Louisville. One writer described it as "a high school masquerading as a college." Its large and comfortable building had been constructed to house the University of Louisville Law School. Its students included the sons of not only professionals but steamboat captains, river pilots, land agents, and tollgate keepers.[35]

He spent six years as a student at the Louisville Male High School, two years in the preparatory division and four years in high school. The preparatory study involved arithmetic, algebra, Latin, physical geography, and English. In all these subjects he scored well, but in "deportment" he received his lowest grades. One can surmise only that he was bored and found outlet for his energies in daydreaming or adolescent mischief. In the high school years, however, his grades showed a growing purposiveness and attention to study. His teachers evaluated his work in the freshman year as outstanding in all subjects but mathematics. In his sophomore year he won the school's Alumni Prize, and as a junior and senior he claimed the Shakespeare and English literature awards. He was chosen salutatorian of his graduating class in 1884 and gave an oration on reform of the civil service system, reflecting his lively interest in the political issues of the day. The demanding course of study he followed—Latin, Greek, German, French, mathematics, natural science, psychology, English literature, physics, and chemistry—belies his later claim that his public school education was inferior.[36]

What the young graduate planned to do after leaving high school is not known. He could hardly have anticipated, in light of the family circumstances, the remarkable gesture made by his eldest brother, Jacob, in 1884, offering to finance a college education. Abraham's entrance into college marked, all the children would agree, a change in the entire family's fortunes. Jacob wrote that it was Abraham's success that enabled the children to rise so far above the level achieved by their parents. Abraham believed, too, that it was the "turning point" for all the Flexners.[37] To Jacob, supporting the brightest and most promising child was an investment in the whole family's future. The debt that Abraham now owed would be repaid many times over in the next two decades, as he gradually took over Jacob's position as head of the family and steered his siblings toward more promising futures.

Jacob's act was the more surprising in light of the new burdens placed on the family by Morris's death in 1882. Many of the father's debts and the support of their mother now fell entirely on the older children. Jacob had married the year of his father's death and had a child of his own. Despite his mother's plea to postpone marriage, Henry, too, had married and become a father the summer that Abraham graduated from high school. The fortunes of all the children were thus uncertain as they continued to help their mother and their younger brothers and sisters. Jacob had prospered most, now owning his own drugstore with the help of his wife's relatives, and had hired Simon as his apprentice. He had been able to save a thousand dollars by 1884; this money financed Abraham's education. While working for Jacob, Simon discovered the magic of the microscope and found his future calling. Bernard, meanwhile, also owed a debt to Jacob for getting him a job at a bookstore, and the other older brothers, Henry and Isadore, were likewise helped to find employment. "We can never be sufficiently grateful to the memory of our oldest brother," recalled Abraham, "for the sacrifices he made . . . when his own needs were pressing."[38]

Jacob's choice of a college for Abraham proved as fateful as the decision to invest in his future. For the rest of his life Abraham would marvel at his brother's prescience in selecting a new school, not yet known in Louisville, that would become perhaps the most influential university of the nineteenth century. American universities were undergoing a rapid, largely unplanned transformation just at this time, but Jacob's choice was especially unusual. How did he happen to hit upon the Johns Hopkins University in Baltimore, a completely new university that had been launched only eight years before? Influential was Jacob's friendship with a rabbi's son who was teaching at the local high school. While living in Baltimore, the teacher had attended the university; the teacher's stories of the new kind of education Johns Hopkins offered fascinated Jacob. Abraham would always remember the June 1884 day he left for Baltimore as the most important day in his life.[39] In many ways, his brother Simon's departure for Johns Hopkins six years later was a similar turning point in Simon's life.

When he moved to Baltimore, Abraham Flexner was seventeen years old. He was an engaging, sensitive, good-looking, articulate young man with fine, almost feminine, features and a full head of dark hair. He resembled his mother in his intelligence, patience, organizational skill, and steely determination, and his father in his friendly disposition, good humor, and easygoing charm. To those who knew him he was thoughtful, kind, mild-mannered, at times playful, and quick-witted. More than he would later admit, much of his personality and characteristic attitudes had already been formed. He was high-minded, energetic, and eager to solve problems. The strong sense of family loyalty, the intense pressure to succeed, the economic turmoil of his growing up all left their stamp upon him. His own success, and then that of all the children, shaped an unshakeable belief in individual effort and a laissez-faire view of public intervention. The liberal Jewish community of Louisville and its early entry into civic life enforced his belief in his own assimilation into national life. It was under these circumstances that he never gave credence to the argument that American anti-Semitism was like that of Europe, or that it was a serious hindrance to Jewish achievement.

But the memory of his family's poverty and the communal struggle against it lay deepest among the motives for his lifelong struggle for place. The fear of failure, of reaching no higher station in life than that of their parents, was a powerful stimulus to all the Flexner children. In middle age, when Abraham and Simon had become two of the most influential men in America, they reminisced about their beginnings and the changes in their lives. "You are right," Abraham told Simon, "in contrasting the childhood of these children of ours with our own. What contrast could be greater than that between the alleys in which we played on Sixth Street and the sidewalk and Court House yard which represented our world when we lived on Market Street, on the one hand, and the school associations and foreign experiences of these fortunate children of ours?" They are certain to be superior in culture and intelligence, he wrote, but would "their fiber be as tough?" And would they "try to get as far beyond their point of origins" as Abraham, Simon, and their siblings had tried to get beyond theirs?[40]

2

A University Like No Other

As the young Abraham Flexner sat in a railroad car heading eastward to Baltimore, he was both excited and apprehensive. Before him lay a new world of experience, new friends, a new city, a new way of life, but also the dreaded entrance examinations. He was by no means sure that he was ready.

Sensitive and dutiful, he likely thought, too, of the family he was leaving behind and the sacrifices being made for him. Not one of his older brothers had escaped the drudgery of work or the prospect of limited lives. He alone was given the chance to finish high school. No other child had traveled more than a few miles from home. Now, again, for another two years, he was exempt from family responsibility. The first unmarried child to live away from home, he was also the first to make arrangements for his own upkeep and the first to enter a university. What a frightening, yet maturing, adventure it must have been for a seventeen-year-old!

And it was all for a purpose. It was the young man's responsibility to stretch his resources over as long a time as possible and to return to help the others in their quest to escape. "I was a mere boy," young and homesick, he remembered, and "as little prepossessing as any boy you can imagine," ready to run away if anyone turned him down. With no money to spend, owning only the suit he wore and a few shirts made by his mother, he spent his days in endless work. Whenever he stopped working, he recalled, he "fell immediately into homesickness." His ties with home, which had been extremely close, were now limited to a single postcard written each day in German to his mother.[1]

There were consolations. The university to which chance delivered him was an exciting place in 1884, full of interesting personalities, unusual classmates, and high regard for the academic life. Indeed, no other American institution had so squarely committed itself to being "different" from the mine run of colleges and universities. Rules were flexible; no set period of study time was required for graduation; classes were not separated by years; and an easy informality marked the life of the institution. The faculty "were extraordinarily kind to me," remembered Cyrus Adler, a future librarian of the Smithsonian Institution and acquaintance of Flexner, "and did everything in their power, waiving many rules." None of the paraphernalia of fraternities, social clubs, student publications, or intercollegiate athletics—hallmarks of the traditional college—existed at the Johns Hopkins of 1884. Nor could dormitories or special houses for students be found among the converted boardinghouses, rented buildings, and newly built laboratories that made up the university.[2]

Students lived in private homes, sometimes as neighbors to faculty members. German-style beer gardens were growing up on the edge of the campus. The library, which stayed open late, was the most popular place to be. In many ways, Johns Hopkins was trying to recreate the contemporary German university—which Abraham would come to admire—while carefully adapting it to American circumstances.

The original plan of President Daniel Coit Gilman made no provision for undergraduate students. Hopkins was to be the first American university to follow the German pattern of concentrating on advanced study and truly "graduate" work. As in Germany, the small research seminar, the learning laboratory, and the formal lecture were to be its characteristic features. Unlike Harvard or Yale, or any other American school, the university was to be faculty centered and its most important output would come in scholarly monographs, scientific discoveries, and superior students. But the vision of an all-graduate university had faded quietly in the face of community pressures for undergraduate instruction and the clear recognition that few well-prepared college graduates were clamoring to come to the new academy in Baltimore. In 1883, just before Flexner arrived, the first strong commitment to "collegiate work" as opposed to graduate study was made by the university. In the sober, heavily academic atmosphere, some of the undergraduates felt as welcome as "red headed stepchildren."[3]

No environment could have been more appealing to the new arrival from Louisville. Unsure of his training, not confident in his relationships with others, unskilled in athletics, yet strongly independent and carrying a mandate to succeed in the shortest possible time, he made the fullest use of the flexible Hopkins system. Confronted immediately with the need to prove himself ready to study by passing the daunting entrance examinations, he promptly failed in mathematics, Greek, and Latin. It was a dispiriting moment. It could have meant the end of his and his family's aspirations. The letters he carried from home, however, convinced the faculty to give him a chance. The mathematician William E. Story scrawled "seems promising" across his application. "Your paper shows that you don't know much Latin," another professor said of his examination, "but [Jacob's friend] says you come from a fine family and we are going to let you in."

His Greek examination was a total failure. After one glance at the questions, he went to Professor Charles D'Urban Morris, seated in front of the class, and told him that it was hopeless. After quizzing him on his background and study, Morris surprised him by offering to meet with him for five minutes each day to guide him in his study. By Thanksgiving, Flexner was ready to enter the regular classes. He was one of forty-seven "special students" who benefited from such flexible arrangements in the year 1884–85.[4]

Surprisingly, considering his weakness in Latin and Greek, Abraham chose these studies as his area of concentration. Hopkins had abandoned the idea of a single curriculum as taught in the traditional college. Nor did it follow the Harvard system of freely elected courses. Instead, the "group system" was introduced to give students some choice but require them to center their choices in a broad area such as chemistry-biology, Latin-Greek, or history-political science. The student was to be prevented from "shirking" systematic study or being "listless and discursive."[5]

Why the young Flexner chose the classics to emphasize is something of a mystery. His strong interests clearly lay in education and psychology, as well as in history and political science. It was these subjects, the former in particular, that he would pursue after graduation and in his later studies abroad. Did he feel the need to prove himself after his initial resounding failures? Or did he simply warm to the generous professors who helped him so greatly at the outset? His Greek mentor, the helpful Morris, he pictured as "one of the most lovable and high-minded men" he had ever known. "When you leave for home," Morris counseled his promising disciple, "buy a complete Homer, the orators, and works of the tragic poets" and spend the next few years reading them. "You will never regret it." A half-century later Flexner claimed that he had taken the advice to heart and that for many years reading Greek was his chief intellectual occupation.[6]

Being in the academic world of Baltimore in the mid-1880s would always seem a "magic moment" in the lives of those who were part of it. The sheer joy of learning in so free and unfettered a place under the spell of savants whose reputations were just then rocketing upward made many of the participants rapturous. It was, marveled the mathematician and journalist Fabian Franklin—one of those recommending Flexner's admission—a rare moment in history seized upon by those "who had been hungering and thirsting" for such an opportunity. For the philosopher Josiah Royce it was indeed a unique time with "the air full of rumors" of the groundbreaking work being done around him. Everyone, he said, was affected. "One longed to be a doer of the word and not a hearer only." Even the most fledgling scholar, he maintained, wanted to contribute at least an "infinitesimal fraction" to the accumulation of new knowledge.[7]

Flexner, too, although only an undergraduate, felt himself a part of the great transforming experience in American higher education. While he had little contact with the towering figures who were shaping the new university, he was clearly aware of their presence. He remembered seeing Woodrow Wilson, a student of history and politics, at work in the political science library. He knew that Walter Hines Page—who had been a teacher during Flexner's first year at the Louisville Male High School—had been a recent fellow at the university. He may have been aware that John Dewey was studying philosophy the year he arrived. "Any body of graduate students that included Woodrow Wilson, John Dewey, and Frederick Jackson Turner," writes historian Hugh Hawkins, "would merit historical attention."[8] And then there was the faculty. Those who impressed Flexner most were the Greek scholar Basil Gildersleeve, the chemist Ira Remsen, the economist Richard T. Ely, and the historians Herbert Baxter Adams and J. Franklin Jameson. Some of them, notably Page and Jameson, later became close associates and friends. His trigonometry professor, Fabian Franklin, one of several Jewish faculty members, was particularly friendly during his stay and invited him to his home for dinner. Fifty-five years later, Flexner recalled feeling "reverence" for all of them. In his memory, they were all "superior beings" whose advice he followed "without question."

For Daniel Coit Gilman, who had brought this magical enterprise to life, his veneration lasted a lifetime. He gave Gilman credit for having started a revolution in American learning. Over and over again, he praised Gilman's dictum that the true concern of a university was study and not training. There was no "froth," he would later say, in the Johns Hopkins University of his time, and "no special schools for the things that cannot be taught anyway," such as journalism, business, and education. In seeking out the ablest scholars and giving them freedom to work out their

ideas, the university ushered in the modern age of learning, Flexner believed. The university, too, was remarkably free of religious prejudice, so
much so that Hawkins has suggested that Flexner's high praise of Gilman
may have been due to his prejudice-free reception. Gilman's influence on
Flexner's work was profound, the younger man said later: it was clear "in
all I have done or tried to do."[9]

His days as a student in Baltimore set a mark for endurance. Since
Jacob's money would cover at most two years of study, he determined to
finish his degree before the money ran out. He enrolled for two, sometimes three, classes at the same hour, then alternated attendance at them.
Rushing from class to class, he barely had time to catch his breath. In his
first semester, he signed up for a prodigious fourteen courses, including
four in Greek, three in Latin, three in German, two in mathematics, and
one each in English and history. Except for mathematics, his grades were
good or excellent in all of them. He was excused from a required physics
course after passing an oral examination, and he persuaded an English
professor to exempt him from writing weekly compositions by showing
him a few brief communications he had planned to publish in the *Nation*. In the second semester he continued the frenzied pace, only to find
that several of the year-end examinations, each six hours long, were given
at the same time. Going directly to President Gilman, he was told to take
the examinations he could; the president would arrange for special examinations for the remainder.[10]

Flexner kept it up in his final year. He enrolled in a total of twenty
courses, doing well in all of them, except a course in drawing where his
work was judged to be "bad." He did especially well in a course on
Demosthenes, where he earned the rare grade of "1+." In his concentration studies in Greek and Latin he completed all the requirements. During the second half of the year, he took two courses with the psychologist
G. Stanley Hall, one in ethics and the other in psychology, and was given
the grade "excellent" in both. According to the course description, the
work in psychology centered on the "practical applications" of new research on the mind and its workings. This seems to have been his first systematic exposure to the emerging ideas about child learning and methods
of teaching children, though he makes no mention of it in his own writing. His own later insistence on children being taught subjects appropriate to their age and teachers understanding the interests of the individual
child surely owed something to this early experience with Hall.[11]

Little is known of his life outside the classroom. In his autobiography he tells us that he found lodging with a Dr. and Mrs. Kaiser, and he apparently became quite close to them. His surroundings in the city he found congenial. Baltimore was not greatly different from his hometown of Louisville. Both were border cities in border states; both were important centers for railroad and water transportation; both had experienced a sharp burst of industrial and commercial prosperity in the post–Civil War years. But Baltimore was older. As Abraham wandered the dockside streets, many of them dating back to the mid-eighteenth century, he encountered such street names as Thames and Fleet and Shakespeare. The city's streets were only partially paved, and drainage still ran off into open gutters.

He formed friendships with Harry and Julius Friedenwald of Baltimore, both of whom became lifelong intimates. They were among the small band of Jewish students at the university. Julius was a classmate, and Flexner was often in the Friedenwald home for supper on Friday evenings, before the Sabbath. Later, both brothers became prominent physicians; Flexner's family consulted them for the next fifty years. His crowded schedule and lack of money left little other opportunity for social life. He remembered going only twice to the theater, in both cases to see Edwin Booth perform Shakespeare.[12] It must have been a lonely and isolated existence.

After his last examination, he left immediately for home without waiting for the formal graduation. He was nineteen years old with a degree in Greek and Latin and no immediate plans. What would he do next? When he had applied to Hopkins, he had said that he wanted to study law, and for a short time after graduation he began reading Blackstone, but Blackstone "did not intrigue" him. In June he applied for a graduate scholarship at Hopkins but was not awarded it.[13] Teaching must have seemed the only possible outlet for a young man with so impractical an education. And there was the need to start repaying the family's investment in him as soon as practicable.

At nineteen many of the traits that became so familiar to a generation of educators—the towering ambition, the remarkable capacity for work, the unbridled confidence, the practical shrewdness, the striking originality of expression, the self-righteous adherence to principle, the remarkable patience and persuasiveness of manner—were becoming visible in the young Flexner. The years of growing up had left him ambitious and optimistic, determined to be the first in his family to break the downward cycle of opportunity. He was intensely loyal and devoted to his family. For nineteen years after leaving Johns Hopkins he would remain in Louisville as the principal mainstay of his family. Those around him saw a serious but good-humored, affectionate, witty, highly motivated, and pleasant young man. He drank no alcohol, did not smoke, and rarely played cards. He had a fondness for practical jokes, often crude, that never left him. On one hot Louisville summer day he convinced his younger brother, Washington, that the floor radiator was the coolest spot on which to lie, then stoked up the furnace to drive Washington from his refuge.

Although he must have been interested in young women, no hint of any relationship either at Johns Hopkins or in Louisville can be found in the recollections of those who knew him. He had a deep respect for women—whom he idealized as he did his mother—and did not see them as did so many of his contemporaries: as only custodians of a "private sphere" of home and family. Like his contemporary John D. Rockefeller, whose beneficence would make Flexner one of the most powerful figures in American education, he became a "surrogate father" to his family on his return from Baltimore, developing, like Rockefeller, "an exaggerated sense of responsibility that would be evident throughout his life." Like Rockefeller, too, he cast his father's memory in shades of high virtue—to his brother Simon's infinite disgust. In actuality, both the Rockefeller and Flexner fathers were for the most part ne'er-do-wells.[14]

The time in Baltimore confirmed Flexner's belief in his capacity for self-expression. Teachers at both the Louisville Male High School and Hopkins had recognized his writing ability and encouraged him to hone his craft. At nineteen he had developed the distinctive, direct prose style that was recognizable a half-century later. "I think I have never written a line," he later wrote, "over which I have not dwelt with the most critical care." Already he held strong views about what he saw as the trivialization and lack of purpose in American schools and was beginning to frame his arguments in increasingly powerful language. Always his public shyness and consciousness of social status caused him to avoid display and to hide behind the written word. The conflict between his inherent modesty and the boldness of his views would strike close observers for the next fifty years.

Flexner's experience at Johns Hopkins had given him a vision of new potentialities and an immense boost to his self-confidence. He had seen up close men who were headed for notable careers in scholarship and science, and he had found himself not wanting. "A half-taught boy, bitterly aware of the fact, who can keep quiet, learn and constantly—without an inferiority complex—compare himself with his superiors," he came to believe, had a bright future. He believed in himself as only someone emerging from poverty and implausible dreams can.[15] Although forced for the next nineteen years to submerge his dreams and sometimes bury them in despair, he somehow kept alive a sense that he was destined for more than just teaching in Louisville.

Flexner returned to a Louisville that offered him few options. His family's circumstances had not improved. Indeed things grew much worse over the next decade, and Abraham's help became at first welcome and then indispensable. Jacob's drugstore was for a time moderately prosperous, but he now had two children and was increasingly unable to help the rest of the family. His brother and clerk, Simon, now a graduate of the local school of pharmacy, still lived at home and contributed most of his weekly income to his mother. Henry, also married with two children, was of no help to the family. Bernard and Isadore were still unmarried, Bernard working in a bookstore and Isadore in a dry goods store. They lived at home with their mother and the three younger children, contributing what they could toward the family's expenses.[16] All the brothers would fall on hard times in the depression years that lay ahead.

Abraham was home only a few weeks when a job opened at his alma mater, the Louisville Male High School. The school was undergoing a crisis as rampant problems of poor discipline, deteriorating morale, and declining quality of staff aroused the community and the school board. Charges of poor management led to the appointment of Morris Kirby, head of the State Normal School at Lexington, as principal in the summer of 1886. A vacancy for a beginning teacher (called an "assistantship") was announced soon after, and the young Hopkins graduate quickly applied. President Gilman was asked for "a few words" on his behalf. Since "college-bred Louisvillians were not abundant," said Flexner, he got the job. The pay was one thousand dollars a year, but the hardworking newcomer was promoted to "full professor" after one term and gained another five hundred dollars in salary. The school board, in approving the promotion, praised the "remarkable energy and ability" he had shown.[17]

When he presented his mother with one hundred dollars in cash at the end of the first month, "her eyes were filled with tears." It was, he said, the largest amount of money that she had seen at any one time since the failure of his father's business. Thus began a pattern of support, soon to extend to the remaining family members, that would not end until middle age.

He found that he had a love of teaching and that he was good at it. His patience and humor found a ready response in pupils unused to a playful and nonjudgmental approach to learning. He genuinely liked children. He began to read widely in the educational literature to find ideas that would help him understand how children learn and how a teacher could help. He taught five different subjects, including Greek, Latin, and algebra, in classes that were as large as fifty students.

Like most of the public schools of the time, the Louisville Male High School employed teachers with no training in pedagogy. Recitations from textbooks were a common method of imparting learning. Sometimes an entire class would recite a passage in unison. In history classes, important dates and patriotic stories were emphasized. In geography, students learned the names of places and the capital cities of states and nations. Greek and Latin were taught with heavy stress on grammar, composition, and memorization. From the beginning, Flexner, fresh from his stay at Johns Hopkins, was eager to try new approaches and new methods.

Discipline was at first a problem. Many of his students had known him as a fellow student only two years before and were eager to give him an early testing. In the beginning Latin class a boy named Davis began an "uproar" that quickly spread to the others in the classroom. Flexner left immediately for the principal's office, promising him that if he helped him this time he would never again ask for support. Principal Kirby strode to the beginner's classroom, entered the room with his stout cane upraised, and asked Flexner to identify the miscreant. When he pointed to Davis, that worthy made for an open window and jumped out. Asked if there were others involved, Flexner said, "No, the others will now behave themselves." No further problems of discipline, according to his recollection, occurred during his years at the high school. In a later account, Flexner made clear that he did not like to rely on force to keep his classroom in order: "I relied then, and have relied ever since, on my love of young people, my interest in them, and the genuine pleasure that my work has given me."[18]

The only real crisis of his first year came in the second term, when he failed an entire class in Greek. So controversial was this action that parental anger and newspaper outcry forced the school board to hold hearings on Flexner's conduct. Kirby strongly backed his teacher, threatening that both would resign if any move was made to reverse him. It was an important lesson for the young teacher in loyalty, defense of high standards, and persistence in the face of opposition.[19]

Flexner was now well known in Louisville. He was easily the most talked-about local teacher. Despite the outcry over the failed students, he was winning impressive support as an unusually energetic and innovative educator with new ideas about how students learn best. He sought to convince Kirby that a complete reorganization of teaching at the school would benefit both student and teacher morale. Instead of each teacher trying to teach all the subjects in the curriculum, he suggested that each concentrate on those subjects in which he had the greatest knowledge and experience. Specialization would encourage higher standards of teaching and prepare pupils better for their futures. Surprisingly, Kirby acquiesced and new teaching schedules were assigned. Flexner was now given the "chair" in Greek and taught four classes of Greek and one of Latin. Teachers unable to meet the new standards were replaced by younger and better-prepared newcomers. "Those were happy days in the old high school," he fondly remembered, when his skills in the field of education were first recognized.[20]

He read further in the growing literature of education and the psychology of learning. The writings of Rousseau and the Swiss reformer Johann Heinrich Pestalozzi were early known to him. Reading Pestalozzi reinforced his belief that the purpose of education was moral, to provide the child with guidance amidst the surrounding anarchy.[21] Over the next few years he became interested in the ideas of Johann Friedrich Herbart, especially his belief that the teacher must know as much as possible about each pupil so that teaching can begin with the child's own level of experience. Teaching at its best was always individual, he came to believe, and every child had distinctive interests and abilities. He was influenced, too, by Friedrich Froebel's stress on the importance of early childhood and the need for "kindergartens" where young children could be gently introduced to the world of learning.

Indeed, Flexner's first published article in the field of education was concerned with the "ultimate importance" of the kindergarten idea. Written only three years after his return from Baltimore, it described the recent introduction of a private kindergarten in Louisville as "a serious and substantial thing" that ought to spread to other communities. "It is an unspeakable gain," he wrote, "to gather in the little ones every morning from their poverty-stricken homes . . . to exchange their uninteresting, if not positively repulsive surroundings for the wholesome conditions of the little kindergarten world."

Flexner believed that the introduction of kindergartens would bring enduring benefits, for education was a process that from the beginning should be conducted with "a clear purpose and animated by a principle of unity." He deplored the recent emphasis on the hard, practical outcomes of education, with the focus on immediate results, and appealed for more attention to the imaginative abilities of children. These were best cultivated at the very outset of learning. When the kindergarten child was absorbed in "imitating the birds, the raindrops, or the snowflakes" or watching an insect in motion, the interest aroused was "not only scientific, but emotional," and "perception is all the truer and deeper for its twofold basis." The "loss of [a] capacity for wonder" through neglect of early childhood education, he maintained, was "a serious misfortune."[22] At this stage in his life, he was clearly swept up in the romantic idealization of childhood that was so much a part of the early progressive movement in education.

His interest in politics also found outlet in publication. In a series of sharply worded letters and short articles, he became a regular contributor to the *Nation* on Kentucky politics and national issues. He commended President Cleveland's courage in opposing his own party on the silver question, in vetoing an overly generous pension bill, and in taking a stand against the tariff. The "silver folly," he wrote, was sweeping the nation because of the sufferance of naive persons who failed to understand how this "madness" could destroy the credit of the nation. The tough-minded Cleveland, he told his readers, was "the most healthful influence" the nation had felt for years. He regularly castigated the Republicans for their stand on protection—"the tariff run mad"—and attacked the Republican stalwart James B. Blaine as "practicing the arts of a politician and a demagogue." The outcome of the 1888 election—Harrison's triumph over Cleveland despite winning fewer votes—was attributed to "ignorance, self-interest, and misrepresentation." He deplored the "race mission" of Great Britain and urged that America not become part of "an Anglo-Saxon crusade." "We are a nation," he asserted, "but not a race; we are the strange product of many mingled races."[23]

In Louisville he applauded an electoral reform, aimed at combatting fraud and intimidation, that would make the ballot more secret. At the state level he decried the baneful effects of the spoils system, which had brought death to two men in a "barbarous" brawl in Lexington. He wrote on revenue reform in the state, on the conduct of the Louisville post office, and on the contest for the speakership in the national House of Representatives.[24] Throughout his two decades in Louisville, his signed accounts continued to appear regularly in the *Nation*. Many of them were marked by forceful argument, close knowledge of the political scene, and references to the Federalist Papers or James Bryce or recent work by historians and political scientists. His prose had an authoritative tone and suggested a degree of political sophistication that belied his lack of experience in the political arena.

While gaining experience as a writer, Flexner settled quietly into the routine of teaching school. He found the job easy; he was at the high school from only eight-thirty in the morning to one-thirty in the afternoon, leaving him plenty of time for reading and writing. His reputation was established as the most effective teacher at the school, and he occasionally tutored a college-bound boy for extra pay. He was now subscribing to educational journals and occasionally attending national meetings of educators. He was making friends and beginning to exert some small influence in educational circles. He opened correspondence with some of the nation's leading educators; some ignored him, but others welcomed the chance to exchange ideas.

His heart was still set on returning to study, but the prospects of breaking free began slowly to dim. In 1889 he asked Johns Hopkins for "a general statement" regarding his work, but no record exists of what use he planned to make of it. Three years later he wrote Gilman that he never stopped thinking about the years he had spent in Baltimore, adding, "I have been eagerly awaiting the opportunity to renew there the life which I left almost seven years ago."[25] Other such outcries followed, but neither his conscience nor the growing urgency of his family responsibilities gave him hope of an early breakout.

For six years he taught his high school classes dutifully. His steady income and dependability made him the anchor of the family's fortunes. For all his boredom at the monotony of his life and his impatience with the school's failure to enforce high standards, he saw no way to escape. When the opportunity came, in 1892, to risk his steady course and try his hand at running a school of his own, he did not hesitate. All the optimism and high-energy determination of the Hopkins years returned with a rush as he planned to make the new school the means of financial escape for his siblings and for himself.

3

Mr. Flexner's School

The new adventure was risky but promised large returns. Flexner was determined to ease his family's finances and to free himself for new possibilities. At age twenty-six, buoyed by the experience at Johns Hopkins and his success at teaching, he was more strongly convinced than ever that his destiny lay ahead, beyond the narrow opportunities in Louisville.

But first he was committed to helping his brothers and sisters. He had started his redemption efforts with his older brother, Simon, just after returning from Baltimore. Simon, who had been sickly and had completed only the sixth grade, was considered the "slow child" and at times the "despair" of his family. While Abraham was away, he had worked at Jacob's drugstore filling prescriptions, helping promote toilet articles and patent medicines, and chatting with the practitioners who made the drugstore headquarters for the latest medical gossip. He became fascinated with a microscope that Jacob had acquired to do saliva and urine analysis for the doctors. He showed a new interest in learning and started reading some of the latest pathology textbooks. Occasionally, he made crude studies of small-animal anatomy, examined the wings of insects, and dreamed of creating his own pathology laboratory. Like his famous brothers, Simon would have a career built on foundations of practical experience, self-taught knowledge, and personal ambition. Never, in the opinion of historian Saul Benison, did a scientific career begin "more inauspiciously." Learning by doing in pathology, he writes, was the "outstanding feature" of Simon's training.[1]

When Abraham came home from Johns Hopkins, he told Simon of the plans to create in Baltimore a new kind of hospital and medical school, one that would emphasize scientific research and original discovery. While still a student, he had heard several lectures by the new pathology professor, William Henry Welch, and he now impressed on Simon his conviction that no other place held such promise for the study of pathology. To even think of studying there, Abraham told Simon, one needed a medical degree. Simon quickly acquired one in two short courses of lectures at the University of Louisville medical school. Most of the practitioner-professors at the school knew him, admired his work in microscopy, and eased his way to a degree in medicine in 1889. "I don't think he ever heard a lecture," recalled Abraham with some exaggeration, "and he never made a dissection or ever saw a patient." It was understood that Simon would never practice medicine. While earning his degree, he even conducted a course in histology and pathology for the other students.[2]

Enthusiastic about the progress so far, Abraham now took as his task the management of his brother's next career move. Learning that a pathology fellowship was being offered at Johns Hopkins, he urged Simon to apply. Simon needed little encouragement. Abraham told him to send with the application a paper he had written on urinalysis, together with slides, some of them of insect wings and eyes. The submission was hardly earth-shaking to Professor Welch, who, for years thereafter, told humorous stories, to Simon's dismay, of how the young doctor from Louisville had submitted "slides of insects' eyes and butterfly wings [of the sort] which young ladies made in finishing school."[3] Simon did not win the fellowship.

Once more Simon began to settle into a career of self-instruction and employment at Jacob's drugstore. The future seemed as bleak as ever. But Abraham now repeated the gesture that Jacob had made to him six years before. He told Simon that he would advance, from the amounts he was giving his mother, the money for a year of study in Baltimore. Neither his mother nor Jacob liked the idea. Simon himself, despite his gratitude, wondered whether a year at the better-known University of Pennsylvania medical school might not serve his interests better. But Abraham was fully convinced and brooked no opposition. Simon left for Baltimore in September 1890.

Forty years later, Simon thanked his brother for his foresight. "Sending me to the Hopkins and Dr. Welch in that far-away autumn of 1890," he said, "has meant more to me than anyone . . . can know. It was not only that you made it possible with money . . . but that you should have possessed the insight that convinced you that Dr. Welch was the master in pathology, that is almost miraculous."[4]

Simon arrived at Johns Hopkins with a diploma but little else. He was essentially self-taught, knew little of the basic medical sciences, and was intensely hungry to learn. Throughout his years in Baltimore, as he became Welch's closest and most prominent protégé, the brothers exchanged frequent letters. Abraham advised his older sibling on his studies, read his papers, cheered his triumphs, and gave him firm advice about job opportunities. When Simon was given the pathology fellowship in his second year, Jacob protested that he could no longer be spared at home, but Abraham offered Simon assurance: Jacob "underrates the value of the fellowship [but] I attach great weight to it." Simon must come back "thoroughly prepared," Abraham told him, able to do original work, and capable of "doing something for the good of humanity." After the fellowship year, he insisted that Simon remain in Baltimore. "One thing is clear," he told him: "You stay where you are."[5]

Time and again, he urged Simon to stay with Welch and to pass up a half-dozen teaching jobs at such schools as Rush Medical College, Jefferson Medical College, and Cornell's school of medicine. "At your age," he counseled Simon, "you should squeeze the lemon dry." "As regards the offer from Rush," he told Simon, "you surely can anticipate my opinion. Under no circumstances, should you permit yourself to be tempted away from Baltimore now. You must play for higher stakes." When Jefferson, a struggling school in Philadelphia, made Simon an offer in 1895, Abraham warned that it was "unwise" to even consider Jefferson. It was "the wrong kind of place"; "that appears to me final." He continued to advance Simon money for books and living expenses, and offered to support a year of study abroad. He advised him not to consider short trips: "I want you to make a long, thorough stay when you go." Nor should Simon worry about him. "I will wait my turn," he wrote, "just as you have had to await yours." Constantly he urged Simon not to cut short his training in order to help at home. "I shall not permit you to sacrifice your future or your ambition to mine," he told his brother.[6]

At times Abraham's tone of noble self-sacrifice grated on his sensitive brother's nerves. He began urging Abraham to break free himself from the family bonds tying him to Louisville. He came close to accusing Abraham of seeking martyrdom through his self-imposed exile. The family, he argued, could if necessary do without him; Abraham's great promise should no longer be sacrificed. He once characterized his brother, not entirely fairly, as "a strong person, very generous, intensely egotistical, with a great capacity for self-deception."[7] Jacob, too, came to resent Abraham's growing assertiveness and his displacing him as the Flexners' surrogate father. The intense responsibility Abraham felt for the rest of the family, however, and a continuing sense of guilt at his own early advantage, as well as perhaps a new sense of importance, left little doubt in his mind that he was the chosen instrument to move his brothers and sisters beyond their limited horizons.

To the younger siblings, Washington, Gertrude, and Mary, and eventually to the older brothers as well, Abraham became in fact a principal means of finding new outlets for their ambitions. In the same year that he began to support Simon's study at Johns Hopkins, he made it possible for his sister Mary to enroll at Bryn Mawr College in Philadelphia. Mary was an unusually bright, personable young woman who had long been the favorite of her brothers. More than fourteen years younger than Jacob, Mary had a hearing problem and was given special treatment. She was especially close to Abraham. His determination to give her what he believed was the best education available to an American woman—he saw Bryn Mawr as the female counterpart to Johns Hopkins—suggests an uncommon view of women's fitness for advanced education. She was one of few Jewish students to attend the exclusive Philadelphia college at that time.

As Simon prepared to depart for Baltimore, Abraham arranged for him to accompany Mary to Philadelphia and obtained a letter of introduction from Daniel Coit Gilman for Mary to take to Bryn Mawr's president. He was proud of his young sister. "I think of her often, indeed often each day," he wrote, "and always with intense gratification on account of her delightful situation and her obvious growth."[8]

His other sister, Gertrude, had meanwhile finished high school and was persuaded by Abraham to teach kindergarten. The job required only a love of children and skill in dealing with them, not special education. In 1890, at age twenty, she began teaching kindergarten at the Union Gospel Mission. She taught there and at other locations until Abraham opened his own kindergarten at his private school in 1897.[9] Mary, having returned from Bryn Mawr, joined Gertrude in teaching at the Flexner school.

Abraham was instrumental, too, along with Jacob, in helping two of his other brothers, Bernard and Washington, start a bookstore and stationery shop. His letters of the nineties are full of references to "the boys," as he called them, and the credits and loans he advanced toward launching the enterprise. Helping them now, he said, would mean "years of life and peace" and "a much needed sense of security" for everyone. With Jacob he made ambitious plans to build two adjoining houses for the family, one for Jacob's family, the other for the rest of the Flexners.[10] At the same time, he told Simon over and over that he planned to get away "next year" to continue his own education, but he spoke with increasing vagueness and decreasing conviction. Perhaps he repeated the plan so often to appease Simon's frequent challenge that he was wasting his talents.

By the spring of 1892 he was thoroughly bored with the routine of teaching his four classes in Greek and one in Latin. For some time, he had been searching for a new outlet for his energies, short of leaving Louisville and abandoning his family. Tutoring some of his pupils had become a good source of new income, and he began seriously to consider leaving his teaching post altogether and devoting all of his time to preparing boys for entrance to college. One troubled father, whose son had been expelled from an eastern preparatory school, was especially insistent that Flexner spend enough time to prepare the boy for Princeton. Seeing his chance, Flexner agreed to undertake the work only if the father could find three or four other boys whose families would support their education in private classes. "If I can make sure of 4 at $400 each I will cast the die," he told Simon. He was very anxious to give the new venture a try. He planned to hold classes from nine to one-thirty each day, which meant that he would be "better off than now," have less to do, and even be able "to take up French in earnest."[11]

He took the gamble, although some of the commitments were shaky. In September he opened classes for five students in four subjects. The classes met in two bare rooms that his mother had located, but these were soon exchanged for larger quarters. He found the small group far easier to teach than his previous classes because there was no need to talk loudly or to hold the attention of many boys at once. He could cover more topics more thoroughly. Now "school board, faculty and janitor, all in one," he enjoyed his new endeavors. He became convinced as he gained success that small classes, personal attention, and hands-on teaching were the keys to effective learning. He would apply these lessons to his later work in medical education, the planning of New York's Lincoln School, and the founding of the Institute for Advanced Study. Not everyone, he believed, was cut out for this kind of personal teaching. It took "considerable familiarity and experience," he said, and no amount of scholarship or learning could take its place. "It is not high teaching," he admitted, but it was far more satisfying than the high school experience had been.[12]

And he was good at it. The first students, troubled youngsters from wealthy families, came to him to qualify for entrance to leading colleges. Many had dropped out of other schools, so his bread and butter depended on his skill with problem students. He was making the effort of his life, he confided, and the pupils were responding. His goal was to teach the boys

self-reliance. "The change in them has come somewhat suddenly," he told
Simon. One boy with a reputation for mischief and poor attention at another school, he wrote, now sat "under [his] eye" and gave him no trouble
at all.[13] To his immense relief, most of them passed the entrance examinations and moved on to eastern colleges. Gradually, as parents learned of his
record in getting sixteen- and seventeen-year-olds into distinguished colleges, he began to attract larger numbers of less troubled youngsters.

He was popular with his pupils and refreshingly unlike the teachers
they had known. Red-headed students in the class were invariably called
"Kentucky Cardinals," after a local baseball team; a good paper came back
with "Hurrah for you" scrawled across the top; a student who was late was
loaned the teacher's watch until he showed up on time. A former pupil
remembered that Mr. Flexner gave many compliments but was "a hellcat
if you were not exerting the best of your abilities." Flexner found that he
could do things very differently than he had in his high school class.
He could use his own wits and ingenuity to stimulate his students. "You
can't make people learn Latin or Greek," he said, "unless they have a bent
for it," for "anything you don't want to do you do in a slipshod fashion."
His success, he insisted, stemmed from the small class size and his bent
for seeing what a particular boy was interested in. "Take hold of a boy
where he's strong," he told a reporter many years later, "not where he's
weak." The important principle in teaching was to focus on the concrete
pupil. "I'd say to myself, 'Now, what the dickens is he interested in?' and
I'd feel my way around until I found out." Beyond learning the ABCs, he
concluded, people learn best by learning things in which "they are interested or can be interested."[14]

By the second year, the number of pupils at "Mr. Flexner's School" increased to twelve and he was forced to take on another teacher. The school
quickly became very profitable. He rented a still larger suite of rooms. In
1895 he accepted the first female students and put out the first catalog.
New teachers were added, including Mary and Gertrude; soon there were
eight faculty members. Instruction was offered in six languages, five sciences, mathematics through trigonometry, history (five courses), and
drawing. He reached out beyond Louisville for students. A year after he
sold the school in 1905, enrollment reached one hundred pupils and the
value of the grounds and building, which he now owned, was estimated
at fifty thousand dollars (perhaps a million and a half dollars in today's
currency). Some of the pupils came from as far away as South America
and Panama.[15]

How did he do it? His graduates were not only being accepted at leading colleges but entering college at a much younger age compared to those from elite private schools. Of the first hundred graduates, all who applied to college were admitted. At Harvard, the phenomenon caught the attention of President Charles W. Eliot, who wrote to ask Flexner for more information about his school's approach.[16]

Eliot was at the head of a national movement to reform secondary curriculum. Like Flexner, he believed that schooling was taking too long. American education, he maintained, was "very confused." He was particularly interested, as was Flexner, in bringing such studies as science, foreign languages, and modern literature into the high school. The old curriculum, which stressed Greek, Latin, and mathematics, was outmoded, Eliot believed. As chairman of the Committee of Ten, created in 1892 by the National Education Association to set a common standard for college admissions, he wielded enormous power. Of special importance for the future was the committee's recommendation that all children, not just the college bound, receive an "academic education." Colleges were urged to loosen their admission requirements; high schools were encouraged to teach students history, science, and modern languages; and all teachers were told to replace memorization and recitation with new, more active teaching methods. Significantly for many in coming generations, the committee decided against treating subject matter differently "for pupils going to college, for those going to a scientific school, and for those who, presumably, are going to neither."[17]

Eliot must have seen in Flexner a kindred spirit. On receiving Eliot's letter, Flexner seized the chance to go to Cambridge and talk to him. He told Eliot, as he remembered it, that it was all quite simple. He treated each child as an individual and "let each go at his own pace." Once their appetites were whetted by finding one area that interested them, he found other areas where interest could be aroused. For students totally lacking mathematical or language ability, he worked at "sheer mechanical techniques" that got them into college.

The unconventional schoolmaster must have impressed Eliot, for the Harvard president urged him to write an article explaining his ideas for a national journal. When the article appeared, Eliot asked to buy forty copies for the governing boards of Harvard University. "Your doctrine," he told the proud Flexner, "should be brought home to every school committeeman, and college trustee in the country."[18] It was the beginning of a long association with the Harvard president, who became one of Flexner's strongest supporters a few years later as a powerful member of Rockefeller's General Education Board.

In his appeal for students, Flexner painted a bright picture of the methods and course of study he followed, contrasting them with those of his competitors, both public and private. The size of his school was a great advantage. The grouping of sixty students into a single class in some public schools, he said, was a disaster. In many cities, superintendents were striving to *reduce* the size of classes to sixty. The "class phalanx," in his view, defied any chance of individual development. Only a radical change—getting rid of the "human staircase" and teaching small groups of twelve children or less with the same teacher year after year—could end the lockstep. No attention was paid in most schools to the rich differences in intelligence, interests, and learning strategies among the assembled mass; the routine was as bad for the bright as for the dull student. As a result, many, perhaps most, youngsters lost interest in schooling and learning for the rest of their lives. Damage was compounded by turning the class over each year to a new teacher, who, like the previous year's teacher, would have to start learning the crucial individual differences among students all over again.[19]

For these reasons, Flexner told parents, he had "utterly discarded" classwork. In its place, he had substituted individual teaching and an individual course of study. Each student was evaluated and materials were selected to fit the student's own capacities. A form of private, tutorial-style instruction was thus available to every child. He was strongly opposed, he said, to "making a distinction in early life" between those who were headed for college and those who were not. Good education was expensive, but the cost was justified by its importance.

Homework was discouraged, especially for those under twelve. Much of the required work could be done at the school, and homework was never so onerous as to limit outdoor exercise, play, or reading for pleasure. Instead of having students read textbooks, he had them read novels and write daily compositions. Science, so far as possible, was taught through observation and experiment. "The thing called nature," he later wrote, "must appeal with living power."[20] He abolished all purely "artificial tasks" such as looking up lists of words in the dictionary, assigning long compositions on unfamiliar topics, and drilling in abstract English grammar.

Discipline was not a problem, he said. A group spirit of respect for each other's work took over, so there was no need for rigid rules. In every possible way, he told parents, he tried to bring variety into the school, assigning different texts in the same subject, taking unexpected outdoor trips, and participating himself in recreation and field projects. To encourage an atmosphere of mutual respect, he banned invidious comparisons, gave no examinations, and bestowed "no marks, honors, prizes or distinctions of any kind." In place of report cards, he arranged parent conferences or sent parents lengthy letters about their child.[21]

Each day was a contest between teacher and pupil to stir the embers of learning. He relied on enthusiasm, cleverness in outwitting students, and good humor. A desire to emulate other students often spurred learning. "I pushed those who showed aptitude for a given subject and was patient when no aptitude existed." While much of his time was spent on the dull and mediocre student, he treasured most those who showed real capacity for learning. "I was never indifferent to mediocrity," he recalled. "I tried hard to do what I could for it with results that were surprisingly good." But it was the able but underachieving child who interested him most. Sometimes he tried new groupings of students to get weaker pupils to follow the example of the stronger. Two or more pupils might compete with one another in algebra while belonging to quite different groups in Greek or Latin. Teaching was thus a continuing strategy to get the best outcome and not just a matter of tutoring or coaching.[22] Parents marveled at his ability to apply practical organizational skills to educational theory in an ongoing educational enterprise.

Flexner was aware that the educational utopia he was creating was expensive and could serve only a very few. "Our efforts," he wrote in the school's prospectus, "are concentrated on a very small number of children, with whom we live on intimate terms, socially and intellectually." He must have known, too, that his own energetic and creative personality had much to do with the school's success. As he came to think about selling the school and moving on to new prospects beyond Louisville he found that it was "too much identified" with him "to be detachable" from him. He had great difficulty in selling the school "without selling [him]self."[23]

As his sisters joined the teaching staff, the school took on the character of a family enterprise. Gertrude Flexner was put in charge of the primary department, which was limited to ten children from six to twelve years of age, while Mary was made assistant to her brother in managing the secondary department. For a brief period, Jacob, too, joined the teaching staff. The presence of women in teaching positions, Flexner believed, would make the school more attractive to female students. Although few girls enrolled (the largest number was six) he made it clear that he favored coeducation. "Whatever argument justifies a given education for boys," he quoted Thomas Huxley approvingly, "justifies its application to girls as well." Within the school, "a decidedly normal and wholesome relation" existed between girls and boys, and he openly pleaded for more girls. He said that he would enroll any girl "who [took] her education seriously" but recognized that most applications would come from those planning to go to college.[24]

The Flexner school was but one of many such experimental attempts at a new kind of education in America's fin-de-siècle years. Educators in scores of communities were interested in new theories of learning, new ideas about teaching, new ways of making schools more useful to an evolving nation of cities and industries.

In Chicago, four years after Flexner opened his innovative school, John Dewey began his famous "laboratory school." Dewey aimed to make education relevant to a society that was no longer rural or agricultural, one whose children were cut off from the lessons of nature and family responsibility. The world of children had changed radically, Dewey taught, and an equally radical change was needed in education. The school must somehow restore the experience with natural things and personal responsibility that were lost with the decline of the farm and small-town life. Learning was no longer a monopoly of the leisure class but a practical necessity in an industrial, democratic society. Schools, Dewey said in 1899, could no longer be passive, mechanically massing children of different talents; they must give individual attention to children in small classes and train creative teachers for a new curriculum focused on the child.[25]

Dewey's theories reminded Flexner of his own developing views. In 1897, two years before Dewey's lectures on "The School and Society," Flexner had written in the *International Journal of Ethics* that education was "essentially a social process" that aims to prepare the child "for an active career in a given social environment." No such thing existed as an ideal educational program. It was for life in a democratic society that the American child must be prepared and the "point of emphasis" was no longer the subjects of study but the child.[26]

After reading one of Dewey's articles, Flexner sent him one of his own papers (he does not say which one) and received "a most cordial reply." Dewey said that he wanted to see the Flexner school and that there was no question in his mind that Flexner's method was "the right one." He complimented Flexner on his unique ability "to state that method [so] clearly and forcibly." If Dewey came to Louisville to see Flexner's school,

no record of the visit remains, but in 1902 Flexner journeyed to Chicago
to visit Dewey. Years later, on Dewey's ninetieth birthday, Flexner recalled
the visit and generously told him that "undoubtedly" some of his inspiration "was due to that visit."[27]

While Flexner saw himself as Dewey's comrade in the emerging "progressive education" movement, he did not share what he saw as Dewey's
utopian view of the school's role in American life. Where Dewey saw the
school as a means of reconstructing a disturbed social order, making the
classroom an agent of social democracy and the reform of urban-indus-
trial ills, Flexner remained firm that school reform should be independent of political considerations. The successes of his own family made him
believe in the laissez-faire economy and the limited state. He favored the
Mugwump doctrines of governing honestly and correcting the glaring ex-
cesses of the Gilded Age, especially the widespread corruption and the
high tariff walls. He believed that with mild reforms the fundamental
workings of the American economy could be made sound.

The purpose of the school, Flexner believed, was to enable individual
children to make the most of their talents, not to bring fundamental
change to American life. His greatest concern was for the exceptional
child lost in a rigid, conventional curriculum of traditional studies. In
Flexner's view far more than Dewey's, it was the teacher's job to "manage
the child-mind," to find areas of interest, to direct students. He was increasingly critical of those whose romantic view of childhood led them to
urge the spontaneous development of children's interests independent of
the teacher. Childhood for many, he was convinced, was a time of overwhelming confusion, clashing emotions, and a struggle for meaning. To
leave children to find their own inner direction at this critical time, said
Flexner, was to abandon them to drift and chance. The good teacher, he
wrote, gave students a sense of direction and possibility.[28]

Steadily, as the years passed, he grew in confidence as an effective and
increasingly outspoken critic of conventional education. His articles appeared in the influential *Educational Review* as well as in such popular
journals as *Atlantic Monthly* and *Popular Science*. By the time he left
Louisville, he had come to reject the idea of schooling as mental discipline
through hard study of traditional subjects. He questioned, too, the usefulness of teaching the classics. In the new world of education, it was
senseless, he believed, to imagine that "hard and unattractive" subjects
like mathematics or Greek trained the mind any better than modern subjects like chemistry or American history.

Although a student and teacher of the classics himself, he labeled their contemporary study "a pathetically futile make-believe." The hold of Greek and Latin on the curriculum was "irretrievably broken," yet the traditional colleges still demanded their study. The only reason to learn a language, he declared, was to use it as a medium of ideas and, in that sense, "honest work in the study of Latin and Greek" was "almost unknown." How could the usefulness of such study be compared to "exposure to science, industry, or manual work or to art, music, or literature?"[29]

According to Flexner, the mindless lockstep curriculum of the average preparatory or high school, tailored to fit a rigid set of college requirements (whether the child planned to attend college or not), made real education nearly impossible. Despite efforts to raise standards in medical school, he wrote in 1899, the medical student would "continue to be a crude and untrained youth" as long as the existing system of preparatory education continued. The American student, unlike the European student, he charged, "knocks at nineteen or later for admission at college doors, with his little Latin and Greek, a bungler in the use of his native tongue, strangely incapable of close observation or thought and generally without marked intellectual interests in any direction." By radical reform, American children could complete their preparation much earlier and, like his own graduates, enter college at sixteen or seventeen. Furthermore, breaking the lockstep in secondary education was the only truly democratic way to treat children, for democracy was the form of society in which "the greatest individual diversity" should be encouraged.[30]

Here again was a theme to which he would often return. Like Dewey, he proposed that the reformed school be made "coextensive" with the child's whole life "for the school is . . . no longer remote from life, it is life." There was no such thing as education in the abstract; in the case of every child it had to be "practical, concrete, and definite."[31]

His very real success as a schoolmaster and the prosperity it brought made him even more the paterfamilias of the Flexner clan. At one time or another he was involved in advising and supporting every member of the family. He became prosperous during a serious economic depression in the 1890s that threatened the Flexners with new disasters rivaling those of twenty years before. Jacob's drugstore, the bookstore belonging to Bernard and Washington, the hat business run by Henry, Isadore's career as replacement for Simon at the drugstore—all were in deep financial trouble by the mid-nineties. The house adjoining Jacob's, intended to house the rest of the family, was surrendered at a loss before it was ever occupied. The Flexner school not only employed three (at times four) of the Flexner clan but staved off disaster for the rest. By Abraham's later estimate, perhaps exaggerated, he advanced or gave outright as much as two hundred thousand dollars to family members during the course of his long life.[32]

In the face of the new financial storms, the family, now largely dependent on Abraham's steady income, borrowed heavily to save the family's enterprises. Bernard and Washington, with Abraham's help, expanded their bookstore into publishing and then into the larger field of lithographic printing. As the economic crisis deepened, Jacob too found himself heavily in debt; he had branched into drug manufacturing and acquired a machine to bottle soft drinks, and he was on the verge of bankruptcy. Abraham came to the rescue. His own plans for further study were constantly postponed as the crisis wore on. His earnings were now entirely devoted to the household. Still, the situation grew worse. He asked Simon in the depression year of 1893 to wait before sending his book bill and inquired how long he thought he could defer paying Mary's tuition at Bryn Mawr. When Simon accused Abraham of finding new excuses to delay his own further education, Abraham asked his brother to believe him when he said that he was "entirely willing to stay on doing one of the indispensable things—providing the family with means to achieve intellectual ends, means which [were] of ever greater importance" to them.[33]

James Thomas Flexner, Simon's historian-son, who read the brothers' exchanges during these years, believes that a number of Abraham's "salient characteristics" came to the fore in the family crisis: a "determination and ability to lead"; a "disdain for moving cautiously"; pride in "carrying off complicated and sometimes secret manipulations"; an ability to accommodate others "to sooth [sic] the impact of his drives"; and "boundless energy," which left him "optimistic in almost any situation."[34] To these should be added a deep sentimentality, usually concealed from others, a genuine gratefulness for the support he himself had gotten, and an almost mystical confidence that delaying his own plans would not matter; his hour would come.

When Simon was hired as an assistant to Welch in 1893, Abraham began to press him for larger contributions to the family. "You and I are the only persons who can help," he told him. He pleaded with his brother to make a commitment to regular support. He assured Simon that he did not want him—nor would he "permit" him—to change his present course but simply wanted him to face their "future responsibilities." Until this time, Simon had been necessarily "out of it," but as his prospects improved, he would be expected to take his share of responsibility. For his part, Abraham would continue to carry the principal burden. "You may say that I ought not to sacrifice myself for the others," he said defensively, "but it is just as certain that I ought not to sacrifice them for me." At age twenty-eight, he said, he had learned not to expect the easy fulfillment of his ambitions.[35]

The concern over money was a constant refrain in the brothers' letters throughout the nineties. "Your hair would rise on end," Abraham told Simon in 1895, "if you could know the inside history of these last years." In the week before the letter was written, five banks had gone under. Others were unlikely to withstand the continuing runs on their reserves. Simon's plea for four hundred dollars for a microscope was rejected. "You cannot easily guess how sorry we all are to be obliged to write in this strain" but "you simply cannot imagine the state of things." Abraham's own hopes were further deferred. He had banished "all idea of an early release."[36]

For all the money Abraham poured into Jacob's drugstore, it continued to flounder. "Jake's condition financially is hopeless," he concluded in 1896. Not only was the business forty thousand dollars in debt, it was still losing money. Bankruptcy—which Abraham had fought so hard to avoid—was now unavoidable. Simon argued that the debt-ridden businesses of Bernard and Washington should also be sacrificed. But Abraham's pride in the family name would not permit further failures, and he advanced still more money to pay off their debts. He pleaded with Simon to forgive him for asking how much support to expect from him in the year ahead.[37]

Abraham now urged the discouraged Jacob, free of the drugstore, to take a rest for several months and then turn to the practice of medicine. The oldest brother could leave behind the "dog's life" he had been forced to lead. Like Simon, Jacob was highly regarded by the faculty at the local medical college, affiliated with the University of Louisville. Jacob just as easily acquired a medical degree. The college required less than a high school education for admission, and two brief courses of lectures for graduation.

After Jacob was awarded his degree, Abraham arranged for him to go to Baltimore and New York for a short period of study before beginning a practice. Simon reported an embarrassing incident when he invited his brother to lunch with the leading figures of the Johns Hopkins School of

Medicine. The quiet and dignified Simon was humiliated by Jacob's loud talk and unpolished manner: "No one else had a chance of a word." He upbraided his brother for his behavior and refused to have him at meals in the hospital. Abraham promptly defended his oldest brother, telling Simon that it was difficult for Jacob, who had made the greatest sacrifice, to be so dependent on his younger brothers. He realized, he told Simon, that Jacob's stay in Baltimore would not make him "a J.H. doctor," but the experience would give him plausibility as a practitioner. Jacob would get his learning, he admonished Simon, "as you got yours, after his work begins, instead of precedent there to, [sic] as in the natural order." It was true that Jacob's bluster and loudness needed to be tamed, he conceded, but while "conceit is intolerable, a certain self-assurance is indispensable."[38]

By the late nineties, conditions began slowly to improve for those remaining in Louisville. Jacob was able to obtain a position as city physician and to begin what became a respected practice. Bernard broke free to begin a distinguished career in law. Like Simon and Jacob, he earned a quick degree at the University of Louisville and then did advanced study elsewhere—in Bernard's case, at the University of Virginia. In time, he would become nearly as well known as Simon and Abraham, winning a reputation as an authority on juvenile law, as a corporate attorney, and as a prominent Zionist during his years as chairman of the Palestine Economic Corporation. His partner at the bookstore, Washington, found new outlets in insurance and printing, moving to Chicago in 1915, where he established the leading financial printing company in the country. The two younger sisters were employed at the Flexner School, and Gertrude was about to marry. The remaining brothers, Henry and Isadore, found secure jobs in the aftermath of the economic downturn.

Although saddled with debts, Abraham could now breathe more easily: the worst was over. The experience left him drained and uncharacteristically pessimistic, however. "I have slowly been drifting to . . . the conclusion," he informed Simon, "that whereas I should never permit anyone else to do what I have done, nevertheless, the obligation is heavy upon all for whom I have given up everything to give up something for me." The pattern of deepening debt had been set with his support of Simon and Mary, he said, and Simon should realize that it was not just his efforts on behalf of Jacob and the others, as Simon seemed to believe, that had buried him so deeply. While the whole story reflected on his "lack of judgment," he still did not know where he could have drawn the line.[39]

One bright ray illuminated the gloom of these years. He had fallen in love with a young woman, once his student, who had graduated from Vassar College. While he did not feel free to marry, he did become engaged in 1896 and began once more to dream of reviving his "early hopes and ambitions" as soon as the debts could be cleared away.[40] It would take another nine years before he was able to break free.

4

Breaking Free

Ten years after his return from Baltimore, Abraham Flexner, now thirty years old, was engaged. The long years of loneliness and single life were about to end. In many ways, he had accomplished much. His private school was highly regarded. He was the mainstay of his family. He was well known in Louisville and was beginning to make contacts in the wider world of education.

But with the passage of time he had grown more uncertain, even downhearted, about his chances of ever starting a new professional life. The weight of family debt suffocated every hope of breaking free. The school, moreover, promised to become more prosperous, making it even more difficult to think of making a "leap in the dark." At times he felt self-pity at the waste of his talents. His health was still good—he was rarely sick—but he complained of fatigue, inability to concentrate, and loss of enthusiasm. Photographs of him in this era show a somber, schoolmasterish man wearing an intense expression behind wire eyeglasses. He had a receding hairline and a prominent moustache. Much of the old spontaneity and wit seem to have wilted. More and more, he moved like a workhorse in harness, shielded by blinders, plodding straight ahead. It was the darkest period in his life.

As a well-known businessman and eligible bachelor who taught some of the children of Louisville's elite, he was sought after in civic and social circles. Dutifully, he attended community lunches, gave the required speeches, and was welcomed into many of the city's homes. Only baseball provided an escape. Frequently he went to see the Kentucky Cardinals play. A visit from a young woman from Cincinnati, a friend of the family, led to a return visit to see the opening game of the Cincinnati Reds. His circle of friends, while small, was close. With his brother Bernard he went to teas at the Semple sisters' home or played whist with other friends. Occasionally he went on picnics, made outings in the countryside, or went to the local theater. His love of the theater was becoming a passion. He received an invitation to share a prominent banker's box at a charity ball. Another time, he spent "a glorious day" at the country estate of a business friend and "climbed by moonlight over rocks and through dense woods"—an "enchantingly beautiful scene."[1]

More often now he was in the company of young women. His earlier shyness and monastic habits gave way to an easier, more relaxed relationship with those he met. He was a pleasant, often funny, attentive companion. He looked forward to the evenings he spent at a "Mrs. Cheatham's," who lived with two attractive nieces. Sometimes the three of them went to a friend's cabin for a "change of scene, good air, and abundant nonsense." More and more, he spoke of "interesting" or "charming" or "attractive" women he met. But it was a woman he had scarcely seen for four years who became his fiancée in the summer of 1896. She had returned to Louisville the preceding year after graduating from Vassar College and had found employment as a tutor and occasional teacher at Mr. Flexner's School.

Anne Laziere Crawford had met her future husband in 1890 when her uncle, a distiller and leading businessman, hired him to tutor her for college. She had grown up in Georgia, the great-granddaughter of William H. Crawford, an 1824 presidential candidate. Her father had surrendered with Lee at Appomattox and then trudged on foot back to Georgia. She had come to live with her wealthy uncle, John Atherton, while still in her teens. On her mother's side, her French grandmother had perished on the voyage to America. Abraham attributed Anne's gaiety, high spirits, and charm to her Gallic forebears.[2]

When she met Abraham, she was a girl of sixteen, taller and more robust than he (he had reached his limit of five feet, five inches), fun-loving, talkative, and clearly very bright. A member of Abraham's family later reported that he found her outgoing and very personable, with a "terrific" personality. At that time, Abraham claimed to have had misgivings about teaching a girl, but he said he had decided that "it might be more fun teaching a clever girl than a dull boy."[3] In a single year she passed all six of the required examinations and left for college. She was one of a handful of Louisville girls, including Abraham's sister, to go east to college in those years.

During her college years Abraham saw little of his former pupil. He remembered sending her a gift when she graduated from Vassar, a volume of the poems of Lord Byron, but the relationship was still casual. On her return, however, he began to see more of her; he hired her occasionally as a tutor, and together they bicycled into the surrounding countryside. The new sport of bicycling was a popular craze in Louisville, as elsewhere, in those years. Romance blossomed. More and more she was mentioned in his letters. He stopped speaking of other prospective matches. They fell deeply in love and a year later announced their engagement. She was twenty-two, eight years younger than her fiancé, when they made known their plans.

The decision to delay marriage was mutual, he said later, claiming that she gladly deferred to his duty to his family. Abraham's nephew, the historian James Thomas Flexner, doubts this, saying Anne was bitter about "being pushed aside while Abraham struggled to shore up the tumbling-down finances of his brothers." To support his version of the delay, the nephew cites the testimony of the couple's daughters, but Jean Flexner, the elder daughter, flatly denied this version of events. In view of Anne's own plans to go to New York to pursue a career in writing, it is doubtful that the delay caused serious friction. To her fiancé she penciled some lines from Robert Louis Stevenson:

> "Hae patience, for they tell't to me aye
> That was the overcome o'life!"
> With what clear courage rings the cry
> Thro' days with disappointment rife
> Above the fever and the fret
> The thrilling voice! "Hae patience yet."[4]

The couple went their separate ways for two years after their engagement. Anne went to New York, while Abraham remained at his post as teacher and promoter of his school. It was the first of many separations that marked a relationship remarkable for that time and place. "We agreed at the outset of our married life," he recalled, "that her interests and work were as sacred as mine."[5] For the next forty years and more, despite advancing age and two children, they enjoyed a companionate relationship that often kept them miles and even continents apart as they pursued independent careers. Their daughters, too—often left for weeks or months with their father—were brought up as strong, independent women. When asked about his unusual attitude toward marriage and family, Abraham gave credit to the example of his mother and the great talent that he believed had been wasted in her.

For Abraham, the late nineties were a time of renewed hope and thoughts of closing his school. "I have never lost sight," he claimed, of "my wish to return to academic walls." He talked once more of spending a year or two in advanced study "prior to doing some of the things" he used to feel he "could do—perhaps even was meant to do." He was encouraged by another letter from Harvard's president, Charles W. Eliot, in which Eliot told Flexner that he not only agreed with Flexner's progressive views but that they were both working toward the same practical ends. Notice the "*we*," Abraham boasted to Simon.[6]

But there were still more delays in his departure from Louisville. New financial threats came on the horizon just as he thought he saw the means of escape. His habitual optimism and self-confidence seemed again to drain away as the lengthening "chain of self-imposed responsibility" stretched into the new century. If he could only get an audience of some size, he complained in 1901, he could make himself "count for something" in the world of education. But the prospect of leaving was more and more difficult. He admitted that it would take courage to finally make the break. At one point, he likened himself to Prometheus "chained to a rock of grinding routine." "I am sick at heart," he confessed in 1903, "when I sit quietly here, planning the deadly work of the interminable 'tomorrow.'" His better instincts revolted, he said, at "the unnatural and useless business."[7]

His despair was heightened by the growing recognition of his brothers' achievements. He felt left behind by those to whom he had given so much. Simon had left Baltimore for a professorship at the University of Pennsylvania in 1900 and two years later was named the first head of the Rockefeller Institute for Medical Research, the first great medical research enterprise in America. This immensely prestigious appointment, Abraham said, brought "the greatest glory the name Flexner has yet won." It was an opportunity, he acknowledged, that came to few in a generation. The spectacle of Simon at the head of his profession, of Bernard "daily enlarging his reputation," of Jacob's growing prestige as a physician in Louisville, and of Washington "with the possibility of great things" clearly troubled the burdened schoolmaster.[8] The brothers were nearing the end of their climb upward; his had not yet begun.

His marriage to Anne, in June 1898, only deepened his ties to his native city. It was a quiet ceremony held in the Episcopal Church and attended by only the families. It was uncommon, especially in Louisville, for a Jew to marry outside the faith. But the Flexners welcomed the lively and gregarious newcomer. The union brought him new contentment and a domestic happiness he had never known. At the same time it made it more unlikely that he could move away. The newlyweds acquired a comfortable house and furnished it to Anne's more expensive tastes. He took on the responsibility of supporting her frequent trips to New York to confer with producers and stage managers. Within a year a daughter was born, for whom a full-time nurse was added to the household. The new father spent more and more time with Jean, as the couple named her, while Anne was away from home.

Jean's childhood memories were chiefly of her father. Her mother, whom she greatly admired, seemed "more distant," less involved with Jean than "with her own career and interests." Her father read aloud to her, took her on outings, and sat with her when she was ill. When Anne was away, father and daughter talked about their need to be "good" until she returned, consoling each other and "vowing" to do their best to "make things go." Both Jean and her sister, Eleanor, born nine years later, would remember their closeness to him and the influence he held on their lives and careers. "It was understood always," Eleanor said, "that my sister and I would have exactly the same kind of education that a boy would have had in that period."[9]

In New York, Anne became immersed in the theater and began to write her own dramatic scripts. Her first original play, "A Man's Woman," a light farce, attracted the interest of America's foremost actress, Minnie Maddern Fiske, who invited her to New York for an interview. It was an exciting trip. She took along Jean, not yet a year old, and her nurse and met Mrs. Fiske at a downtown hotel. The great lady, described by the critic Brooks Atkinson as "a red-headed, mettlesome actress," was a formidable force on the New York stage—by far the most independent and original figure on Broadway. Anne was overwhelmed by her dramatic personality. She said she liked Anne's play but thought it unsuited to her own talents. Then, to Anne's surprise, she asked whether Anne might be able to adapt a novel she admired, A.E.W. Mason's *Miranda of the Balcony*, for the stage. Without hesitation, Anne agreed. Proudly Abraham told of a long letter from Mrs. Fiske that showed a "confidence and intimacy" that were "visible in every sentence."[10]

Anne's play was the first to be performed in a theater newly remodeled by Mrs. Fiske's husband, the wealthy Harrison Gray Fiske, who had inherited his millions from his father. The hugely expensive reconstruction was aimed at breaking the stranglehold of the infamous Klew and Erlanger "syndicate," which controlled theater bookings throughout the city. The play, finished in less than a year, was thus assured the attention of the New York theater world. But while critics praised the theater, Mrs. Fiske, the sets, and the costumes, they were at best lukewarm about the play. The *Herald Tribune* called it "amateurish," with "a trite theme" full of "eclectic caprice," although admitting it was doubtful that another writer could have done better. The play ran nevertheless for ten weeks and Mrs. Fiske seemed not to have been disappointed. It was, writes James Thomas Flexner, "by far the most glamorous event in the history of the Flexner family," and Anne's future was bright.[11]

Her next play marked a turning point in her career and that of her husband. Her inspiration came from her membership in the Author's Club in Louisville—a group of seven or eight aspiring women writers—where she heard a reading by a friend named Alice Hegan from a comical novel called *Mrs. Wiggs of the Cabbage Patch*. Hegan published the work in late 1901 and it quickly became a bestseller, reaching sales of forty thousand copies a month. Her fame spread. From the White House came an invitation from Theodore Roosevelt to come to lunch.

Mrs. Wiggs of the Cabbage Patch is the story of an indomitably cheerful woman from Louisville's most run-down neighborhood, called the "Cabbage Patch," who manages a large family with folksy good humor and slipshod improvisation through a series of comic and pathetic events. Her husband is a ne'er-do-well who is "just as bad as a poor man could be." Whatever the failures and dangers around her, Mrs. Wiggs never wavers in her belief that "everything comes right if we just wait long enough."

It struck Anne that the story would make a wonderful play. Despite Alice Hegan's doubts, she began work, sending the result to a leading literary agent. Her husband—"the most hostile and least partial of critics"—loved it. It was quickly picked up and it opened in Louisville in the fall of 1903, with the Flexners and Alice Hegan sitting in the box of "Marse" Henry Watterson, the powerful editor of the *Louisville Courier-Journal*.

The success of the play far exceeded all expectations. For seven consecutive seasons, beginning in 1904, it was the biggest hit on Broadway. At times three road companies were carrying it across the country. In London it was moved to a larger theater and played to full houses for two seasons. A special matinee was arranged for two thousand scrubwomen and their families. A London critic wrote of the play's characters: "If there are not such people in the world, there ought to be." In time the play would be staged throughout the world and be made into two Hollywood motion pictures starring such well-known figures as Zasu Pitts and W.C. Fields. Even Mae West appeared in one of the stock companies.[12]

By the time of Anne's success, her husband was much closer to a decision to leave Louisville. He had begun making plans to sell the school in 1903 but was unable to find a buyer. He began nevertheless to write to professors at Harvard about work he planned to do there, which included reading the writings of and studying with the German-born psychologist and philosopher Hugo Münsterberg. He also managed to see the philosopher Josiah Royce when he came to Louisville on a recruiting trip.

Simon Flexner kept up the pressure on Abraham to give up his ties to Louisville and stop trying to provide for the whole family. Abraham's caution, Simon tried to explain, came from a fear of failure that was compounded by an "exaggerated" duty to those he loved. His brother, now thirty-seven, must act now and "detach himself from everything" except what he wished and hoped to do, Simon wrote. Abraham himself admitted that he was aware of "very human doubts and fears" about making so long delayed a move but told Simon in the spring of 1904 that he was resolved to "cast prudence to the winds" and break loose the following year. If he did not act this time, he said, he would never forgive himself for selling his ideals "for a mess of worldly comfort."[13]

The rousing success of *Mrs. Wiggs* made money suddenly less important. In her diary Anne wrote: "When we get away [from Louisville]—if we get away—I am most anxious that no time shall be wasted." There would be more time together, less time spent in traveling, and "the margin of time over and above" her work could be used "in a really scholarly way." In the first year alone the play brought in about fifteen thousand dollars—an immense amount—and was now the "main peg" in their future.[14] The following years brought in similar amounts. Anne was unwavering in support of Abraham's dream to break free and realize his long-suppressed ambition.

Just as important as the family's bright financial prospects was Abraham's dread of further long separations from his wife. "I am not willing under any preventable circumstances to leave Anne again," he announced. "It's too big a price to pay." On the other hand, he did not want her to "limit or abridge" her own ambition to enlarge her achievements.[15] Most of all, he wanted a job in New York, close to her work.

The school was sold on favorable terms in the early months of 1905. "The struggle is over and won," he said, but he was "keenly conscious" of how empty his intellectual life had become. The couple began planning

their move to Cambridge. When the time finally came in the summer of
1905, nineteen years after he returned from Johns Hopkins, he was in his
thirty-ninth year, well into middle age, married with a child, worn down
by routine, little known outside a small circle of educators, and bent on
finding a job in education that he was not sure even existed. But his old
confidence was returning, and an eagerness to begin anew was apparent
in all his letters.

He was leaving Louisville, as Simon had left it fifteen years before,
without expecting to return. The years behind him now took on a rosy
glow as he faced the future. "The discipline of our growing up," he told a
skeptical Simon, had been responsible for the "remarkable successes of all
the children." The experience had been valuable for the "largeness of
spirit" it fostered. His own inner confidence, he felt certain, had come
from the nurturing environment of home, school, and community and the
strength of his mother. His years as an underage student at Hopkins and
young schoolmaster had given him a chance to try out bold and unconventional ideas. At Mr. Flexner's School he had learned by experience what
did and did not work in the classroom. "If I ever embody my present conviction in a real work or institution," he said before leaving Louisville, "this
long and dismal routine will be responsible for it."[16] He had been a teacher
and schoolmaster longer than he would hold any other job.

The long apprenticeship in Louisville was followed by some of the happiest years of his life. Freed from all responsibility, he immersed himself
for three years in study, reflection, and enjoyment of periods of unwonted
leisure. First there was a year of graduate study at Harvard, then came a
somewhat longer sojourn in Berlin and Heidelberg, and finally there
began a year of writing and searching for a job. He was now convinced
that he would never become a professor; he was much too old to begin,
and he lacked the temperament for narrow research and specialized study.
What he was seeking, he came to believe, was a career in educational administration and planning. Even this was improbable, since college presidents and deans normally rose out of the academic ranks of professors.
It seems unlikely that he would have been aware of any possibility for
himself in the new educational foundations of Carnegie, Rockefeller, or
another wealthy donor, but Simon may have given him encouragement
to at least begin considering such an outlet for his talents. He seldom
mentioned any particular goal for his new studies, considering them impracticable for most useful employment.

During the summer before the Harvard classes began, the family spent three months in the Berkshire mountains in a rented cottage once belonging to the writer Richard Watson Gilder. He wrote that it was "a peaceful spot, absolutely barren of excitement and interest," one that gave him a chance to get back to intellectual interests. He was reminded of the English lake country, he said, "minus the lakes and the exquisite finish of lawn and hedge." He made one trip to Cambridge to become familiar with the surroundings and to find out about preliminary reading for his fall courses. The change of pace from the crowded years in Louisville was remarkable. "I have the emptiest and strangest feeling about myself," he said, "like a tree, torn up, that doesn't yet know what to do with its roots and tendrils."[17] Much of the time was spent reading, relaxing, and romping with Jean and Anne over the rolling countryside.

In late September they moved to rooms in a Cambridge boarding-house. While her father found the arrangement "comfortable and commodious," Jean recalled only "a tall, gloomy house of a forbidding old lady" whom she came to loathe. From this house Flexner made his way to Professor Münsterberg's office for an initial interview about his course of study. The professor knew of him, had read his article on the preparatory school in the *Atlantic,* and was much impressed by his kinship to Simon. He advised Flexner to work in psychology and not to worry about immediate immersion in pedagogy. In his excitement about a new life, Flexner little appreciated how unrealistic his hopes for study must have appeared to a scholar like Münsterberg. The new student was shaken by the professor's insistence on the importance of laboratory training and his "radical advice" to forgo lecture courses in favor of small seminars. He told Simon he now realized "with fourfold intensity" how badly equipped he was to start out.[18] Münsterberg did approve of his enrolling in a lecture course on Immanuel Kent given by Josiah Royce.

The first month was discouraging. He had trouble following lectures, he often fell asleep, and he dreaded the mornings in Münsterberg's laboratory. At night he was awake at all hours and when he fell asleep found "Kant and Münsterberg chasing themselves phantasmagorically across [his] brain." The weight of new knowledge and experiences was overwhelming. For several weeks he could feel his "skull-sutures in the very act of loosening up." He wrote three papers on Kant, including one on his treatment of the ego, which Royce judged variously to be "thoroughgoing," "admirable," and in one case "too remote." There could be no thought of the future. What importance his studies might have on his future work he "absolutely never" speculated. The future was "non-existent."

To return to teaching was unthinkable, yet he had nowhere else to go "except in revolt."[19]

Of all his teachers he found Royce the most memorable. Royce's lectures, after the first week, began to "lighten up"; he felt that he was beginning to understand current philosophical and pedagogical thought. Without question, he said, the soft-spoken Royce was "a great intellect: clear, ready, coherent, with a great sweep and marvelous powers of elucidation." In the Royce seminar he began taking a prominent part, relating to Simon his contribution to a discussion on the meaning of scientific experiment. "A scientist experimented with a 'problem,' he did not go on a 'voyage of discovery,'" he told the seminar; "he need not have a definite theory, he may be switched off by suggestion as he proceeds, he may 'shamble' on something unexpectedly." But there had to be an initial purpose behind the experiment, or else there would be "chaos." His thinking, he confessed to Simon, was based on his brother's example. Personally, he found Royce "a dear, most kind, considerate and patient."[20]

In Münsterberg's laboratory, on the other hand, he was constantly frustrated by his lack of technical know-how and the strong sense that the detailed, empirical world of the scientist was not for him. He was more interested in concepts, in learning about experimental methods that would enlarge his understanding of how learning takes place. After a few months he abandoned the laboratory altogether, reminding the professor that he had told him at the outset that he lacked the background to carry on a worthwhile experiment. To his astonishment, Münsterberg agreed. "Was he disappointed in my work," he wondered years after, "or relieved that I was leaving?"[21]

The forty-year-old graduate student devoured the opportunities open to him. He sat through scores of lectures beyond his own classes, scoured the literature of education, and was sometimes invited by teachers, often younger than himself, to teas and dinners. He came briefly to know William James and to treasure his "brilliant personality and bristling intellect." "I have no idle moments," he reported, "but I live like a lotus-eater, without care." Anne sparkled in the new environment and facilitated his entry into social circles that would normally have been closed to him. At one social event she handled an amusing incident with such disarming composure that her proud husband promptly wrote Simon about it. She had fallen into discussion with "a clever Bostonian" who was a great theater fan and together they had reviewed a number of recent plays. "The worst play I saw last season," he told Anne, "was 'Mrs. Wiggs.'" It was "awful" and "I never wanted my money back so badly in all my life." She quietly continued to egg him on without showing the least sign of her own involvement. But afterward, said Abraham, "how we did laugh."[22]

The university where Flexner studied was still under the firm hand of Charles W. Eliot. Since his inauguration in 1869, student enrollment at Harvard had quadrupled and the faculty had grown tenfold. More than three thousand students now walked the pathways and filled the buildings around Harvard Yard. The surrounding town was little more than a village. A graduate school of arts and sciences, in which Flexner was enrolled, had been created in 1890, and graduate schools of engineering and architecture had also been added. The professional schools of medicine and law, previously independent, were modernized and folded into the university. The elective system for undergraduates, which Flexner saw as the bane of student training, was at its apex. Harvard was clearly in the forefront of the university movement in America, and Eliot was deeply involved in the reform of secondary curriculum as well. Did Flexner meet with the Harvard president during his year in Cambridge? Did they talk about the wave of changes taking place in schools and colleges across the nation, or did they discuss Flexner's own plans? Almost certainly they did, although there is no written record of their coming together.

Abraham left Cambridge long enough to spend a few weeks in New York, visiting schools and Simon's institute. His brother arranged a short indoctrination in the anatomy of the human brain, which Abraham had been told was essential to the study of psychology and education. He also attended sessions of the American Psychological Association, which was meeting in Boston, to get some impression of the men of "standing and prominence" in the field but was most taken by a woman, Mary Calkins, a professor at Wellesley College and president of the Association. He was particularly struck by her professionalism, he said, and "the absolute unconsciousness of sex" in the sessions at which she presided. Back at Cambridge he finished the year's work with grades of "A" in virtually all of his studies and was awarded the M.A. degree in philosophy in June 1906.[23]

What next? He had long been aware of the many Americans who had gone to Germany for study, and he had counseled Simon to do advanced work there. Now he discovered that his Harvard professors, especially Münsterberg, believed that his own plans for a life in education were best furthered by at least a year of study abroad. He wanted to study education itself but found he would have to be content, aside from the history of education, with further work in psychology and physiology. With these subjects under his belt, he could then venture to try out his own ideas in the field of education and learning. Anne liked the idea of going to Germany. They had spent a brief honeymoon in England and Scotland, but neither had been to the continent. Soon after Abraham finished the last course at Harvard, the three Flexners set sail for England on a slow steamer that was part cattleboat. Anne was the center of social life on the ship. Every afternoon she played hostess for a tea party on the bow, "everyone squatting or sitting on a steamer rug laid flat on deck."[24]

Once in England, the family toured familiar landmarks and Abraham made visits to Oxford and Cambridge as well as to the renowned preparatory schools at Rugby and Eton. He was trying, he said, to get a glimpse into educational organization but had little time for more than a brief overview. Of the English public schools like Rugby he thought only their "discipline and manners" worthy of praise; enforcement of these traits made originality "well nigh impossible." Their curricula were narrow and heavily classical, neglecting modern studies. They catered to only the "best boys" and could not produce the graduates "that modern society most urgently" needed. On the tours around England, he told Jean about the history of such places as Warwick, Chatsworth, and Haddon Hall. But they were all anxious to get to know the country where they were to spend the coming year. After only a week in London, they began making their way "with throbbing hearts" to Berlin.[25]

Berlin made a profound impression on Flexner. The busy imperial city was approaching two million in population. German science and scholarship were at the peak of their influence. Here he found what he had missed at Harvard: informative, stimulating lectures on psychology, education, and philosophy by men with world-class reputations. As an informal student, he went to scores of lectures, engaged professors in lengthy discussions, and spent time visiting other universities and secondary schools. He had no difficulty understanding German. Of all the professors he met, none made a deeper impression upon him than the austere Friedrich Paulsen, the leading authority on German university education. A man of "swarthy complexion, flashing eye and eloquent voice," much admired by Americans, he offered a course on the rationale, organization, and ideals behind the German school system. To Flexner he seemed "a wise, gentle, learned soul, kind and helpful to the last degree." Old-fashioned and conservative, Paulsen, he believed, was an antidote to his own "radical tendencies." It would do him no harm "to see the situation [in education] as others see it who see more ground for satisfaction than dissatisfaction" than he did.[26]

The lectures of Karl Stumpf, the leading German psychologist—a "prince of teachers"—he described as the best he had ever heard: "I raise my hat to him—clearest, keenest, and most modest of men." Stumpf, a champion of the scientific method in psychology, burst through the complexities of a dry subject, said Flexner, cutting "a broad swath, and turning it into a garden as he goes."[27] When time permitted, he "drifted" into a classroom where lectures were being given on Faust. He heard lectures too, by the "scrappy" sociologist George Simmel—"a brilliant restless man"—which Flexner found like "the opening of a new world."

This experience in Germany took him back to his time in Baltimore, he said, except that he was now forty instead of seventeen. He confessed that he had to be careful that his advanced age and hardened views did not lead him to seize upon every suggestion or observation "because it fell in with [his] views!" He kept notebooks for lectures on Nietzche, Santayana, Dewey, Darwinism, ethics, and the philosophy of culture. Unfortunately, the notes, written in a kind of Yiddish-German, tell us little of what he found important or relevant to his own interests.[28]

On long weekends and holidays, often accompanied by his daughter, he left the family's pension on the Tauenziehenstrasse in central Berlin for visits to high schools or gymnasia in other parts of Germany. The seven-year-old was kept amused by her indulgent father, who stuffed his pockets with toy animals and read to her from German fairy tales. He liked the schools' tone of high seriousness and emphasis on scholarly training. The gymnasium, he felt, had no counterpart in American high schools or preparatory schools. For all its virtues, however, the German high school was narrow in its conception, an "effective engine for the production of a preconceived life." He had seen boys from nine to nineteen "hammered, driven, pounded, thumped, [and] kneaded." No concern was evident for "what was going on in the boy's mind." He did not approve of the severe discipline imposed on the schools' secondary students. The older boys, as one might expect, looked "driven, listless."[29]

The German university student was far more serious and driven than the American student. Never had he seen such "earnestness" when he was at Harvard. To see more than seven hundred men march into a lecture room at six o'clock in the morning to follow a philosophical argument, he told Simon, "undoubtedly does signify something." What he saw and experienced in his German travels left a mark on his later work and convinced

him of the value of seeing things for himself. He was learning a good deal
and enjoying it. "There's nothing like work," he said, "for making life seem
a game actually worthwhile to play." For the rest of his life he was an in-
veterate traveler and inquirer after how things worked—"*ambulando
discimus*," he called it—and he was constantly on the road to see for himself.[30] No educator relied more on personal impressions of persons and institutions in a search for answers to his questions. Next to Johns Hopkins
and the Flexner school, the sojourn in Germany did the most to shape his
ideas on education.

The legacy of Berlin and the gymnasia in Flexner's mind, however, remained mixed. While he admired the seriousness of German schools,
praised the universities extravagantly, and approved of the strict separation of general education from advanced learning, he was loud in his criticism of the rigid curriculum, the classical core of the gymnasium, and the
heavy reliance on the classroom lecture. Repeatedly he denounced the
class-bound nature of both the gymnasium and the university as reflections of German life. Learning should not be an end in itself, especially
at the high school level, he asserted, but should be directed toward social
and individual needs. What he saw in Berlin was important for his own
intellectual growth, but Germany would not be his model. Clearly his vision of the future would lie closer to Charles Eliot's, Daniel Coit Gilman's,
and John Dewey's than to the excessively formal structure of German education. Indeed, as we have seen, he thought of himself as a "radical" in
comparison with conservatives like Friedrich Paulsen.

Outside the world of schools and universities, he found Berlin society
repressive and unpleasant. "How queer Berlin is anyway," he wrote, "with
its incongruous combination of intellectual preferences in music and
drama with a grotesque lack of taste in so many other directions."[31] Nor
was he attracted by the martial displays and aggressive tone of so much of
German public life.

The last summer was spent in Heidelberg, where he began to put down
some of the impressions he had gained in the twenty years since leaving
Baltimore. These thoughts became the basis for his first book, *The American College*, written largely after his return to America. What consumed
him now was how to attract the attention of educators and to find a job. In
his letters he was alternately hopeful and pessimistic that anyone would
hire a forty-one-year-old schoolmaster with a smattering of advanced work
in psychology and education. What would he do on returning to America
with neither a residence nor a job? The savings on which the family had

lived for two years were running low and would have to stretch still further. The "featureless expanse" of the future lay ominously before him.

On arriving in America in the late summer of 1907, the family split up for a time. Anne and Jean went to stay with Anne's parents in Atlanta, while Abraham returned to his family in Louisville. Anne then took Jean to her uncle's cottage on Campobello Island in Passamaquoddy Bay, between Maine and New Brunswick, Canada, before joining her husband in an apartment he found on East Seventy-Seventh Street in New York.

New York would be his home for the next fifty years. When he arrived, the city was in the midst of a dramatic transformation. The population was soaring; more than a million immigrants came through the great port each year. More than two of every five inhabitants were foreign born, and Jews were the largest of the immigrant groups. "It is a seething human sea," declared a Jewish newcomer named Abraham Cohen. Within a decade, one of every three New Yorkers would be a Jew. New manufacturing, shipping, and entertainment businesses, including a film industry, were flourishing. The last of the horse-drawn streetcars were being removed the year he arrived, and a vast network of subways was spreading across the expanding city. Resting on steel frameworks, the first dozen skyscrapers were altering the skyline of New York. "It is as if some mighty force were astir beneath the ground, hour by hour," said a writer in *Harper's Weekly.* No city anywhere was more exciting and vital than the Flexners' new home.[32]

The family settled in for a period of intensive work, Anne on a new play, her husband on his book about the American college. Jean remembered perfectly the huge antique desk where her mother worked from nine until one every day with "no interruptions!" Her work was important to the whole family since it was now the family's only means of support. In the small apartment the atmosphere was "masculine and intellectual." A maid took care of housekeeping and meals, and reading aloud was the favorite evening pastime. "I never saw my Mother make a bed, or cook an egg, or wash a dish or sew," said Jean.[33]

The birth of a second daughter, Eleanor, in October came as a complete shock to the nine-year-old Jean and perhaps to her parents as well. She recalled vividly her envy and resentment of the newcomer, who now claimed much of her parents' attention. Her father made things worse by admonishing Jean to love her "little pet lamb." But he did try to assure her of his love by walking her to school each day, taking her to Central Park and the

Metropolitan Museum, and buying books for her. He encouraged her and later her sister to learn foreign languages and for a time insisted that their recreational reading be in either German or French. But the friction that was born when Eleanor arrived persisted into early adulthood.[34]

Flexner began work on *The American College* in the fall of 1907 and finished it in June 1908. At first he thought it might be a long article, but he gradually began to set his sights on a "brochure" or small book, which would get more attention than a mere piece in a magazine. Simon found him a place to work at the Rockefeller Institute; there, Abraham could work in private and consult with his brother.

During this period, a plan was formed for Abraham to seek employment at the new Carnegie Foundation for the Advancement of Teaching. Whether the idea came from Abraham or Simon is not known. Simon knew the foundation's president, Henry S. Pritchett, and several of its board members and was almost certainly aware of talk about the foundation's conducting a series of educational surveys, including one on medical education. Abraham surely knew, too, that President Eliot was a powerful member of the board and Pritchett's close friend. It was, then, no coincidence that Pritchett was quoted approvingly at length in no fewer than five different places in the Flexner book. Pritchett, it seemed, agreed with Flexner's principal impressions about the weaknesses of the American college, especially the vagueness of its goals, its lack of intellectual standards, and the confusion brought about by its absorption into the university.

The book, published by the Century Company, is an unrelievedly critical attack on the emerging American settlement in higher education. The American system of education, he argued, was a disjointed amalgamation of poorly defined preparatory schools, loosely organized colleges, and amorphous universities made up of undergraduate, graduate, and vocational studies. He held to this judgment for the next fifty years.

Just what purpose did the general college serve? It did not prepare students for the university the way the German gymnasium did, nor did it provide truly university-level study like that of European universities. The college graduate was "neither a trained nor a serious worker." Even the English college, parent to its American counterpart, was separate from the great English universities devoted to advanced study and research. In America, the old classical college, conservative and dedicated to fortifying Puritanism, was dead and had been replaced by a college with cafeteria-style freedom of choice from a wide range of new offerings. But the student coming to college was not prepared to make such choices. "Isn't it absurd, on its face," he asked in a letter to the *Nation*, "to maintain that an American boy should be free to choose which he shall know—the history of Greece or the history of his own country, the Constitution of Kleisthenes or the Constitution of the United States?"[35]

A college degree meant no more than that a student had spent three or four years in more or less indiscriminate study. A typical graduate, Flexner wrote, "may have adhered closely to the traditional classical scheme; or . . . may have entirely ignored the humanities in favor of physical science; or . . . may have ignored all the sciences but one; or . . . may have cultivated philosophy or modern literature; or done none of these."[36] The diploma thus did not indicate what its recipient had studied. Only the quantity of college output in America, not its quality, had increased. Astonishingly, he said, no real differences existed among the leading colleges. All of them, without exception, were "deficient in earnestness and pedagogical intelligence."

Worse, the colleges rigidly controlled the curriculum of secondary schools through entrance examinations so that the confusion over the purpose of college was extended down to the high school. The college deprived the school of discretion and shaped its offerings. Any effort at experimentation to make the secondary school fit individual talents was sharply fettered to get the student into college. How did four years of Greek or Latin or mathematics, he asked, prepare one "to find his way intelligently in totally distinct realms of activity and interest?"

If Latin was not required in college, why should it have been demanded in high school? Constantly cramming for examinations set by the colleges, the preparatory student was "under no constraint to uncover or develop a purpose." Whence came the requirements set by a college such as Harvard anyway? From an uneasy fusion of academic politics and outside pressures, he said. The requirements were "in the main, simply the old fixed curriculum that is deemed to have been replaced: an arbitrary [mix] of unrelated and jarring items: English, for example, enters for practical reasons; Latin and Greek is a concession to the educational Tories; science, an offset to placate the radicals; and mathematics offers homage to 'drill.' Every item is a separate scrap; the whole is a patchwork, suggesting . . . a political platform rather than a rational educational program."[37]

Such a broadside attack from a little-known unemployed writer could scarcely win Flexner friends among those who were running America's colleges. Flexner did not temper his language to please readers—a quality that was to become typical of Flexner's style. He was as tenacious as a bull-dog in holding to his positions.

He seemed not to be awed by the formidable figures whom he encountered, many of whom would become lifelong adversaries. As early as 1904, he told Simon that he had no illusions about the forces that would be arrayed against him as his ideas gained currency. These forces, he wrote, particularly those of President Nicholas Murray Butler of Columbia University "and his cohorts," were "never more compactly massed and drilled . . . And my little pea-shooter rattles its toy bullets off their armor as harmlessly as Russian shells fall away from a Japanese man-of-war."[38] He clearly enjoyed intellectual combat. He was becoming a puzzling figure to his contemporaries, who alternately admired and feared him. The powerful language that marked his forays into all fields of American education made him particularly controversial—and effective.

A number of Flexner's strictures against the college have echoed through the writings of later critics. He was one of the first to notice the role of the "faculty adviser," who steered the uninitiated student through the maze of courses and options that was the elective system. But who was the adviser? The adviser, wrote Flexner, was a professor, "with lectures to give, researches to supervise, investigations of his own." The average adviser was neither interested nor trained in guiding impressionable youngsters. Most advising, therefore, was only "perfunctory assent" by the professor to random choices made by the student and was "little more than a joke." He found fault, too, with a practice that became the target of generations of critics. Teaching in the "liberal arts," which presumably aimed at a broad audience, was increasingly directed to the narrow interests of a particular department of knowledge. An elective system in which the teachers were specialists existed for specialists and not run-of-the-mill students. How could such a college continue to call itself "liberal"?

In the classroom, where formerly there were discussions and "recitations," lectures now ruled, totally destroying all contact between student and teacher. The lecture enabled the college "to handle cheaply by whole-sale" a large body of students that would be otherwise unmanageable and gave the lecturer time for research. The actual contact with students came more and more from graduate student teachers who were "young and therefore without much experience in teaching."

It was this blind amalgamation of the undergraduate college into the research university that disturbed Flexner most. By using the same teacher to conduct beginning lectures and graduate seminars and by allowing graduate students to enroll in the same classes as young undergraduates, the college was "insidiously sacrificing" its own interest to that of the university. Any financial accounting of the use of endowment and tuition funds would show that the graduate program inevitably "got the better" of the undergraduate college, since graduate students were few and most endowment funds were intended for college students. The strength of the inordinately expensive graduate programs varied with the amounts siphoned off the undergraduate enterprise.[39]

His solutions, as reviewers were quick to note, were sweeping and largely impractical. The priority of the college, he advised, needed to be "vigorously reasserted"; the preparatory school needed to be given more freedom and "reconstructed"; the college curriculum was in need of "a core of organized knowledge"; and the college had to be more sharply differentiated from the university. But how were these grandiose plans to be realized? How were the historical currents that had brought these changes to be reversed? To critics, many of them part of the enterprise under attack, *The American College* seemed unrealistic, dogmatic in tone, too quick to assign blame, and unbalanced. A writer in the *Educational Review,* which Nicholas Murray Butler led and edited, chided Flexner for his naiveté and for writing about things beyond his knowledge and experience. Others flatly denied that there was organizational chaos in American colleges. Still others defended the opening up of the colleges as wholesome and democratic, charging Flexner with using the class-bound schools of Germany as a model for America. For the bulk of American educators, the book fell flat. It made an impact on "no university president," Flexner himself admitted years later.[40] Yet it set the pattern for his future work on medical education, secondary schools, and universities.

Was Flexner motivated by his desire for employment or by his longstanding urge to make a difference in American education? Was he chagrined by his late start in life? What prompted him to take so curmudgeonly a stance when more moderate language might have served his interests better? In the long sweep of Flexner's career, his motives in writing *The American College* seem a familiar mix of idealism, pragmatism, and love of argument. He did feel strongly about the direction American schools and colleges were heading; he did want a job with the Carnegie Foundation in New York; and he did want to incite a national debate by his strong language. But he had little immediate success.

Even before the book appeared, he had launched his campaign to find a job at the Carnegie Foundation. Meeting with Henry Pritchett, he carried

with him a letter of introduction from Ira Remsen, who had succeeded
Gilman as president of Johns Hopkins. At the first meeting, Pritchett, a
trim, hard-driving former president of the Massachusetts Institute of Technology, explained that the foundation was considering a series of studies
of professional education—law, medicine, engineering, theology—that
would set national standards and move the foundation beyond its original
purpose of creating a pension system for college teachers. He may have
mentioned that his hope of beginning with legal education had been
dampened by the profession's reluctance to cooperate and that he had
begun preliminary discussions with representatives of the American Medical Association. They talked about Flexner's book, and Pritchett asked to
see the proofs of the work.[41] At their second meeting, in all probability,
Pritchett mentioned the possibility of Flexner's doing the survey of medical schools. Flexner was caught by surprise, asking Pritchett if he were not
confusing him with his brother Simon, but Pritchett told him he knew
Simon well and that he wanted an educator, not a medical man, to do the
study.

But the matter was far from settled. Pritchett encountered resistance
from members of his board to both the survey and Flexner. Some were reluctant to begin an undertaking that was sure to be controversial, while
others were not convinced that a layperson could make the kind of survey that was needed. And some members of the board, notably Nicholas
Murray Butler, were hostile to the idea of Flexner's doing the work.[42]
Most of the board members were university presidents who were scarcely
enamored of giving a platform to a man who had criticized them so mercilessly.

But Pritchett dug in his heels. He told the board, Flexner recalled, that
he had to be free to choose his own associates and that he alone assumed
responsibility for their competence. Almost certainly Flexner had the
strong support of President Eliot, who may even have suggested his name.
While he awaited the outcome, Flexner called on David Starr Jordan, the
president of Stanford University and a member of the Carnegie board,
who was in town. Jordan told him he was much impressed by Flexner's
ideas about college organization and tentatively asked him if he would be
interested in coming to Palo Alto to reorganize the curriculum. Armed
with this tantalizing proposition, Flexner went back to Pritchett. The
foundation president told him that he would not stand in his way but that
the executive committee had approved Flexner's appointment. An elated
Flexner wrote Simon that at last "the long campaign" was over; he would

"go to bed the proud earner" of his own income. In his letter of appointment, it was made clear to Flexner that this was a temporary assignment of about two years and that Flexner would work not only on the medical survey but on surveys in law, graduate education, and possibly theology. He would be paid three thousand dollars a year and given a generous expense account.[43]

Why did Pritchett hire Flexner? It was one of the strangest appointments in education history. Later Carnegie surveys relied on trained experts. Flexner himself admitted that he had never been inside a medical school. But Pritchett had clear and detailed views of his own on medical education and had already outlined them in a paper that foreshadowed the coming Flexner report. Pritchett was counting on the American Medical Association's Council on Medical Education to be interested in reform and eager to cooperate behind the scenes. Having laid out the road map, he knew that the council would help in educating whomever he picked.

Still, why Flexner? In all likelihood, he picked Flexner because he was impressed by his personality and self-confidence, by his willingness to criticize the status quo boldly, and by his ability to write clear, trenchant prose. Beyond these personal characteristics, Flexner, he knew, had the admiration of the president of Harvard University and good connections, through his powerful brother, with the medical education establishment centered at Johns Hopkins. Whatever the reasons, the two men formed a close partnership that would outlast strong differences in opinion and Flexner's departure from the Carnegie Foundation four years later. For the next quarter-century they conferred regularly on educational surveys, current grant proposals, and interfoundation cooperation. They exchanged personal visits and their families became close. When Pritchett died in 1939, it was Flexner to whom his widow turned to write his biography.

5

A Legend Is Born

The study of medical education for Henry Pritchett changed Flexner's life. By the time this exciting period ended, his existence had been turned upside down. He was suddenly famous. Overnight his name and picture appeared in hundreds of newspapers and magazines. Stories dealt with his Louisville upbringing, his wife's career on Broadway, his well-known brother Simon, and his days as an innovative schoolmaster.

His bold attack on medical schools was grist for every editor seeking color and sensation. The *New York Times* featured the report under the banner headline "Factories for the Making of Ignorant Doctors." The "startling" report, said the *Times,* showed that "incompetent physicians" were "manufactured by wholesale in this country." The *World's Work* queried threateningly: "Do You Know Where Your Doctor Was Trained?" Flexner was highly praised in *Collier's Magazine* for his "searching and brilliant exposé." America's medical schools, said *Harper's Weekly,* had never been subjected "to so severe a scrutiny."[1] The report was front-page news everywhere, especially in communities whose medical schools were under attack.

In the world of medicine, Simon told him, the excitement was profound. At a luncheon with Wallace Buttrick, the genial and influential secretary of Rockefeller's General Education Board, Simon found the secretary unable to talk about anything else. Buttrick said he was reading the report "with absolute absorption" and praised it as "most courageous." Even Frederick T. Gates, the stiff-spined, lordly chief of all the Rockefeller philanthropies, was deep into it, according to Simon. From his European travels even Columbia's Nicholas Murray Butler, no fan of Flexner's, wrote Pritchett with enthusiasm about the report.[2]

What had happened? How did this obscure, forty-four-year-old schoolmaster, unlettered in medicine and lacking in professional authority, create so much furor around so improbable a subject as the training of doctors? He had never been inside a medical school. Why such remarkable interest in medical schools anyway? For one thing, medical schools, unlike law schools or engineering schools, trained persons who dealt daily with matters of life and death. Their graduates held the power to alleviate human suffering and to improve health. Few persons escaped contact with these graduates. Flexner's blistering indictment of medical schools challenged people's faith in doctors and educators, groups normally portrayed in only the gentlest and most respectful terms. If American doctors were not well trained, what was the cost in wrong diagnoses, barbarous treatments, and missed opportunities?

In Flexner's day, more than 150 schools, enrolling some twenty-five thousand students, dotted the landscape across the United States and Canada. They were the survivors of some 457 medical schools that had sprung up willy-nilly in North America over the preceding century and a half. Illinois alone had been the "prolific mother" of thirty-nine; forty-two had sprung from the "fertile soil" of Missouri; and New York had produced forty-three. Cincinnati was the site of twenty largely extinct colleges of medicine. While the number of schools had begun to decline, the roster of those studying medicine continued to climb. Nearly twice the number of students were enrolled in 1910 as had been ten years earlier. Nearly half of the world's medical students, in fact, were crowded into American schools.[3]

Important reforms were under way. A dozen universities offered quality instruction, and another twenty stood out from the rest. Still others were making valiant efforts to improve. But change had not reached a large number of the marginal schools. These schools were typically housed in a single building, often in poor repair. Classrooms were bare, except for chairs, a table, and perhaps a blackboard. Laboratories were tiny or nonexistent. Equipment was sparse. The smell of formaldehyde and decaying bodies permeated the atmosphere; the pall of smoke from countless cigarettes and cigars, intended to conceal the odors, hung over the rooms. The schools' faculties, chiefly local doctors, lectured at stated hours but were otherwise not to be found. Many of the students, most of them much younger than medical students today, had less than a high school education—some far less. They obtained their practical experience on a catch-as-catch-can basis in a neighboring clinic or hospital. And they graduated without serious testing of their knowledge or skills. Perhaps half of all medical schools fitted this troubling description.

Each day students were subjected to interminable lectures and recitations. After a long morning of dissection or a series of quiz sections, they might sit wearily in the afternoon through three or four or even five lectures delivered in methodical fashion by part-time teachers. Evenings were given over to reading and preparation for recitations. If fortunate enough to gain entrance to a hospital, they observed more than participated. Even in New York a student asked plaintively why he and his comrades could not at least "do some of the work, left entirely to the nurses, such as the taking of temperature [or] the counting of pulses."[4] Small wonder that, diploma in hand, many began medical practices with fear and trembling.

The special schools for women and black students, founded to give opportunity to those turned away by conventional schools, were especially vulnerable. Fourteen such schools for women and a like number for blacks had opened their doors in the laissez-faire years after the Civil War. But the gradual spread of coeducation and the recurring financial crises of the black schools had reduced that number by 1910 to three schools for women and seven for blacks. Most of these, especially the black schools, had tragically meager facilities, no endowment, no connection to a university, almost no equipment, little access to a hospital, and poorly prepared students. Now, with the escalating costs of study and the rising standards of accreditation, their very survival was at stake.

Powerful changes were transforming a score of the better schools, and the current of reform was running swiftly, but in many parts of the country the outlook was still bleak. Flexner judged two-thirds of the schools he visited to be "utterly hopeless," including the three women's schools and all but Howard University in Washington and Meharry Medical College in Nashville among the black institutions. The special schools for homeopathy, eclectic medicine, and osteopathy were especially weak. The difference between the osteopathic schools and the rest, including the homeopathic colleges, Flexner told the New York legislature, was that while the latter were both good and bad, "the osteopathic schools were all bad."[5]

Eighty-nine of the nation's schools, about 60 percent of the total, required for admission only the rudiments or the "recollection" of an elementary education. Only one in eight required two years of college. Many students were woefully unprepared. In Chicago, three evening medical colleges—offering a full medical course to students who worked all day—managed to keep their doors open despite almost universal condemnation. "These sundown institutions," charged the prominent Chicago physician Frank Billings, made it possible for "the clerk, the street-car conductor, the janitor, and others . . . to obtain a medical degree." A Philadelphia professor, asked for his opinion about admissions standards, responded: "Well, the most I would claim is that nobody who is absolutely worthless gets in." A dean of a marginal school whose physiological laboratory Flexner asked to see sent a young woman to bring back a small box the size of a safety-razor case containing a blood pressure device.

Worst of all, many of these questionable schools were being run for a profit. They were, Flexner charged, "essentially money-making in spirit and object," multiplying "without restraint," and "conferring degrees on any man who had settled his tuition . . . whether he had regularly attended lectures or not."[6] While the number of schools had dipped since its peak in 1906, few observers were sanguine that the worst was over.

Repercussions from the controversial report appeared almost at once and persisted across the years. In time, the report would acquire mythic status. After ninety years it is still the best known of all such surveys. Flexner was given credit for eliminating "more bad schools in less time than any other time in the history of the world." He was likened to Martin Luther in starting a new era and creating "violent storms of protest, approbation, and argument." He was praised for "shak[ing] American medical education to its very roots." He was said to have "hasten[ed] the schools to their graves and depriv[ed] them of mourners." Not all of this credit was deserved—the reform movement was farther along than Flexner acknowledged—but its constant reiteration made Abraham Flexner a formidable figure in the history of American education.[7]

Timing was all. Flexner became the unwitting agent of powerful forces that had been building in medicine for nearly half a century. The stunning nineteenth-century achievements in laboratory science had brought a new sophistication to the understanding of the physical and chemical makeup of the human body, and to the treatment of disease. Physicians could now treat diphtheria and syphilis, operate with little fear of causing infection, and prevent many communicable diseases. "The baffling and terrifying world of illness," writes historian Kenneth Ludmerer, "was finally becoming intelligible and comprehensible." For the first time in history, it could be said that "a random patient, with a random disorder, who consulted a physician chosen at random, had a better than 50–50 chance of benefiting from the encounter."[8]

These hopeful changes, in turn, demanded a more comprehensive standard for the training of doctors, especially in their premedical preparation and scientific study. Many American doctors who had gone to Germany in the 1870s and 1880s to learn the new medical sciences were now agitating, with increasing success, for a more thorough, science-based curriculum. At Johns Hopkins University, where Simon had been a pioneer worker, standards were particularly high. The student was required to have a college degree before entering; two years of laboratory study in the medical sciences were followed by two years of hands-on experience in the university hospital. The idea that a university like Johns Hopkins was the most suitable home for medical teaching had taken hold in such institutions as Harvard, the University of Michigan, and the University of Pennsylvania.

Particularly important for Flexner, newly made fortunes, especially those of Andrew Carnegie and John D. Rockefeller, were being put to use in supporting scientific work in universities and research institutions. "So long as medical schools are conducted as private ventures for the benefit of a few physicians and surgeons," President Charles W. Eliot of Harvard had warned, "the community ought not to endow them."[9] But now it was Rockefeller money that was supporting such organizational initiatives as Simon's Institute for Medical Research, and it was money supplied by Carnegie that was financing Abraham's study of medical education.

When he embarked on his study of medical schools in 1908, Flexner thus stood at the vortex of swiftly moving scientific, educational, and philanthropic currents that strongly favored reform. Shrewdly, Henry Pritchett saw in the medical study a means of making the Carnegie Foundation an arbiter of the new standards not only in medicine but in the professions generally. The time was ripe. The American Medical Association, through its reform-dominated Council on Medical Education, saw in Pritchett's willingness to cooperate a way of getting independent and presumably disinterested support for its efforts.

According to the council's aggressive, hard-charging head, Chicago surgeon Arthur Dean Bevan, in 1908, medical instruction was a "farce" as it was taught in many schools, "without laboratories, without trained and salaried men, without dispensaries and without hospitals." Some of these schools, he said, were no better equipped to teach medicine "than is a Turkish-bath establishment or a barbershop." By this time the council, dominated by men from the stronger medical schools, had set an "ideal standard" for training doctors: a high school education, two years of laboratory science, two years of clinical work, and a year of hospital practice or internship. Even against this minimal standard the council rated half of America's schools as less than "satisfactory," despite the standard's having been "exceedingly lenient." Unable to demand that all schools comply at once for fear of splitting the association, the council moved to "obtain the publication and approval of [its] work by the Carnegie Foundation for the Advancement of Teaching," a step that would "assist materially" in bringing about change.[10]

At Flexner's first council meeting, he heard Pritchett agree that while the foundation's study would be "guided" by the council's previous investigations, the council itself would not be mentioned so as "to avoid the usual claims of partiality."[11] Further, the council's most recent survey of medical schools would not be released until Flexner had finished his work. Flexner himself, less than four weeks into the job, was silent. He must have felt intimidated by the powerful figures around him and by the task before him. Most of the discussion centered on an outline that Pritchett had prepared anticipating the structure of Flexner's final report. Almost certainly Pritchett had gone over the outline with his new employee, but it is unlikely that Flexner contributed much to it.

Pritchett's plan called for a study divided into two parts. The first would describe the historical evolution of medical teaching in America and lay down the minimum requirements for study, equipment, and finances in a modern school of medicine. In this part of the report, Pritchett suggested sections on sectarian schools—the schools of osteopathy, homeopathy, and eclectic medicine, and those for women and blacks, and, very importantly, a concluding set of recommendations on how American medical education could best be reconstructed. For Pritchett, as for Flexner, this was the heart of the planned study: to formulate an ideal system for training modern doctors in population centers with good universities that would ensure high standards. The second part of the report, of more interest to the American Medical Association, would survey each medical school in the United States and Canada, following in the footsteps of the Council on Medical Education, with a view to rooting out those with weak or inadequate programs.[12]

A sharp difference of opinion broke out immediately over Pritchett's claim that in the conditions then existing, only a minimum and flexible standard for medical instruction was possible. "An absolute uniform procedure," he warned, was "inadvisable and impossible" because it would create a doctor shortage and because "a competent practitioner" could still be produced in some of the weaker schools. "A certain amount of diversity," in fact, was desirable for it would give "leverage, interplay, and stimulus" to the reform effort.[13] But the eager reformers of the council considered a flexible standard of measurement the very cause of their current difficulties; holding out any hope for its continuation would only mire the reform effort deeper in uncertainty.

Why should the United States not hold to a single standard of training doctors, as was the case in Germany? This argument revealed that none of the participants knew very much about German or European physician education. Pritchett then suggested that once Flexner completed his investigation of American medical schools, he join the secretary of the council, Dr. Nathan P. Colwell, in making a survey of schools in Germany, France, and Britain. Since a similar idea had already been put forward in a private session of the council, the proposal was quickly approved.[14] Following the current study, Flexner would depart for Europe (as it turned out, alone) to do his second study of medical education. As yet, he had not even begun the first.

As 1909 dawned, Flexner was still an unknown figure in American medicine. He had few friends in educational or medical circles. His old enemies in collegiate circles, on the other hand, had not been idle. He had scarcely begun his forays across the country when Pritchett reported "a good many criticisms" concerning Flexner's appointment. Most of them, he said, indicated that he was "erratic and hard to get along with and somewhat uncertain in his judgment." To two friends at Harvard, Pritchett wrote that there were "some intimations that there was friction with respect to him during his stay at Harvard." Pritchett asked for frank and confidential reactions to the anti-Flexner campaign. Only the somewhat equivocal response from William T. Councilman, professor of pathology at Harvard, has been found. Councilman, Simon's old friend and fellow student at Hopkins, said he did not know Flexner well but had "liked what [he] saw of him." Flexner might be "somewhat erratic and probably hasty in judgment," but he was "a very able and valuable man for all that." As for Harvard, it was easy to understand why he was not popular there after his sharp criticisms of the college in his 1908 book. Councilman knew of no friction during his year at Cambridge and, on the contrary, had "heard him very well spoken of by Münsterberg and others."[15]

Pritchett was apparently satisfied, since he made no further mention of the criticisms. By the time Pritchett got Councilman's reply in late January, Flexner had already visited fifteen schools in six states and had begun reporting on his findings. Pritchett was much impressed by his energy, his succinct, precise reports, and the insight he showed into what a good education in medicine required. After his early visit to the Southwestern

Homeopathic Medical College in Louisville, Flexner wrote that the total budget was $1,100, that no laboratories "worth speaking of" were found, that the small building was "wretchedly dirty," and that there was no sign of "recent dissecting." Here and at other schools, he met with deans, faculty members, and sometimes students. He looked carefully at the facilities and asked about equipment. He examined books and catalogs. Pritchett's confidence in his new researcher grew as the two men met to discuss Flexner's findings on his return trips to New York, where he would write up his notes and begin preparation for the next trip. Flexner was even able to turn aside a suggestion from some board members that an advisory committee of physicians be appointed to work with him on the survey.[16]

How was Flexner able to master so much information on American medical education so quickly? By any standard, his grasp of the subject was astounding. To be sure, he had been interested in medical education since his encounters with William Henry Welch at Hopkins and had shown a great deal of insight into the subject when he was advising Simon and urging him to go to Hopkins. In the month between his hiring and the start of his first survey in early January 1909, moreover, he had done a prodigious job of familiarizing himself with the literature on medical training, reading such classics as Theodor Billroth's *The Medical Sciences in the German University*. His immense powers of concentration and organization were brought to bear on a wealth of sources.

Flexner found time to visit Chicago to go over the reports on individual colleges by the Council on Medical Education. He met with the knowledgeable Simon a number of times, and he spent enough time in Baltimore to impress the leading figures of the Johns Hopkins School of Medicine with his probing intellect and quick grasp of what needed to be done. Even the tough-minded, impatient anatomist Franklin Mall, who was at first skeptical of the survey, was converted and became a close ally of Flexner's in shaping the direction of the report. When Mall died eight years later, Flexner praised his contributions as "the most helpful . . . I received. I went to him for advice and guidance. I read his articles until I knew them by heart."[17] For the rest of Flexner's life, Mall would remain one of his heroes.

Even in these early weeks it was becoming clear that here was no pliant hired hand doing what he was told by the foundation or the American Medical Association. Flexner showed himself to be fiercely independent, often quarrelsome, an abrupt man who had definite ideas of his own. He had a knack for seeing quickly the critical weaknesses in a school and summarizing them in a few sentences. He learned as he went along, and his confidence steadily grew.

How much did he depend on the advice and suggestions of Dr. Colwell, who accompanied him on some trips? While professing publicly his debt to Colwell and his admiration for the American Medical Association secretary's experience, he privately made almost no mention of him. How often did Colwell actually join Flexner in his journeys? The evidence is unclear since Flexner makes so little mention of him in his letters, and neither the foundation nor the association was anxious to publicize the association's role in the surveys. Flexner himself gave varying estimates of how many trips he made with Colwell. In his autobiography, he wrote that Colwell and he "made many trips together," but later he took issue with an association publication that claimed they had visited every school together, saying, "I do not remember the precise number, but it could hardly have exceeded half a dozen."[18] Whatever the number, it is clear that Flexner felt free to follow his own instincts in conducting and evaluating the trips he made to all 155 medical schools in the United States and Canada.

Why Canada? The council had included the Canadian medical schools in its second tour of medical colleges, but why did Canadian officials consent so readily to outside inspection? Bevan explained only that Canadian schools furnished "so many medical practitioners to various states" that they had to be included; he makes no mention of any effort to gain consent or cooperation. Only two Canadians served on the council's "Committee of One Hundred" to frame a new standard curriculum. The Canadians may well have opened their doors to Flexner, as did many of the American schools, in the belief that the Carnegie survey would be followed by Carnegie gold. Even so, it is somewhat jarring to find Flexner, as a representative of a private American foundation, making recommendations about "the proper distribution of medical schools" in a neighboring sovereign state. "Canada reproduces the United States on a greatly reduced scale," he wrote matter-of-factly; "Western University at London is as bad as anything to be found on this side of the line; Laval and Halifax Medical College are feeble; Winnipeg and Kingston represent a distinct effort toward higher ideals; McGill and Toronto are excellent." Canada, he concluded, needed no more than five schools.[19]

The pace of Flexner's trips to distant cities over a period of sixteen months staggers the imagination. In an era of railroad travel, supplemented by primitive automobiles and horse-drawn carriages, Flexner criss-crossed the continent dozens of times, stopping at ninety-eight cities and making 174 separate visits to medical schools (some more than once). In April 1909 alone, he inspected thirty schools in twelve cities.[20] During the summer of 1909 he took time out to do further research and to begin writing the report. His final visits came in April 1910, and by June the report had been printed and circulated.

In his letters, we get an occasional glimpse of Flexner hurrying from a railroad station, consulting his timetable for the next trip, stopping overnight in a nearby hotel, penning a quick note to Pritchett, taking his meals alone in the hotel dining room, arriving unannounced at a medical school, bending over student records, glancing at microscopes for signs of use, asking that doors be unlocked, or stopping a student to ask a question.

How thorough were the inspections? Critics then and since have stressed how little time—a day or sometimes only a few hours—he spent at each school. But Flexner had prepared himself with remarkable care for each visit and immediately on arrival began to check the claims in the school's catalog and its reports to the American Medical Association. Were the entrance requirements enforced? A half-hour spent looking through student records could determine the answer. What was the actual size and training of the faculty? A review of class assignments and faculty records could provide a good idea. Could the size of the endowment and the income from student fees be verified? A stroll through the rooms assigned to laboratory work gave a quick impression of the adequacy of the space, the amount of equipment, and the degree of use the equipment was getting. What access did the students have to patients in neighboring hospitals, and how much control did the faculty exert over teaching in them? "A few inquiries made clear," he wrote in his autobiography, "whether the faculty was composed of local doctors . . . or the extent to which efforts had been made to obtain teachers properly trained elsewhere." In the anatomy room, "a 'whiff' told the inside story regarding the manner in which anatomy was cultivated."[21]

Since many of the schools were small, confined often to a single building, and records were not extensive, it was possible to gain an overall impression in a day or less. Flexner's findings, furthermore, were sent to each school, which was given an opportunity to correct any misstatements of fact. When one compares his inspections to a modern accreditation visit at a university of perhaps forty thousand students, spread over a hundred or more buildings, and carried out by a half-dozen visitors in two or three days, it is clear that Flexner got a much closer view of actual conditions in the medical schools of 1910. The dean of the University of Maine Medical School spoke for many when he responded to a faculty member's criticism that Flexner had spent only one day at the school. "That is where we were lucky," said the dean.[22]

It was the pungency of his reports on the weak schools that captured the attention of contemporaries. The California Medical College at Oakland he described as "a disgrace to the State whose laws permit its existence"; the St. Louis College of Physicians and Surgeons had only "a make-believe laboratory for experimental physiology" and "the dust-covered tables [did] not indicate use"; in Georgia the anatomy room at the College of Eclectic Medicine and Surgery was "indescribably foul" and its pathological laboratory contained only three microscopes and "a few dirty slides"; Chicago, with its fourteen medical schools, was "the plague spot of the nation"; at the Kansas Medical College in Topeka the anatomy room contained "a single, badly hacked cadaver" and was also used as a chicken yard; the admissions policy at the College of Physicians and Surgeons in Memphis was "to accept students and try them out"; at Vanderbilt University, anatomy was "bad—the work being conducted on antiquated lines in a foul-dissection-room."

No state or city escaped these damning indictments of the way American doctors were being trained in scores of small, intensely practical, and often commercially inspired schools of medicine. Only the Johns Hopkins School of Medicine, whose laboratory facilities were "unsurpassed" and which provided "ideal opportunities" for clinical teaching, won unstinted praise, while a number of other schools, especially Pennsylvania, Michigan, Yale, Western Reserve, Toronto, and Harvard, were lauded for the progress they had made.[23]

Even as he raced back and forth across the country, Flexner, with Pritchett's approval, sought to begin the process of reconstruction. He encouraged consolidations, promoted ties between medical schools and universities, and suggested ways to improve clinical facilities. His imagination and quick insight into organizational possibilities won commendation from Pritchett. In Chicago, during his second visit, he brought together the presidents of Northwestern, the University of Chicago, and the University of Illinois to plan a common clinical program at the Cook County Hospital. "For the present," he wrote Pritchett, "the momentum of the scheme will carry it along some distance." In Iowa City, he counseled university authorities to hold off on plans for a new wing of the medical building because it "failed to provide for their real needs" for more laboratory space. He urged them to seek a dean with broad experience to build a modern medical school. From the secretary of Yale University, Anson Phelps Stokes (a member of the Carnegie board), he received a letter thanking him for his advice that Yale had "an unusual opportunity" to build "a small university Medical School of the highest standards." He had urged Yale in the report to develop its research potential and to increase its clinical opportunities. In Cincinnati, he told President Charles Dabney, a future close friend, that to have a first-rate medical school, the faculty must have a controlling role in appointments at the city hospital.[24]

Other schools intent on reform welcomed Flexner's counsel and suggestions. At Vanderbilt University Flexner struck up a warm relationship with Chancellor James H. Kirkland, a friendship that would transform the medical school after he convinced Kirkland that the school's future lay in building the strongest institution in the South. Similarly, Flexner advised Washington University in St. Louis that it could be a magnet school for the Southwest. He warned that "heroic measures" were necessary, since no current member of the Washington University faculty was "preeminently fitted to undertake the work." He criticized sharply the number of part-time teachers at the St. Louis school, the "wretched condition" of clinical teaching, and the isolation of the wards from the laboratory work of the first two years. Hospital beds were not well used for teaching, and the school dispensary did "more to demoralize than to train" students.[25] Board chairman Robert Brookings, indignant at the preliminary report and at not being called on by Flexner, hurried to New York to confer with Pritchett, an old friend and former professor at the university.

Flexner was summoned and agreed to Pritchett's strong suggestion that he make a second tour of the Washington University facility, this time with Brookings as his guide. On this visit he quickly convinced the reform-minded Brookings of the enormous work to be done. The chairman began immediately to raise money for a development plan that Flexner had begun to prepare. Pritchett, meanwhile, apologized to the university's chancellor for Flexner's tendency "to sometimes put things in a more sharp way" than necessary. The chancellor replied that Flexner's report was what he wanted: "The fact that he speaks out his mind sharply pleases me." Asked by Brookings to help find the right man to lead the department of surgery, Flexner urged Harvey Cushing, the Johns Hopkins neurosurgeon, to come to New York to meet with Brookings.[26] Cushing, who had acquired a towering reputation during his twelve years at Johns Hopkins, was interested but was already thinking of positions at Harvard and other institutions. After giving the offer serious consideration, he declined it. Flexner then played a role, as did Pritchett, in recruiting David Edsall, another future Harvard luminary, to head the reorganized school. In at least a half-dozen other cases, Flexner was asked to recommend deans or professors even before he finished the report.

The eighteen months Flexner spent on the report energized him and boosted his self-confidence immensely. He was encouraged by his unexpected acceptance by university presidents and deans, despite his meager background and Jewish heritage. In an age when social origins counted heavily, his intelligence, good humor, and ingratiating personality (he was ingratiating when it suited him) won him unusual acceptance not only by academics but by some of the leaders of business and society. It is difficult to think of another Jew who in these years moved so easily across the boundaries of scholarship, philanthropy, and government. The Carnegie assignment was the opportunity for which he had waited so long, and he meant to make the most of it.

He spared no effort to make himself useful and then virtually indispensable to Pritchett and the Carnegie Foundation. Even as he immersed himself in the medical report, he took on new assignments. He wrote a draft of a study of legal education; he undertook a survey of college advising and sabbatical leaves; he prepared for a study of divinity schools. In an article in the *Atlantic Monthly*, he attacked the growing emphasis on research in the hiring and promotion of college teachers. He spoke to the American Association for the Advancement of Science, telling its members that the American college was "almost wholly unorganized." The elective system had indiscriminately piled up huge numbers of courses at the behest of research-minded faculty members, but how were students to choose among these courses, and why? College courses had become interchangeable with graduate school courses in many cases. The proper concern of the college, he wrote, was broadly on "human and disciplinary, formative and cultural" matters, not research or specialized knowledge.[27]

The writing of the medical report took precedence, of course, over all other activities. Even before it was finished, Flexner understood its potential. Pritchett had told him after reading the opening chapters that if he "could keep to this level," the result would be "epoch-making."[28] Simon and Mall likewise encouraged him to persevere. The bulk of the writing was done during four months in the summer of 1909 at the same

Tyringham Valley house in the Berkshire Mountains where he had stayed the summer before he went to Harvard. It was a pleasant time for the Flexner family, reunited for an extended stay in a roomy cottage surrounded by bucolic vistas. They were all glad to get away from the cramped apartment on Seventy-Seventh Street in New York. Flexner's study contained many windows and bookshelves and looked out over an extended garden. It was here that he "wrote, cut and pinned up sections of the medical report." Anne likewise had her own study, with a private entrance, and upstairs were four bedrooms and a large attic. Eleanor was only seven months old when they came to Tyringham, and in good weather she was "parked in her perambulator in a shady spot under the window of [her father's] study." He liked nothing better than "to hear her gooing and gurgling" as he worked.

The summer was one of unusual sociability. Anne's parents came for several weeks, as did Flexner's secretary from New York. They became very friendly with a family next door, which likewise had young children. In the evenings, the Flexners read together by lamplight either aloud or, more commonly, each in his or her own book. Often they went to see the moon rise across the road in an open field. On weekends they sometimes rented a horse and buggy and took a picnic basket to the neighboring towns of Lee, Lenox, and Stockbridge. For Jean, the summer was the most pleasant part of her childhood.[29]

Throughout the summer, as Flexner finished sections of the report, he would send them to Pritchett and Simon, and occasionally to Mall at Johns Hopkins. Pritchett and Mall were sparing in their comments; Simon proved the most reliable and helpful critic. "I appear to have no compunction about imposing tasks on you," Abraham told his brother as he sent another chapter, "when as a matter of fact, I have a good deal." But Simon was the only one who could keep him "from saying absurd things in a 'green' way"—and, he told Simon, "Mr. Pritchett relies largely on your opinion on the medical side." He also asked Simon for help in getting information from the surgeon general on the statistics of those taking the examination for medical officers. Later in the summer, he described to Simon his work on the medical curriculum. "I could fill a bigger book with what I don't know," he confessed, "but I'll brass it through—and with a straight face, if possible."[30]

That fall and winter he finished his tours around the country. He was tired of travel and grew anxious about how his work would be received. Between his trips away from New York, he labored feverishly to complete the final study. He was now eager to see the report in print. Pritchett wrote the introduction in April, and Flexner read the proofs during April and May. By early June, copies of the report were being sent to universities, medical schools, and newspapers across the country. Pritchett promptly raised Flexner's salary to five thousand dollars a year.

The report became famous for its biting reviews of individual schools, but its enduring importance, as both Flexner and Pritchett recognized, lay in its critical analysis of what a good medical school should be. It codified, as Pritchett had hoped it would, the essentials of a modern medical education and laid out a plan for the reconstruction of American medical schools. It created a single model of medical training and rejected the idea of an alternative, practical school of medicine. All physicians should be well-educated, highly trained diagnosticians and problem solvers who understand the laboratory basis for scientific knowledge of the body and have become skilled, through extensive clinical experience, in recognizing and treating disease. Medical education should thus be a union of the scientific and the practical, the laboratory and the clinic, both art and science. From his experience at the Flexner school, he was convinced that students should be active participants in the learning process and not merely passive recipients of knowledge. "On the pedagogic side," he wrote in the report, "modern medicine, like all scientific teaching, is characterized by activity. The student no longer watches, listens, memorizes; he *does*. His own activities in the laboratory and in the clinic are the main factors in his instruction and discipline. An education in medicine involves both learning and learning how; the student cannot effectively know, unless he knows how." To this method of learning the historian Kenneth Ludmerer has given the name "progressive medical education."[31]

The heart of Flexner's conviction about medical study lay in the belief that experimental science had made the union between science and medicine both inevitable and irreversible. Inductive teaching in medicine and science—"learning by doing"—was the key to a pedagogical revolution that was sweeping through medical schools. The fledgling physician must himself see, feel, hear, and test in the laboratory, in the clinic, and at the bedside. Only in a university that joined investigative science to practical training, as at Johns Hopkins, could a modern doctor be educated. The laboratory movement in America was already well advanced and "gave no slight cause for satisfaction." Its future, "even its immediate future," was not in doubt. But there could no longer be two types of medical schools, he argued, one for medical scientists and one for ordinary practitioners, if the aim of medical education was the production of "alert, systematic, thorough, critically open-minded" physicians. Medicine as science, he had come to believe, "could not be separated from medicine as useful human service."[32]

Flexner believed that time spent in practical, hands-on training in the hospital, if supervised by up-to-date, research-minded clinicians, was just as important as time spent in the laboratory. He thought it "absurd" that laboratory teachers should think their work more "pure," more "scientific," than the observations made by a careful observer in a clinic. The essence of science, after all, was its method—"the painstaking collection of all relevant data, the severe effort to read their significance." This was as true of the clinic as of the laboratory, since both were dependent on people's "defective senses." In the strictest sense of the term, both were laboratories: "It makes no difference to science whether usable data be obtained from a slide beneath a microscope or a sick man stretched out on a cot." For the student, the learning experience was to collect and impartially evaluate facts that were "locked up in the patient." It was with patients' illnesses that the vast majority of students would be concerned for the rest of their lives. Good clinical teaching therefore meant bringing "the student into close and active relation with the patient: close, by removing all hindrance to immediate investigation; active, in the sense, not merely of offering opportunities, but of imposing responsibilities."

This was not possible in a faculty of busy, indifferently trained practitioners. To ensure good teaching, the medical school must control all teaching in the university hospital as it was controlled in the laboratory. The faculty must *be* the staff—"solely and alone"—of the hospital, and the professor of medicine must be its physician-in-chief. In the future, clinical professors should be hired on the same basis as other university professors, that is, based on their university salaries and not on practice. Teaching students was too important to be left to part-time practitioners or consultants. "There is no inherent reason," he declared, "why a professor of medicine should not make something of the financial sacrifice that the professor of physics makes."[33] This early recognition of the importance of full-time clinical teaching would lead to one of Flexner's most controversial and hard-fought battles.

Unlike later critics, Flexner was keenly aware of the importance of the physician's role in society. "The physician is a social instrument," he insisted, whose "function is fast becoming social and preventive, rather than individual and curative." The health of the public, sanitation, and preventive health measures were of "overwhelming importance" to schools of medicine and the profession generally. Much of the new knowledge available to physicians was not being used to better the public's health. The "sick man is relatively rare for whom actually all is done that is at this day humanly possible." The medical school had a responsibility as "a public service corporation" that was chartered by the state and made use of public hospitals. It could not escape close scrutiny and regulation. The same law "that protects the public against the unfit doctor should in fairness protect the student against the unfit school." In time, he foresaw the creation of "a national organization" that would guard the public's health against "the formidable combination made by ignorance, incompetency, commercialism, and disease."[34]

The report condemned educators and schools that put private interest or commercial profit above the welfare of the public. Like contemporary critics of the selfishness of American businessmen and politicians, Flexner believed that the self-aggrandizement of commercially inspired medical educators should be "crushed" along with their schools—schools "that trade on ignorance and disease." The Flexner report transformed the reform of medical education into "a broad social movement" akin to the antitrust and workers' protection drives of the Progressive Era.[35]

Flexner found particularly offensive the argument that standards should not be raised so high that the "poor boy" no longer had a chance to become a doctor. The drive to raise standards and limit enrollment to the well prepared meant inevitably that students in the future would spend more time and money in preparing for medicine. The costs of medical education thus threatened to drive all but the most thriving of the middle class out of medicine. Flexner said that he had the utmost sympathy for talented but poor students; after all, he had once been one. But while these students should be encouraged to go into medicine, Flexner believed, they, like other students, must come prepared to absorb the new sciences and knowledge that made up modern medicine. "It is right to sympathize with those who lack only opportunity," he wrote, "still better to assist them in surmounting obstacles, but not at the price of certain injury to the common weal." The "poor boy" had no right to practice medicine unless it was "best for society that he should." In actual fact, he argued, every student, even the poorest, had to pay the school's fees—they were "not cheap"—and it was the weakest schools that provided the least student financial assistance.

The low entrance requirements, in truth, existed for the benefit of "the poor school, not of the poor boy." It was the commercial medical school, run by and for its proprietors, that through unethical advertising enticed the unprepared youth, often poor, into enrolling in medicine.[36] He offered no solution for educating those in the working and lower-middle classes who would now effectively be barred from medicine. Like many in his generation, he believed that the dedicated, hardworking youngster could still succeed, as he had, in spite of the overwhelming changes in American life.

The many weaknesses of American medical training could not be overcome, in his judgment, if "all or most" of the contemporary schools were to survive. To continue to exist, such schools would need to enroll students "far in excess of the numbers" they would graduate; and they would have to "graduate them far in excess of the number of doctors needed." So they would need to continue to entice "their clientele of ill prepared, disconnected, drifting boys, accessible to successful solicitation on commercial lines."[37]

What America needed, Flexner argued, was fewer and better schools, located in population centers, attached to universities and teaching hospitals. Strong legislative action by states, supported by public demand, was required to drive out the weaker schools. Through stricter requirements for licensure, he wrote, "the entire field may be lifted; for the power to examine is the power to destroy." The 148 schools in the United States (the rest were in Canada) should be reduced over time to 31 strategically located schools and the number of graduates cut nearly in half.[38] Nineteen of the schools would be located in large cities, eight in large towns, and four in smaller towns. The reformed schools, he recommended, should demand two years of collegiate preparation, then require two years of preclinical work in medical science followed by two years of supervised clinical experience.

Teaching in these schools should be increasingly personal, carried out by full-time teachers in laboratories and clinics, and less time should be spent in lectures before large classes, which he thought the least effective way for students to learn. "Bedside teaching has consequences," he once told the classical scholar Gilbert Highet; "it destroys planned lecture presentation of clinical subjects for the patient determines the subject to be discussed."[39] Similarly, student work in the laboratory changed the focus and importance of large, formal lectures in the medical sciences.

He knew that his sweeping recommendations could be attacked as favoring elitism over democratic access to medicine. The strong, established institutions, if his plan were followed, would drive out the weak, more accessible medical schools. The special schools for African Americans and women, like the majority of schools that lacked endowment, university connections, and strong support, would succumb along with the rest. The women's schools, he argued, were no longer necessary since 80 percent of women students were now in coeducational schools, while "the negro needs good schools rather than many schools." Howard University and Meharry Medical College, in particular, needed "immensely greater support" if they were to become first-rate schools.[40]

Critics would charge, he knew, that democratic individualism was threatened by a meritocratic profession that welcomed only the well prepared. But such control over standards, while it denied freedom to some, brought greater freedom at a higher level, for it resulted in better health care for the many. Was this a setback to democracy? In building his case, Flexner denied that the reorganization of medical training meant "the weakening of democratic principle," because it tended to "provide the conditions upon which well-being and effectual liberty depend." The "danger of democracy" was that it would "fail to appreciate excellence." But, rightly understood, "an aristocracy of excellence" was the "truest form of democracy."[41]

The issue continued to trouble him. The year after the report's publication, he wrote in the *Atlantic Monthly* that achieving high standards in a democracy was much more difficult than doing so in an autocratic system. In Germany, a firm framework of government kept "society and the distribution of social functions" at a high level, while in America the loose state controls over education made for a more plastic system in which all people were free to find their own place. Germans "drill the mind as they drill the body," Flexner wrote; their schools were aimed at the maintenance of the status quo. The son of a workman was rarely able to reach the university. But in America the "reassignment of the individual on his own merits" was the very purpose of universal education. Organizing a universal system, however, would be difficult in America's democracy. "We have in America," he wrote, "no way of achieving rational ends except by voluntary submission to rational ideals." To gain such voluntary compliance would take persuasion, publicity, strong leadership, and the kind of philanthropic support being supplied by the Carnegie Foundation.[42]

Pritchett was awed by the power and range of the report. He praised its "extraordinary quality" to the Carnegie board, showed board members letters of praise from Welch and others, and predicted that the demand for it would far outstrip that for any of the foundation's earlier reports. He authorized the distribution of fifteen thousand copies of the report—an unprecedented number for the foundation—to universities, medical schools, physicians, medical journals, the lay press, and influential individuals, and more copies would follow. Summaries of the report were released to such journals as the *Atlantic Monthly, Science,* and the *American Review of Reviews,* often under such attention-grabbing titles as "Fewer and Better Doctors" and "The Plethora of Doctors." Charles Eliot wrote Andrew Carnegie from Cambridge that the report was "a very valuable investigation" that would "excite the wrath of all the quacks, vendors of patent medicines, [and] teachers in cheap medical schools."[43] Pritchett and Eliot hoped secretly to convince the canny Scot to furnish the monies necessary to rescue America's medical schools, but the report, curiously, had the opposite effect. Carnegie told Flexner: "You have proved that medical education is a business," and "I will not endow any other man's business."[44]

Especially encouraging to Flexner, however, was the warm reaction of Welch, who thought it "one of the most remarkable and influential publications in educational literature."[45] All in all, the response was remarkably favorable from those whom Flexner and Pritchett wanted most to reach—reform leaders, the medical profession, medical educators, state boards of medical examiners, and the popular press. All that was needed was some means of putting the reconstruction plan into effect.

In retrospect, the report was a tour de force. In striking prose it set down in one place the accumulated lessons of four decades of reform effort. It brought together most of what proponents of change had been arguing for piecemeal since the Civil War. It drew on a generation's experience with German study, with progressive ideas about learning, and with the early success of the Johns Hopkins School of Medicine. It dissected a tangled problem and set out a remarkably clear road map for the future. Flexner's writing embodied the passion for order and efficiency that were hallmarks of the Progressive years, a time when social and political changes were everywhere crowding for attention.

The praise he received confirmed his conviction that he had found his place in the educational world. He would be a critic, a provocateur, a master of the educational survey, a source of learned opinion about the whole enterprise of education. He would find a secure berth in one of the educational foundations, and from there he would project his influence on the reconstruction of American learning.

As expected, a torrent of criticism poured forth from the injured medical schools and local medical journals. Pritchett thanked Eliot for his warm support at a time when he was "getting so many stones thrown" in his direction. The report was variously described as "unfair," "hasty," "flippant," "aristocratic," "full of errors," and "a piece of monumental impudence." Flexner was "a self-constituted censor," "self-satisfied and destructive," "too much the crusader," and "an ignorant layman" with "conceit of Herculean proportions." A prominent Chicago physician regretted that Flexner "had not been kicked down the front steps" of at least one medical school, saying that the failure to do so was "a reflection on medical manhood." Nor were the leaders of the strongest schools satisfied with the report. "Lesser and more prudent men," writes the medical educator Carleton B. Chapman, "would almost certainly have hesitated to invite the disapproval of Harvard's medical Brahmins, Arkansas deans, and Chicago's commercial entrepreneurs all at the same time."[46]

The national press, however, generally praised the report. Pritchett and Flexner were prepared to exploit the publicity and welcomed the public controversy. Within a few months, many of the schools under attack were quietly writing Pritchett, asking what they could do to ensure their survival.

With the report's notoriety, the Louisville schoolmaster had achieved what he had set out to do. He was now a well-known, even famous, figure in the world of education. His talents were sought after by educators and foundation officials anxious to carry out similar surveys of social and educational problems. Within two years of completing the medical report, Flexner would undertake and complete three further investigations—of medical schools in Europe, prostitution in Europe, and clinical full-time teaching at Johns Hopkins—which together earned him a reputation as one of the preeminent social investigators of his time. While he still had no permanent job, he could begin to feel confident that permanent employment would soon be forthcoming.

Since his return from Germany in 1907, his personal fortunes had undergone a profound and dramatic change. Never again would he experience the deep doubts about his capacity that had plagued him during his last years in Louisville. Those closest to him noticed a new self-certainty that bordered at times on cockiness or arrogance. "As success and power came to Abraham," said Simon's son, the historian James Thomas Flexner, "the lack of self-confidence that had held him back until he was almost forty was replaced by its opposite."[47]

The long absences from home put a strain on his marriage. He had seen little of his wife and children for weeks at a time, and both Jean and Eleanor, from their later accounts, missed his comforting presence. Anne, for her part, found that the burdens of parenthood were falling heavily on her just as she was struggling to create new plays to match her initial success. Even before the medical report was printed, Flexner was getting ready to leave for an extended tour of the medical schools of Europe. He would take Anne and the children with him for the summer, but there would be further long separations over the next two years. Like his father, he longed for a period of quiet home life and complained of the loneliness during the long months apart. "Sweet little Eleanor," he wrote after the family left him to return to America, "how I hate to miss the steps in her development . . . [and] to think of being away from home on Jean's birthday two successive years!" "I'll be with you soon, I hope," he wrote wistfully, "and thenceforth, a long together may we enjoy!"[48]

6

Master of the Survey

The strain on the Flexner marriage was eased in the summer of 1910, when the family was reunited for a vacation in the Bavarian alps at Berchtesgaden. They had left New York in late May aboard a small Hamburg-American liner that took ten days to arrive in the port of Cuxhaven. Flexner saw that his daughter had a "marvelous" time in the ship's gym, riding mechanical horses and camels, and being tucked up in steamer chairs on a wind-protected deck. They saw whales spouting, dolphins leaping in the spray of the ship's bow, and four-masted schooners loaded with grain or lumber. From the deck they caught a glimpse of Halley's Comet in its pilgrimage across the sky. In the evenings he and Anne waltzed in formal dress to the strains of romantic music. When young Eleanor became ill, the family had the good fortune of being attended by a leading New York pediatrician, Alfred Hess, who was a fellow passenger.[1] It was a relaxed, happy time. Flexner basked in the warm reactions to his first major triumph.

In Berchtesgaden, they stayed in a small pension and made excursions into the surrounding countryside. They went by carriage to the Königssee, visited the palace of King Ludwig II, and toured Salzburg's palace and cathedral. They descended into the nearby salt mines, crossing an underground lake by boat.[2] But Flexner was not entirely at ease. He was already preparing for the European study and had brought along a collection of books and studies. He made several forays into Munich, where he met Franklin Mall, who was spending the summer there. He saw much of Mall and found him a generous and helpful critic.

It was Mall who counseled Flexner on the strengths and variety of German medical education. Together they visited laboratories and clinics and attended lectures. Flexner was particularly impressed with the brilliant lectures of Friedrich von Müller, the most celebrated clinician of the day. While the audience at other lectures "melted away" toward the end of the semester, Müller's were so crowded that they had to go early to get a seat.

Müller became Flexner's beau ideal of what a university clinician should be—a superb teacher and a first-class researcher. Flexner cherished his time with Mall, including the relaxed hours they whiled away at his rooms after a day in the laboratory or lecture hall.[3] Together the Germanophile Mall and the more skeptical Flexner talked over the best way to educate a doctor. A close friendship sprang up between the two men.

The European tour was clearly going to be different from the strenuous visits he had made to American and Canadian medical schools. Here the schools were all "substantial" in comparison with American schools and Flexner had no mandate to reform them. His purpose in Europe, he agreed with Henry S. Pritchett, was simply to portray the broad principles and structures underlying the various systems so that American educators might adapt what was useful to their circumstances. There was no need to visit every school of medicine, as there had been in America. When it was suggested that he go to the famous Italian school in Pavia, he responded that he could not limit an Italian visit to Pavia without mentioning Italy's other universities and medical schools, "mostly wretched and poor." He likewise rejected suggestions that he go to Budapest or Stockholm since his intent was not to pick out first-rate schools but to describe medical education as a whole. He would carefully limit his survey to a fair sample of entire countries.[4] Unlike in the American study, he had no importunate American Medical Association looking over his shoulder, pressing him to go on the attack.

After preliminary work in Munich and a stop in Paris, he traveled in October to England to begin his first country study. On his arrival, he discovered that his American report, already known, earned him entry into medical and educational circles. The president of the Royal College of Surgeons, Henry Butlin, told him he needed no formal introductions to the principal figures in British medicine. "I've read your report," he said, "it's masterly. I am preparing a memorial to the Royal Commission on London University and you are my authority—see here, here's your Report—every margin filled with pencil comments showing how you have analyzed our difficulties for us." It was an auspicious beginning for what proved to be an unexpected role for Flexner: reformer of British medical education. It emboldened him to take a much stronger position toward the schools he visited. Fifty years later, a British medical dean gave him credit for "the present evolution of British medical education."[5]

The training of doctors in Britain, as in America, was in turmoil, especially in London. Flexner learned of the dissatisfaction with the many ways that doctors could be licensed in England and Scotland. He found, too, that the rigidity of the seniority system in British hospitals frustrated those trying to reform hospital teaching. Britain's slowness in developing laboratory study and scientific research, moreover, had produced a sense of crisis in those aware of developments in Germany and the United States. A year before Flexner's arrival, William Osler, who had recently left the Johns Hopkins School of Medicine for the Regius Chair of Medicine at Oxford, had sharply criticized the neglect of laboratory studies in British medical schools.[6]

The Royal Commission that Butlin referred to was established to address the tangled relationship between the degree-granting University of London, which offered no courses, and the largely independent colleges that actually carried out instruction in the city. It was a peculiarly British arrangement with no parallels to the situation in America. The twelve medical schools in the city, largely the outgrowth of its major hospitals, were not to be included in the study. Curiously, it was Flexner's presence in London and his intention to study British medical schools that stirred up interest in medicine in the commission.[7] Through William Mc-Cormick, manager of the Carnegie philanthropies in Britain and a member of the commission, Flexner met the chairman, Secretary of State for War Richard Haldane, and helped persuade him that medical study should not be left out of the commission's work.

Excitedly, Flexner wired Pritchett of this development and asked for permission to appear before the commission. He spent a weekend with Osler, going over a draft of the statement he proposed to make. "I feared it might be regarded as too direct," he informed Pritchett, but Osler "approved it unqualifiedly," arguing "that only by thus making a sharp issue" would the commission be assisted. Osler came to London to give him further support and later testified himself. Flexner remained concerned that his intended criticisms, coming as they did from a foreigner, were so sweeping that a "huge howl was inevitable."[8]

Flexner's stunning testimony became the point of departure for the hearings. With the same brutal frankness that marked his statements on American medical schools, he told the commissioners that medical teaching in London was not "fully modern" and that even the preclinical branches lagged far behind the schools of the Continent and the better schools of America. Anatomy was still being taught by busy consultants; pharmacology could be found in only one of the twelve London schools; nowhere was scientific teaching adequate for sound medical training. Clinical teaching in London was the haphazard responsibility of visiting practitioners whose chief interests lay elsewhere. Nowhere could he find the close interaction between the preclinical sciences and the medical clinics that he was convinced was the sine qua non of a modern medical education.

What London and Great Britain lacked, he boldly told the commission, was a university model to "break the existing level of mediocrity." A university system, he warned, meant radical change: reconstituting the teaching staffs, breaking up the seniority system in making hospital appointments, and providing adequate salaries to medical professors so they could spend all their time in teaching and investigation. Asked by Haldane whether the ideal model could be found in Baltimore, Flexner replied simply, "yes." For all his devastating criticism, he did offer the consolation that clinical training in Britain was still better than clinical training in the ordinary medical school in America. Following his two-hour testimony, he learned from several of the commission members, as he reported, that he had "scored." Would he permit his statement to be given to all those asked to testify, so as to provide common ground for all the hearings? Without hesitation, he agreed. Looking back on the hearings a quarter-century later, he confessed that he was appalled by his "absolutely colossal nerve."[9] His testimony brought him instant attention and a growing corps of supporters and enemies in Britain.

As expected, much of the subsequent testimony before the Haldane Commission was in strong opposition to what Flexner proposed. The former president of the Royal College of Surgeons, Sir Henry Morris, objected to the "crispness, dogmatism . . . and cocksureness" of Flexner's testimony. "I am not aware," said Morris acerbically, "that Mr. Abraham Flexner is either a clinician or a science teacher." What the American was proposing, in Morris's view, was "simply the rigid German system under a modern American name." Others feared that the Flexner plan, with its stress on having only well-prepared scientific and clinical teachers instruct students, would sacrifice the great strength of the English system of reying on medical clerks and surgical dressers—medical students who learned while doing clinical tasks under the supervision of visiting consultants. The hostile testimony confirmed for Flexner that the real difficulty lay not in understanding the plan but "pushing it thro', over the certain hostility of the local profession." For years members of the London profession had spread the idea that their "practical" schools were the best in the world. Now they were afraid, he said, that a move to scientific training would destroy their practical value.[10]

The commission's report was largely an endorsement of Flexner's testimony. For the sake of the critics, the importance of retaining the clerkship system under professional direction, which Flexner never questioned, was also emphasized. Indeed, Flexner regarded the clinical clerk and surgical dresser as the heart of the English system and urged their wider adoption in the United States. Their education, however, in his judgment, must come under the direct supervision of university professors and not hospital consultants, as in London. The main features of the report, said Haldane in 1913, recognized that Britain had fallen behind the United States and Germany in university education. As Flexner had proposed, the report recommended that the standard for clinical teachers match that of other university professors in requiring them to spend most of their time in teaching and research.[11] Seven years later, the Rockefeller Foundation provided the funds to create a university medical center in London with full-time "units" in the medical schools.

Flexner was jubilant. He wrote later of the Haldane Report that "no more incisive document on the subject" had ever been written. Simon congratulated him for having exerted such a powerful impact on the outcome. He had played a role in changing minds and making possible "the regeneration of medical teaching in England." "It is splendid," he added. The influential M. Carey Thomas, president of Bryn Mawr College and Simon's sister-in-law, who was in London, told him that she was impressed by the high regard with which his work was held in England. It was the first time, she complimented him, that an American report or usage had influenced English education "in this direct way."[12] All in all, it was an unexpected triumph for Flexner and a remarkable beginning for the European study. The friendships with Haldane, McCormick, and other members of the commission became some of the closest of his life, and the fondness for British academic life acquired during the visit was an enduring feature of his later career.

As a whole, he found British medical training superb in its practical aspects but woefully lagging in bringing experimental science into the curriculum. The typical school of medicine was no more than an apprenticeship program in a hospital supplemented by haphazard courses in the preclinical sciences. Students did not normally go to a university before entering medical school at age 18 or 19. None of the schools was a full-fledged university school of medicine or had close ties to work in basic science. The equipment and researchers needed for the critical study of disease were everywhere in short supply. Only physiology of the underlying medical sciences was found in the typical English hospital school. As in the United States, in Britain, students entering medical school lacked a good secondary education. The rigid class system allowed few prospective doctors to study at the elite private schools and academies. The requirements for admission to professional training were mechanical and minimal. The very basis of English medical training was therefore "indisputably low."[13]

The commercial spirit contaminating American medical education was also widespread in Britain, Flexner asserted. It was "personal pecuniary and professional interest" alone that kept alive eleven of the London schools, as well as a number of the "struggling, poorly attended schools" elsewhere in Britain. Who resisted most the improvement of scientific instruction? It was the "financially-interested teachers" of London. The real hope of English medicine, he asserted, lay in the laboratories, where men with "sound ideals" could be found. But they would fail in having much impact, unless they were able to destroy the commercial impulse in medical teaching.[14]

Conditions in France he found so similar to those across the English Channel that he frequently combined his discussion of medical education in the two countries. As in Britain, in France instruction of students at the bedside was "excellent," while teaching in the preclinical sciences, carried out in large lecture halls, was at best perfunctory. Physiology was taught in Paris in the huge amphitheater of the Faculté de Médecine in the École Pratique. Lectures there were supplemented by demonstrations before hundreds of students. Almost no provision was made for students to do their own experimental work. The bond between medical teaching and research was particularly weak, even looser than in Great Britain. The French school of medicine, like its British counterpart, was essentially a clinical school centered in a hospital.

In drawing conclusions about French teaching, Flexner was much influenced by the Lyon surgeon Alexis Carrel, who was now a colleague of Simon's at the Rockefeller Institute for Medical Research. After visiting seventeen of the twenty-seven British schools of medicine, Flexner, on Carrel's counsel, went only to Paris, Lyon, and Lille. In Paris, the overwhelming concentration of students made it virtually impossible to give hands-on training to students in either the laboratory or the clinic. In neither Britain nor France was there a single example of the university school of medical education that he favored for the emerging American system of educating doctors.[15] At the Pasteur Institute he met with the

immunologist Elie Metchnikoff, who discussed French medical education "for me rather than with me" for an hour. He was not impressed.

Only when he entered Germany and Austria did he encounter the kind
of system that he believed would produce the kind of doctors that would
be needed in the future. In the universities of Germany, unlike those of
France or Britain, were imbedded both the preclinical sciences that were
the foundation of medical learning and the teaching clinics that provided
practical training. It was this contiguity of the scientific laboratory and
the hospital clinic that was the heart of the German achievement. "In the
eighteenth century, the professor of medicine and the professor of physics
both talked," he wrote; "in the nineteenth, the former got his hospital,
the latter his 'institute,' and both thenceforth produced as well as talked."

But the German medical school, too, had its weaknesses, especially in
the overloaded curriculum and the overemphasis on lectures and class
demonstrations. Because of the expansion of German student bodies after
1890, learners were being deprived of a chance to gain much individual
experience in either the laboratory or the clinic. Once the expansion
began, it was no more difficult to arrange a lecture for three hundred students than for thirty. From an educational point of view, he said, the German practice was "surely mistaken." Even the most brilliant demonstration was "less educative" than a "more or less bungled experiment" carried
out by the student. In the clinic, the ability of students to touch and treat
patients at the bedside in huge schools like Vienna and Berlin, admittedly
extreme examples, was virtually lost. Flexner feared for the future of clinical teaching in such places and contrasted conditions there with what he
had seen in the hospitals of Britain and France.[16]

A more "traumatic contrast" than Vienna and London, he told Pritchett, could scarcely be imagined. In teaching bedside skills, the English
method had much to offer to both Germans and Americans, while the
scientific and clinical work in Vienna made the English hospital look "absolutely dead." The "close juxtaposition" of these two visits, he believed,
made the approaches seem more complementary than contradictory.[17]

The clear lesson for America was to combine the best of British clinical experience with the university organization and scientific laboratories
of Germany. This had already begun to happen at the Johns Hopkins
Hospital and Medical School, and in a few other places. It would need to
be the distinguishing characteristic of future medical education in America, Flexner believed. This conviction, now firmly implanted in his mind,
best explains the policies he followed later as chief dispenser of medical

philanthropy at the General Education Board. "My head fairly reels with my experience here thus far," he confided to Simon. He was eager to apply the lessons he had learned to America. To be a part of it, to have a hand in "modelling and determining it"—this is what "stirs the imagination."[18]

Looking back, Flexner wondered how he had kept up so exhausting a pace for so long a time. As in America, he hurried from school to school. "I may succeed in doing Köln and Düsseldorf in one day," he wrote Anne, "in that case I may do Marburg instead of Frankfurt, say Friday and Saturday." By now he had been traveling constantly in America and Europe for two years and there was more to come. In recalling his travels, he was struck by the "unremitting zeal" and torrid activity that "now seem to me . . . half mad."[19]

But the success of the European survey brought him closer to the place of power he sought. These were "glorious days," he said in retrospect, for "I was young [45!], enthusiastic, and strong," and each day brought him into contact with outstanding persons. He spent his evenings writing up notes "till the small hours of the morning," for he had no secretary and no one to whom he could dictate.[20] "I have had another 9 to 6 today," he wrote Anne, "and the end is not yet, for at eight I am to witness an examination in medicine before the conjoint board of the Royal College of Physicians and Surgeons."[21] By February 1911, after seven months abroad, he was back in New York completing the report in a rear office of the Carnegie Foundation.

All during the stay in Europe he kept a close watch on developments in America. Constantly he advised Pritchett on how to deal with the aftermath of the American report. The "unconscionable" medical school at Memphis, he told Pritchett, was planning new ventures—could he not "do something?" The "consolidating sentiment" was strong in California, and he asked Pritchett to encourage it. In Chicago, the fourteen schools he had visited a year before had been reduced to eight, and more shrinkage, he felt certain, was possible. Leaders at the school in Louisville dropped a professor whom "they appeared to be very fond and proud of," and that puzzled Flexner. While in Europe, he helped with efforts to recruit the Viennese pediatrician Clemens von Pirquet for the Johns Hopkins School of Medicine.[22]

He also kept up a running battle with A. Lawrence Lowell, Eliot's successor at Harvard, who resented Flexner's sharp criticism of Harvard's "old-boy" network of clinicians, in which teachers were promoted on seniority rather than merit. The two men quarreled, too, over Lowell's fondness for classical studies as a preparation for medicine and other professions. The Harvard president was not convinced that more study of modern science and foreign languages should be allowed to crowd out classical literature or mathematics. "I think it is extremely kind of you to take such pains to enlighten me," he wrote Lowell, but "your proposition seems to me, on its face, in the highest degree improbable."[23]

He began writing the European report in the early months of 1911. In June he moved to Tyringham and continued writing until October. His pattern followed that used for writing the American report. As he finished each chapter, he sent it to Simon, to Pritchett, and to Franklin Mall. Mall offered the most detailed criticism and suggested the largest number of changes. "I hope you will continue to keep me on the defensive mercilessly," he told Mall after the latter had dissected his chapter on British anatomy.[24] More and more, as he worked on the report, he confided in Mall his hope of realizing a radical change in the American medical curriculum. What was needed in America, he said, was a logical curriculum, leaving plenty of "leeway" for individual differences, giving students as much freedom as possible to pursue their own interests, and concluding with a rigorous examination. This would remain his goal over the coming years, even as the organized profession moved in the opposite direction, limiting flexibility and establishing firm standards.

As his study neared completion, Flexner began to feel certain that it would be a powerful supplement to the American report. In three hundred and fifty pages of solid analysis and careful reporting—almost double the analytical portion of the earlier study—he had put together the most comprehensive survey of Western medical teaching in any language. Simon was overwhelmed at his brother's achievement and had little to suggest in the way of criticism. Neither did Mall contain his enthusiasm for the forthcoming work: it was "far superior," he said, to the American report.[25] Pritchett, too, was enthusiastic and ordered a printing equal to that of the earlier report.

More than forty thousand copies of the two Carnegie reports were eventually distributed across America, Britain, and the Continent. A flood of editorials in medical and popular journals—135 of them in response to the European report alone—appeared across western Europe and the United States. Leaders of medical schools, heads of universities, and medical spokesmen read and digested the details of the lengthy academic studies. Hundreds of letters addressed to Flexner arrived at the Carnegie Foundation offices in New York. The only criticism of the report, the secretary of the foundation wrote him, was that "somehow it has been read by a good many people as indicating that everything German is perfect and everything else is not."[26] By the time of the European report's publication, in the summer of 1912, Flexner's work was nearly as well known in Europe as in America.

While at work on the European report, Flexner was approached about undertaking two further surveys that would lead finally to the position of power he sought. Within a few weeks of each other, John D. Rockefeller Jr. and Frederick T. Gates came to Flexner for help on two very different projects. The quiet but effective Rockefeller son was now the direct representative of his father in overseeing the family's philanthropies, while Gates, a hard-driving Baptist minister, was the chief administrator and adviser on the distribution of the fast-accumulating Rockefeller fortunes. Together they represented a level of philanthropic power never before seen—and they both wanted Flexner to undertake a delicate and important investigation on their behalf. In Flexner's mind, and almost certainly in the thinking of Rockefeller and Gates, the undertakings were also an unspoken trial of his ability to work effectively in the Rockefeller organization.

Of the two assignments, Gates's was by far the more congenial. Gates was a convert to the idea that medicine must become far more scientific before it could overcome its empirical, catch-as-catch-can heritage as a practical art benefiting relatively few people. From his reading of William Osler's pioneering textbook on medicine, he was struck by the need to begin anew an effort to establish therapeutic medicine on a foundation of scientific study and experiment. He had played a strategic role in founding the Rockefeller Institute for Medical Research—which Simon Flexner now headed—and regarded it as the most important of the Rockefeller philanthropies. For him the work of the institute bordered on the spiritual. "There have been times," he wrote in his memoirs, "when, as I have looked through these microscopes, I have been stricken with speechless awe. I have felt that I was 'gazing' with unhallowed eyes into the secret places of the Most High."[27]

In early January 1911, Gates wrote to William Henry Welch in Baltimore, asking him what it would cost to double the size of the entering class in medicine to one hundred students and, as "an ultimate ideal," to pay the clinical professors enough that they would not be permitted to charge for their work with private patients. While the first estimate was not difficult, Welch wrote back, the second was much more complex because of the tradition of part-time clinical teaching in America and the attitudes of the clinical teachers themselves. Gates persisted, citing the strong criticism of clinical teaching in Flexner's American report and insisting that some idea of the costs involved was necessary before a plan to reconstruct medical education could be put together. When Welch finally turned over some rough estimates to Gates in late January, Gates pleaded his inability to carry the negotiations further. The job of making sense of the several proposals, he told Welch, "is too big a one for me to tackle at this period in my life."[28]

On March 11, Gates invited Flexner to lunch and told him that his 1910 report was a plan for future action as well as a critique of existing conditions in medical education. What he wanted from Flexner was a detailed report on the costs of beginning the transformation of medical teaching at Johns Hopkins, presumably by moving clinical medicine toward full-time university status. Flexner was not unprepared for the assignment. He had been alerted by both Simon and Mall to the Welch-Gates discussions and knew that he was likely to be asked to play a role. Nearly a month before the meeting with Gates, Simon had suggested a way of approaching the "clinical situation" in Baltimore by breaking down the time each clinician spent in teaching and research as opposed to private consultation and practice. To Mall, Flexner wrote that he could not give him some data he wanted on teaching assignments because "for the present" his name needed to "be kept out of the discussions." This "mysterious request," he told Mall, "won't be mysterious very long."[29]

So the story told by Flexner in his autobiography and repeated by countless others that Flexner's being sent to Baltimore was the result of an offhand question of Gates as to what he would do if he were given a million dollars to improve medical education is clearly misleading if not apocryphal. Gates may have indeed posed such a question, and Flexner may have replied that he would give it all to Welch, as he said, but both men knew what the real purpose of the luncheon was. There was no one for whom Gates had deeper respect than Simon Flexner, and he knew that Welch regarded him as his finest disciple, so that asking Simon's brother, who he knew shared Simon's views on scientific medicine and full-time teaching, to act as negotiator was a logical and sensible step.

Gates had been interested in the full-time idea in clinical medicine for at least a decade. In conversations with Welch, who headed the board of scientific advisers of the Rockefeller Institute, and with Simon, he had become convinced that clinical research to benefit patients would come only with financial incentives for full-time clinical teaching. The good teacher, he believed, was also a good investigator, and students taught by such a teacher would be better doctors. In 1902, he was approached for support of a full-time plan by the Hopkins-trained Lewellys Barker, then at the University of Chicago. Barker had just made a stirring speech arguing for more research in the clinical branches of medicine through creating full-time positions corresponding to those in the preclinical sciences. But Gates was at the time preoccupied with the creation of the Rockefeller Institute and had neither the time nor the resources to begin a new undertaking. Barker's colleague at Chicago at the time, Mall, was also arguing for more scientific colleagues in clinical medicine. Such colleagues, he told Barker, must be "an entirely different breed of man" than the current practitioner-teachers. The latter, he predicted to Barker, "will be at you in full force for you are meddling with their pocket-books." The full-time clinical plan was thus on the minds of all the key players well before Abraham Flexner was sent to Baltimore in the spring of 1911 to confer with Welch and his colleagues.[30]

It came as no surprise to Flexner that the strongest voice for full-time clinical teaching in Baltimore was Mall's. The two men had been close since their time in Munich in 1910 and had already exchanged preliminary ideas about how such a plan might work. When Welch planned a dinner to discuss the overture from Gates, he invited only Mall and the research-minded surgeon William Halsted, who was already engaged nearly full-time in teaching and research. For three weeks, with the warm approval of Pritchett, who saw the assignment as the first fruit of the Carnegie surveys, Flexner accumulated data, spoke with faculty members, visited laboratories and clinics, and stayed in close touch with Mall and Welch.

He was struck, he wrote to several of his correspondents, with the failure of the Johns Hopkins faculty to maintain the school's wide lead over other schools of medicine. Tension was growing between the preclinical faculty and the teachers of clinical subjects. Mall was particularly critical of the clinical faculty, their lack of scientific commitment, and their wide-ranging consultative and private practices. "We are told that medical and surgical professors cannot take interest in medical problems and the sick unless they are paid for each move," he wrote at the time of Flexner's visit; "it falls to us to demand of the last two years of medicine what they demanded of the first two and I think the day of reckoning is at hand."[31] By the spring of 1911, other voices were being raised across the country in favor of bringing clinical teaching more closely into the orbit of the university, with its commitment to science, research, and full-time engagement.

Flexner's recommendations were never in doubt. After praising the devotion and contributions of the preclinical faculty, he described the clinical faculty as "on the whole less productive and less devoted." Too little of their time was spent in scientific work or teaching. Only a few of them devoted any "considerable part" of their lives to science. Their work as researchers and teachers was being "sacrificed to private professional engagements." They turned their classes over to assistants in order to leave town to see patients, "not because they [we]re scientifically interesting, but because they [we]re pecuniarily worthwhile." The chief interest of the clinicians, he bluntly charged, was not science or education but profit.[32] His analysis, intended as a confidential report to Gates, was devastating and sure to ignite hostility if it became public.

Although the report listed other options for the use of a Rockefeller gift—creating additional laboratories, setting the size of the school at four hundred students—creating full-time clinical appointments was his clear recommendation. Such an effort, estimated by Flexner to require one and a half million dollars, would establish the school as a model for the entire country. Clinicians would at last become true university teachers, barred from all but charity practice, in the interest of teaching. For Flexner, as for Gates, Mall, and, at some remove, Welch, the crushing of the commercial impulse in medicine had become a moral imperative. The commercial impulse represented, in the eyes of its critics, a "dynamic malignancy" that was blocking the creation of a clinical science of medicine in the United States.[33] At some deeper level, Flexner's distaste for commercial motives in medicine may have derived from his parents' strong preference for "honorable" professions rather than commercial pursuits.

Gates saw Flexner's twenty-five-page report as a model of its kind. Characteristically, it cut through all the ambiguities and shades of opinion on the subject and ignored the sure hostility of most American clinicians. In a telephone call, Gates told Flexner, "I am more than satisfied . . . I have occasion to read many reports, but when I have read anything like that I cannot recall." Would the Johns Hopkins faculty, he asked Flexner, have the backbone to make so revolutionary a change? It would be Flexner's job, Gates informed him, to steer the proposal to its final realization.[34] The impulsive Gates was ready to endorse the proposal immediately, but Flexner counseled him that the initiative should come from Baltimore and be worked out with the medical faculty and the university. This course of action meant that the Flexner plan would become the subject of public discussion as university trustees and medical faculty members alike debated whether to have full-time instructors.

The confidential report itself was leaked by someone in Baltimore, and a battle-royal followed not only at Hopkins but in clinical circles across the country. William Osler, who was initially attracted to the idea of full-time university service, was put off by Flexner's attack on the clinical staff at Johns Hopkins. From Oxford he entered the fray, advising the university president, Ira Remsen, that "pure laboratory men"—he was undoubtedly referring to Mall and possibly Welch—were misleading the university about the full-time issue. It was simply not true that the clinical faculty had been less productive than their scientific colleagues, he protested, citing the original work done by such protégés as the neurosurgeon Harvey Cushing, the clinical investigator William Thayer, and the surgeon J.M.T. Finney. Furthermore, a completely scientific clinician, without constant resort to patients, would be no more than a "clinical prig" confined to the wards of a hospital, "practising the fugitive and cloistered virtues of a clinical monk." How could such a man train others for a "race the dust and heat of which he knows nothing and—this is a possibility!—cares less?" The hospital itself, furthermore, would lose its identity as "a place of refuge for the sick poor of the city" and a consultation center for the whole country.

It was a pity, said Osler, that the Flexner report had gone out as it had, for it showed "a very feeble grasp of the clinical situation." He called the report's author an "Angel of Bethesda" (a Biblical angel who brought healing to a pool in Bethesda) who had done "much good in troubling [medicine's] fish-pond" but who was "irritatingly ignorant" of hospital practice and clinical training. He was bent on demolishing what so many had sacrificed to build in Baltimore. Flexner responded that, given Osler's take on the report, he was glad to be called "any kind of angel." To Mall he confided that he did not think Osler's stand added much to the discussion but that he regretted any suggestion that he was criticizing Osler's own service, of which he said he knew "nothing."[35]

Welch welcomed the blunt report but had not intended it to reach the whole medical community. He prepared a more emollient version for faculty members and trustees. In response to the objection that depriving clinical teachers of private practice would deny them valuable teaching and personal experience, Welch recast Flexner's proposal to permit clinical teachers to do limited consultations and see paying patients at the Johns Hopkins Hospital, provided that the fees paid by such patients went to the hospital or the university. He also made clear his belief that the requirement of full-time obligation to the university, while necessary in current conditions, might be loosened somewhat as the plan developed.[36]

In a visit to Gates and Flexner in early June, Welch said that he supported the modified plan, but he unnerved Flexner with the suggestion that some of the clinical faculty, such as Lewellys Barker (who had moved to Baltimore from Chicago to succeed Osler in 1905), might be named "clinical professors" with full access to the pay wards. Barker himself had sharply modified his earlier views on the full-time status requirement, writing Flexner that a "judicious compromise" would preserve the "opportunity for increase of material reward" for outstanding teachers. Alarmed, Flexner opened a sharp exchange with Barker and fought hard to buttress Gates's stand against a more flexible definition of full-time service. After one exchange, Simon commended his brother: "You have in a few sentences not only blown up Barker's fortress but you have also, I fear, cut off the possibility of his retreat."[37]

It was now clear to both Flexners that Barker would leave the chair of medicine if he lost the case for greater flexibility. Barker had family obligations that would not permit any sharp diminution of his income. To Flexner it appeared that Barker's whole attitude was infected by "his Jesuitical efforts to find a good reason for resisting what in his heart he approves." From his discussions with Welch and Gates, Flexner was convinced that if Gates stood firm and made the offer, it would prevail. By mid-June, he was persuaded that Gates was not going to flinch. The Rockefeller lieutenant was determined, he said, that patient fees "not go to the individual under any circumstances."[38]

It took another two years before agreement was reached on inaugurating full-time clinical medicine at the Johns Hopkins School of Medicine. Welch insisted on moving slowly to gain acquiescence, making it "unnecessary to hurt feelings by the use of force." While the preclinical faculty and the trustees were quickly won over, a number of the clinical faculty harbored deep resentments and concerns about their futures. Several of the professors with large incomes, Gates wrote to John D. Rockefeller Sr., would "either have to resign from the institution to private practice, or else their incomes [would] be reduced to half and in some instances perhaps one-tenth" of what they had been. Some of them, said Gates, were prepared to make the sacrifice, but others would "take their places, not with the sheep, but with the goats." They would continue to practice medicine as a commercial pursuit, dissociated from the college.[39]

The dispute ignited a storm of conflict across the country. Clinical teachers and practitioners generally opposed the plan. Leading the attack was Arthur Dean Bevan, chairman of the American Medical Association's Council on Medical Education, who thought it "unethical, immoral and wicked." To Pritchett he wrote that the plan was "absurd" and must have come from men "not familiar with modern clinical medicine." But leaders of medical schools, especially those at Washington University, Yale, and Harvard, were quick to seek Rockefeller support for their own schools even before the gift to Johns Hopkins was made final. Flexner, although still an employee of the Carnegie Foundation, was involved in all of these early negotiations. By the time he joined the General Education Board in late 1912, Flexner had become so closely identified with the full-time principle that, quite erroneously, he was credited with originating the idea. He would spend much of the rest of his career trying to explain and defend his role in what has been called "the most important single movement in modern medical education."[40]

But these battles lay in the future, and Flexner turned to the other assignment brought him by his growing fame as a master of the educational survey. While still writing the report on European medical education and simultaneously carrying on negotiations over the full-time arrangement at Johns Hopkins, he also began to consider how to carry out the remarkable assignment given him by John D. Rockefeller Jr. Flexner approached it with deep misgivings. Probably only the realization that its successful completion would bring him even closer to a permanent position in the Rockefeller charities overcame his initial hesitancy. By the time Rockefeller approached him in January 1911, he was convinced that the Carnegie Foundation held no promise as the source of the monies needed to reform American education and that only the General Education Board, with its seemingly unlimited resources, could carry out worthwhile projects.

The unlikely subject of Flexner's fourth investigation in as many years was prostitution. The younger Rockefeller had been asked the year before to head a special grand jury to probe the politically controversial issue in New York City. The Tammany Hall administration of the city, accused of complicity in spreading the vice, saw a high-level investigation under the mild-mannered Rockefeller as a way of diffusing the growing criticism. But Rockefeller, anxious for a public role that would deflect public criticism from his family, threw himself into the probe with a zeal that frightened the Tammany leaders. "I never worked harder in my life," he wrote. "I was on the job morning, noon, and night."[41] Under his leadership, the grand jury returned fifty-four indictments and recommended a permanent commission to monitor vice in the city. When the cornered Tammany Mayor, William Jay Gaynor, flatly dismissed the recommendation, Rockefeller created his own commission, called the Bureau of Social Hygiene, to continue the investigation.

To gain perspective and learn how prostitution was dealt with in other countries, the bureau early determined to study prostitution and its control in Europe. Both Pritchett and Simon Flexner recommended Abraham Flexner as the best person for the job. When first approached by Rockefeller, Flexner declined the proposal, and only Simon's persuasion, he later wrote, caused him to yield. He saw himself as "absolutely without qualifications," but perhaps no less so, he said later, than he had been for the studies of medical education. On February 9, 1911, Rockefeller formally gave him the job, having secured Flexner's temporary release from Pritchett. He was charged with making "a thorough and comprehensive study" of the prostitution problem and how it was handled in Europe. He was to be paid six thousand dollars a year and, since the job was temporary, a bonus of one thousand dollars on completing the work.[42]

He could not begin the new study until the fall. As he worked feverishly to complete the European medical report and pushed forward the negotiations with Johns Hopkins, he was given still other tasks by Pritchett. As Flexner was preparing to leave for Europe for the prostitution study, Pritchett asked him to confer with a half-dozen medical authorities abroad who had agreed to read the proofs of the foreign study, warning him that occasionally "he might be asked to visit some institution or attend some meeting." It was clear that his efforts to please Pritchett, and now Rockefeller and Gates, begun in 1908, would continue for at least another year and that his status as a temporary employee often on loan to others, was not to change. Another two years of his life were mortgaged, he wrote in his autobiography, with still no idea as to his ultimate destination.[43]

The continuing uncertainty about the future and the prospect of still further absences from Anne and the children weighed heavily upon him. He was now forty-five years old, he had no permanent job or home, and his wife and children, now twelve and three, were becoming used to his being away. Both Jean and Eleanor felt the growing strain in their parents'

marriage. Both missed their father. And he dreaded the continuing separations. "It's ghastly business, this being alone," he had written Anne on
his last trip abroad, and here he was about to start again on a lengthy tour
of European cities.[44]

Once aboard the *Lusitania* en route to Britain, he poured out his loneliness at the thought of what was to come: "The hours are dragging slowly
by and leave my heart bruised and empty." He shrank from the months
of effort ahead, with their many new faces, "into which I shall in vain try
to wish you."[45] In all, he would spend the better part of four years on the
road working on the various surveys as he struggled to find a secure berth
in the burgeoning world of educational philanthropy. It was a new and
closed world, and he was as yet an outsider.

Before leaving for Europe, he consulted with social workers and police
officials but found little help on the subject of prostitution. Most of them
had a "general notion" that prostitution in Europe was somehow regulated and that the risk to public health was thereby minimized. But the
exact relationship between prostitutes and police was a mystery. He determined to follow the informal method of his previous surveys—*ambulando discimus*—traveling to major cities, talking to officials and prostitutes, gathering what data existed in public reports and private studies.
Although he found a great deal of literature about prostitution in France
and Germany—much of it focused on how to address this deeply rooted
problem—it provided no clear guidelines. On one side were those who
believed that the danger to public health from prostitution was best controlled by inspection and regulation; on the other were those who were
convinced that public control engendered a false sense of security and actually spread disease.[46] Only gradually did he come to conclusions of his
own on the best course for America to follow.

His foreign tour began in London and ended in Budapest. With interruptions for family vacations in Europe and brief visits home, he spent
more than a year visiting twenty-eight cities in twelve countries, chiefly
in western Europe. Prostitution, he early determined, was overwhelmingly an urban problem that depended largely on a city's size. In the "huge
floating populations" of the great cities, the family was frequently shattered; thousands of detached, more or less isolated, youngsters poured
into these "modern Babylons" under conditions that destroyed character
and ambition.

People did not know their neighbors; anonymity was the rule in social
life; it was virtually impossible to recognize a prostitute. "Neither by garb,

appearance, abode, or apparent manner of living" could the majority of women subsisting on prostitution be recognized. In places where registration was required, the law applied only to "professional prostitutes" and not to the larger number who worked only part-time in the trade. In Zurich, of nearly twelve hundred women with venereal disease, less than 8 percent were identified by the police as prostitutes. Although the Paris police registered six thousand prostitutes, Flexner estimated the real number to be fifty thousand. The vast majority of those selling their sexual services were active for only a short time; they tended to oscillate "to and fro across the dividing line." Nor was prostitution confined to women. In such cities as Berlin he found hostelries that were closed to women. Flexner attended one homosexual ball in the German capital at which one hundred and fifty couples, all male, were counted.[47]

He was particularly disturbed that prostitution was viewed from the perspective of only the women involved. It was patently absurd, he wrote, to talk about prostitution as if it were only a woman's act. He found Europe, more than America, "a man's world—managed by men and largely for men, for cynical men at that—men inured to the sight of human inequalities, callous as to the value of lower-class life, and distinctly lacking in respect for womanhood, especially that of the working classes." Nowhere did he find any systematic sex education in schools or other community institutions. The poorly prepared school graduates came to the cities, where they encountered the "glitter, luxury, the mad rush for amusement, the stage, the café, the tavern"—all of which aroused sexual appetite.

Who were the prostitutes? Overwhelmingly, they were the daughters of the lower working classes, especially the unmarried women of those classes. It was rare to find a streetwalker with education, social standing, or personal charm. Many were young girls who had simply left home. They turned to prostitution not only for economic reasons but to escape humdrum lives.[48] To secure protection, the majority of them allied themselves with pimps, who frequently became their lovers and masters.

In every city he visited, he talked with government officials, police officers, physicians, and prostitutes. He inspected venereal disease clinics and reviewed the legislation and social histories of prostitution. He became a habitué of red-light districts and brothels at three or four o'clock in the morning. He carried out long conversations with streetwalkers and pimps. He must have been a persuasive conversationalist, observes a recent writer, "as adept at extracting inside information from a streetwalker as at inspiring the generosity of a millionaire."[49]

In a letter to Anne he described taking to dinner an attractive young English-speaking woman and then accompanying her back to her Montmartre apartment for an hour-long talk about her life. A serious middleaged man in intimate conversation with an attractive, provocatively dressed young woman, he must have been tempted, despite his straightlaced background, to abandon his role of scientific investigator and succumb to his natural feelings. The woman, too, must have expected more, for when he gave her several gold pieces for her time, she asked: "Is this all?" When he said "yes," she answered: "Why, you are not a man; you are an angel." "No," said Flexner, "I am a man all right."[50]

This woman became his unofficial guide to places in Paris that the police did not wish him to see. They became good friends. When he was ready to leave the city, he asked her if there was anything he could do for her. "Yes, there are two things," she told him. "I should like to dine with you some evening like a lady and afterwards go to the Opéra." And so, for the only time on the tour, he donned evening dress to take her to the Café de Paris and then on to the Opéra to see *The Sorrows of Young Werther*.[51]

He wrote constantly to his family, to Pritchett, and to Rockefeller about what he was finding. "London has been a hard job," he told Anne. "The whole thing is so fragmentary, so elusive, so riddled with contradictory opinions, that it will require careful sifting and weighing before I formulate anything." From Germany, which he thought particularly insensitive to the problem, he wrote, the "morality of Germany must be nil!" He was growing weary of the topic and regretted that he had given up education for such a task. Education was the great hope. What could not be solved by education was "hardly soluble at all: prostitution, among other things." With Rockefeller he kept up a steady exchange of reports, queries, and anecdotes about his experiences. The philanthropist sent him reports he requested, raised questions about the prevalence of syphilis, and thanked him for suggestions about courses in sex hygiene. Carefully, he read drafts of material Flexner had written and offered detailed comments. "I have only recently found time to read your Seventh and Eighth Chapters," he wrote in July 1913. "The Seventh [on regulation and disease] is horrible but convincing . . . pages 14 and 15 are magnificent. Of course the chapter is long and yet I do not see how it can be abbreviated."[52]

As the months dragged on, Flexner's homesickness and anxiety about his marriage increased. "I have had ages of time in which to think in the whirlwind that has passed since I left," he wrote Anne in January, "and my throat closes a lump as I endeavor to realize the distance and the totality of your apartness for the time being." He hoped that the separation might somehow "unify" them and teach "the priceless beauty and satisfaction of a life that, whatever else may be true of it, is lived together." He wrote with envy of the "unabashed fondness" that the wife of a prominent official had displayed toward her husband, expressing the wish that Anne might openly "betray some such admiration" for him. Soon he was lamenting the lack of letters from her. When a letter did arrive, he wired her that the "whole universe look[ed] different."[53]

Throughout the spring he continued to complain of her infrequent and "perfunctory" letters. Of course, he knew she was busy with her work, clubs, servants, and other matters, as she said. "The only thing of moment that could not be squeezed in was *me.*" Particularly upsetting was her failure to respond to his invitation to join him for the summer. Again he asked for "some praise, some pride" in what he was doing: "Never in all my experience have I needed support and confidence and affection as in this maddening task." Anne, too, was apparently experiencing feelings of low esteem, for he wrote her encouragingly in April, "I know that you have it in you to be one of the notable women of your generation." By May she had brought the children with her to Munich—where they had such "beautiful memories," he noted—and the world began to look brighter.[54] Some of the tensions of the early part of the year began to melt during the summer they spent in Germany, although both daughters recalled this period as a time of storm and stress in their parents' marriage.

As the long exile in Europe came to an end, Flexner reached a number of conclusions about the management of prostitution. Despite claims to the contrary, he found that regulation by police power across the Continent did not improve order in the streets. It was more of a hindrance than a help that police were forced to make constant discriminations between legally registered prostitutes and those who worked outside the law. Amsterdam, Zurich, and Liverpool, where prostitution was not regulated, were freer of problems than was Paris or Berlin, Flexner believed.

As for the prevention of disease, the government-run inspection clinics were often scandalously unhygienic. In Paris, he saw all day long "a dismal succession of groups of abandoned women" filing into bare rooms where the physicians plied their repulsive tasks: "with open jaws and protruding tongue they march rapidly past; the doctor uses one spatula for all, wiping it hastily on a soiled towel from time to time." In one instance

he saw a doctor's finger covered by one woman's "abundant suspicious se-
cretion" used unwashed in the next examination. Public regulation, far
from limiting disease, actually encouraged it by promoting a myth of sexual cleanliness. The public was deceived into believing that a diseased
woman could be distinguished from a healthy one. And because the object of inspection was not to heal them but to protect the male patron,
proper treatment was rarely given. Only in Scandinavia, where venereal
disease was viewed as a public health and not a police concern, and where
the aim was to treat all sufferers, men and women alike, did he find a policy worthy of emulation.[55]

In his 450-page report, he was clearly pessimistic about the European
experience in dealing with prostitution. Not only was the extent of prostitution vastly underreported and its social roots far deeper than believed,
it was not helped by police regulation, which in the main was "positively
harmful" in spreading venereal disease. If prostitution was due to such social evils as bad homes, illegitimacy, alcohol, or wretched industrial conditions, as he believed, then "only a transformation wrought by education, science, sanitation, and national policy" could make a difference.[56]
For America, the course was clear. Neither police controls nor clinics for
prostitutes nor registered bordellos but more and better education and en-
lightened social policies offered the hope for better conditions.

Rockefeller and the Bureau of Social Hygiene quickly accepted
Flexner's findings—Rockefeller wrote a glowing foreword to the study—
and the report found its way into the mainstream of thinking about prostitution in America. Four years after the study was published, General
John J. Pershing ordered two hundred copies for use in American camps
in France and urged that it be translated into French. The French government conferred on him the Croix of the Chevalier de La Legion
d'Honneur. The book was widely cited over the next decades. A reviewer
in the *American Journal of Sociology* called it an "authoritative study" that
had turned the tide against segregated vice districts in America. It was
translated into German and Czech. In 1936, the *Journal of Social Hygiene*,
praising the book's "world-wide influence," called it a "complete source
book" for public policy.[57]

For Flexner, the long and close association with John D. Rockefeller
and the men around him was the most important outcome of the prostitution study. It was clear that Rockefeller was impressed with his work
and would try to find a place for him within the Rockefeller philanthropies. Frederick Gates, too, had come away from his experience with

Flexner in the Johns Hopkins assignment with a strong sense of his usefulness. Within the General Education Board, Secretary Wallace Buttrick had also come to know Flexner and kept in close touch with him during his time abroad. For his part, Flexner had begun to think of a "General Education Board devoted to medicine" that would carry out what governments did in Europe—develop policies and furnish incentives to stimulate their acceptance.[58]

Henry Pritchett still hoped to retain him and to convince Andrew Carnegie to supply the monies needed for a thoroughgoing reform of medical education. He persuaded the Carnegie board to make Flexner his principal deputy and put Flexner in charge of the foundation in Pritchett's absence. Carnegie himself, arriving in Britain, was told by Osler of the likelihood of a Rockefeller offer to Flexner. "We must not think of letting Flexner go," Osler advised. But in October 1912 Flexner was offered the position of assistant secretary of the General Education Board at a salary of seventy-five hundred dollars. It was apparent to Pritchett that the offer dwarfed the potentialities as his deputy and that Carnegie would never match the amounts that the Rockefellers were planning to devote to education. It was Flexner's duty to education to accept, Pritchett generously told him, for now he would "be a greater power in education" than would ever be possible at the Carnegie Foundation.[59]

To Simon, Abraham wrote of his immense gratification. "And so," he told him after describing the thrilling events, "opens a new chapter!"[60] Four years of constant deadlines, travel, and insecurity, striving for a position he was not sure even existed, were over, and the next fifteen years would be spent at the center of the most influential educational foundation the world had ever seen. Only Abraham Flexner could know how truly remarkable it was that he had come so far since leaving his school in Louisville.

7

A Secure Berth—At Last

Having won a position at Rockefeller's General Education Board in his forty-seventh year, Abraham Flexner was in the place he had long wanted to be. His hour had come. Education—how it could change lives, as it had his, how it could be molded to fit a new and different age—had always been his greatest interest. Education was important because it changed human expectations. It lifted sights and spurred ambition. It awakened a child's potential. Through education, and education alone, he believed, human beings might solve their moral and societal dilemmas. For two decades he had had firsthand experience with children as a schoolteacher and innovative schoolmaster, had reflected seriously on the reform literature, and had written about how children learn and why the conventional school needed to change. Repeatedly he had attacked the rigidities of the old-time college and the wastefulness and overlap of the emerging university.

His strength, he knew, was his ability to gain quick insight into complex problems, formulate ideas and concepts, and carry out plans for large-scale change. He had proven himself a master at surveying large amounts of data and turning them into lively reports that demanded action. He had impressed a wide range of leaders in philanthropy and education with his organizational skills. An outsider, he had learned to move surefootedly in the corridors of universities as well as powerful and wealthy foundations. With each new triumph, his self-confidence had grown. He knew that he was happiest when thoroughly engaged in tackling a problem. Now he saw unlimited opportunities to make a difference in the unfinished and rapidly changing world of education. And in the congenial association with John D. Rockefeller Jr., Frederick T. Gates, and his immediate boss at the General Education Board, Wallace Buttrick, he found the support and the resources he needed.

His ideas about education were by now well formed. He believed that education was a lifelong and active process, that students learned best by combining doing with studying, that the old ways of indoctrination and passive absorption of knowledge must be swept away. Education, he was convinced, must have a much larger and better-supported place in America's future. He had been profoundly stirred by the atmosphere of serious learning he had found in the universities and preparatory schools of Germany. In America, he was troubled by the casual attitude toward schooling—the lack of financial support, the teacher-dominated classrooms, the large number of pupils in each class, the lack of imagination in the curriculum, the persistence of the classics, and the failure to bring fresh knowledge into the student's experience. Above all, he missed the enthusiasm for learning that he had discovered in Europe.

He wrestled with the problem of meritocratic learning in a democratic society. Convinced that democracy must enable all people to reach their full potential, he nevertheless believed strongly that some types of learning were appropriate for only the brightest students. Whether in medical learning, university education, or public schools, if America was to realize its potential, excellence must be the final measure against which to test all performance. "I was never indifferent to mediocrity," he wrote in his autobiography. "I tried hard to do what I could for it [but] I realized early the impossibility of combining a tender regard for mediocrity with a real enthusiasm for learning."[1] And enthusiasm for learning and the conditions that make it possible was the propulsive force behind his many-sided interests in education.

The nation, he believed, was ready for change. He took office as the Progressive movement in American politics reached its zenith. On every front, widely heralded efforts were under way to confront the problems of poor living conditions in crowded cities, harsh conditions in the workplace, and the suffering of needy families. Flexner was convinced that education must be part of the response. Like most intellectuals, he shared in the "recovery of conscience" and optimism about the future that characterized the outlook of the Progressive years. The reform spirit made easier the task of foundation leaders intent on bringing change.

Abroad, too, America's changing position in the world affected the views of those in the foundations. The outbreak of general war in Europe in 1914, watched with fascination and horror by Americans, formed a jagged line across the pages of modern history. It separated a century of isolation for Americans from a long era of violence and insecurity. Flexner, with his wide experience and contacts in Europe, was looked to by colleagues for advice and counsel about events abroad and their effect on foundation policies. Torn between his closeness to British friends and his fondness for British academic life on the one hand, and his admiration for German achievements in science and education on the other, he came more and more to sympathize with the British in their struggle to avert catastrophe. By the time America entered the war in 1917, he was intensely partisan to the Allied cause, though resisting calls to put blame for the war entirely at the feet of the Germans.

With his volcanic energy and wide experience, Flexner made himself indispensable, as he had at the Carnegie Foundation, to his new associates at the General Education Board. Not one of them had much direct experience with public education, universities, or professional schools, and most had not spent much time abroad. Both Gates, chairman of the board, and Buttrick, secretary and executive officer, were Baptist ministers educated at the Baptist Theological Seminary of Rochester, New York, who had come to education as dispensers of Rockefeller philanthropy. The board met infrequently and depended on Buttrick, and now Flexner, often in consultation with Gates, to propose plans to carry out its broad mandate of promoting education, especially in the South, and developing "a comprehensive system of higher education in the United States."[2] The General Education Board, only ten years old, was struggling to determine how best to carry out its mission.

No one was certain how philanthropy could be best used. Both Henry Pritchett and Gates were feeling their way carefully in a new and uncharted world. They were seeking, in the words of historian Steven Wheatley, "to mediate between their patrons' hesitation, their own understanding of the nature of knowledge, and the opportunities which were presented to them."[3] Pritchett, as we have seen, was guiding the Carnegie Foundation for the Advancement of Teaching toward holding America's universities responsible for high standards in professional and graduate education. Gates was committed to a program of general support for schools and colleges, especially in the South, and was particularly interested in the potential of medical research. Both wanted a role for their philanthropies that would bring long-term benefits, raise educational standards, stay clear of politics, and, if at all possible, avoid controversy.

From the beginning of his new life, while still working to complete the study of prostitution, Flexner was immersed in the whole range of General Education Board activities—programs for farm demonstrations, aid to struggling elementary schools for southern blacks, plans to develop

more high schools in the South, and the selection of colleges and universities to receive endowment gifts. Without hesitation, he took on task
after task. He volunteered to write the history of the board since its creation in 1902 as a way of becoming acquainted with the board's activities; he accompanied Buttrick on tours of black schools in the South; he
undertook surveys of the public school systems in a number of the southern states; he created a plan for a model progressive school; and he was
intimately involved with the board's actions in the field of medical education. He was in effect given what he came to describe as "a roving commission."

Within the board, he very early played a prominent, even decisive, role
on a range of educational policies. The sixty-year-old Buttrick, an outgoing and friendly man, treated his new associate, in Flexner's recollection,
"first as an equal and then afterwards as a son."[4] In only a few months his
salary was boosted to match Buttrick's. At the end of the first year, he was
elected to serve on the policymaking board of trustees. Three years later
he was named secretary of the board when Buttrick replaced the retiring
Gates as chairman. His foothold on the ladder of educational planning in
America was now secure.

His sympathies for the least advantaged in American life began to
deepen. In his trips with Buttrick he showed a new empathy with Southern blacks struggling to get an education in the most backward parts of
the nation. During his Louisville years he had shown some sympathy for
efforts by blacks to gain an education, but he played no role in supporting them. Now, after firsthand exposure to learning conditions in black
schools, he became an influential backer of efforts to improve education
for African Americans across the South. He became friends with leading
black educators. "It is indeed a sad sight to see a whole race heavily hand-
icapped and struggling to get a decent foothold in life," he wrote his
daughter Jean in his first year at the board. It was "amazing" and an "example of human wretchedness," he said, to find a state superintendent of
schools who "argued against educating negro children, because they are
black!" There were people, he told his daughter, who were "trying hard to
improve matters for the unfortunate"; "when you grow up, you must be
among them."[5]

He was made a member of a board committee on education for blacks
and prepared the agenda for a national conference in 1915 of black and
white educators. His was the guiding spirit at the conference. The General Education Board, he told the assembled group, "is not interested in

alms-giving"; its aim was to develop "a long-headed policy" to improve education for African Americans, and this policy would take years to implement. Support by the power of the state was the goal; "anything else is a makeshift." As public schools got under way, with the encouragement of the board, many of the struggling private schools for blacks would eventually disappear, as the black medical schools had done.[6] He urged closer ties with public school leaders in developing state school systems for blacks, helping such relatively strong institutions as Tuskegee and Hampton institutes train teachers for rural areas, and raising the level of support for higher education for blacks. As an officer of the board, he took a direct part in efforts to create and improve schools for African Americans. More forcefully at times than his fellow officers and board members, he urged the extension of the curriculum in these schools to liberal subjects beyond the standard vocational fare. Repeatedly, he argued for measures to improve the preparation of black teachers and professionals.

Such efforts were limited, however, by having to work within the castelike social and political structure of the southern states. Time and again, board members and officers stressed that one must first gain the support of state and local leaders in government and education before taking any action. To succeed in helping blacks, they believed that they had to reassure whites and include opportunities for rural whites in their plans. To challenge the doctrine of white supremacy or to antagonize white leaders, they felt certain, meant the end of the board's ability to carry out programs benefiting African Americans. In a letter to Charles Eliot, Frederick Gates laid down the basic policy: "As to Negro education, I favor our activity there only when, where, and so far as, we can place our means for Negro uplift in the hands, and our spirits in the hearts of the Southern white man, with whom the Negro has to live, and on whom his destiny for good or ill does certainly depend."[7]

Flexner, too, recognized the realism of this approach but chafed at the stubborn racism that made bold efforts at change so daunting. "I was deeply stirred, as I always am," he wrote after one trip, "by the splendid and courageous spectacle of a race striving away from centuries of slavery. I could curse the man—or men—who puts obstacles in their way." He was disturbed by the federal government's indifference to what was happening. Sitting in a classroom at the Tuskegee Institute, he said that he could not think very kindly of President Wilson, who, "with his tardy concern for Armenians and Balkans," had failed and was still failing to "take cognizance of the greatest race problem of all—and [America's] race problem at that."[8] While still nominally a Democrat, Flexner was increasingly critical of Wilson, especially his failure to challenge Southern leaders on race and what he saw as Wilson's lack of understanding of ethnic problems in central Europe.

At times, he despaired of the slow pace of change for African Americans. He told Buttrick, in 1919, following a visit to some forty schools and colleges: "The truth is if I see much more of Negroes and Negro schools, and the way they are throwing themselves into it and trying to squeeze 100% value out of what there is, I am going to drop the Whites and devote the rest of my life to Negro education." In the history of the world, he wondered, had any race done "what the Negroes were doing with their meager resources." He deplored the distortions of the black role in the post–Civil War South in the pioneering film *The Birth of a Nation.* While the photography was "far superior" to anything he had ever seen, he said, historically it was "utterly worthless trash."[9]

As his daughters moved into the educational system, his sympathy for women's efforts to gain an equal chance at learning began likewise to deepen. He had earlier helped his sisters complete their studies and had encouraged his wife to prepare for an independent career. In 1910, in his report on medical education, he had argued that women had "so assured a place in medicine" that their fight for an equal chance at learning "was predestined to an early success." None of the existing separate medical schools for women, however, in his judgment, was likely to acquire the full-time faculty, the endowment, and the close connection with a university that would enable it to offer a first-rate education.[10] For him, coeducation was the only sensible answer to gender equality in education.

To M. Carey Thomas, Bryn Mawr's president, whose college prided itself on offering a liberal education equal to that available to men, Flexner wrote a strong letter in 1911 questioning why, if women were to be given an equal chance at education, they were still required to take Latin when many men's colleges offered degrees "without wasting any time in acquiring the elements of Latin." Why should women not be able "to get an academic education upon precisely the same terms as men?" To a Harvard professor who asked his advice about admitting women to the medical school, Flexner replied that the presence of women had "been a good thing" and expressed the hope that Harvard would "let down its bars." Was it logical, he asked, to extend women's opportunities in civic and social life, "and then to deny them this, that, or the other professional opportunity?" When Jean began to study at Cambridge University, in 1921, Flexner was visibly upset when he learned of her cold reception and the opposition of male students to granting women degrees. "It is most important," he wrote, "that [women] get all the opportunities men get," yet "this is the moment chosen by Cambridge students to create bad feelings and raise obstacles." Philosophers might argue that there was no Satan, but "there [he] is—and he is busy, insensitive, and most efficient!"[11]

With his appointment to the General Education Board, his private life took a turn for the better. The years of uninterrupted travel were over. Although he still made frequent business trips, he was now home much of the time. He spent more time with his daughters and became again the one to whom they turned for attention and counsel. Anne remained constantly busy during these years, to the extent that Eleanor complained that she was "uninterested" in her. It was her father, she said, "who really carried on into young adulthood." If she were sick or having some difficulty, it was "always" her father, not her mother, who came to her aid. Her mother's indifference she attributed to her faltering career, begun so spectacularly with *Mrs. Wiggs,* but now stymied by the theater's growing preoccupation with serious, socially responsive themes. Anne did have some success with her lighthearted play of 1916, *The Marriage Game,* described by a critic as "clear and sparkling," but it did not come close to *Mrs. Wiggs* at the box office. The play features three married couples, all drifting apart, who are brought back together by being shown the importance of "a soft polish" in their mutual relations and being "exceedingly careful not to let anything scratch or mar" the sensitive surface.[12]

She remained hard at work on plans for new plays, becoming ever more deeply involved in the Broadway theater world. She seemed always to be on the road, negotiating, seeking talent, trying out plays, and searching for producers. In 1919 she was elected vice-president of the Society of American Dramatists, a group she had helped organize. Her husband sent her notes of encouragement, made suggestions, attended her rehearsals, and tried to counter the opinions of critics. He described for Jean a typical day in her mother's life: "Mother went to a rehearsal at 7:30 last night and left the theater at 2:30 this morning. I have not seen her this morning, but left word that she is to call me by telephone when she gets up."[13]

The tension that had marked the marriage during Flexner's last tour abroad began to abate during the years with Rockefeller. The letters between them in these years were long, playful, and affectionate. In the summer of 1914 they were brought even closer by the sudden diagnosis of a probable malignancy in Anne during a business trip to Boston. She discovered a lump in her right breast and called for a doctor, who happened to be on the staff of the Peter Bent Brigham Hospital. She was operated on immediately. "The lump was the wrong kind," she wrote her husband, "and much healthy tissue had to be sacrificed." The tone of the letter was remarkably cheerful under the circumstances. She was writing him, she said, only because he would no doubt hear of it from another source. During the long convalescence that followed, they spent a great deal of time together. She became depressed at the slowness of her recovery and discouraged that her efforts at writing and producing plays were not better received. "Achievement always disappoints," he tried to console her; "no one can achieve enough and well enough to keep happy on the basis of achievement alone." Happiness, if it came at all, "was the result of serenity of spirit, going about one's business in a calm, unquestioning . . . way, meeting problems as they arise and in the main keeping one's eye on a goal."[14]

In the year after the operation, Abraham wrote some of the most tender love letters of their long and sometimes rocky marriage. He gave her credit for all the success that he had achieved, asking, "What could make for the most beautiful relations between man and wife than that the husband should be thus beholden to his beloved?" Love, he continued, "ought to make people so deeply and inextricably indebted to one another that payment or return is utterly impossible. The only legal tender that can discharge debts incurred through love is—love itself." In another letter he told her: "You are entitled to all the love and appreciation I can pour upon you . . . for what you have been to the children, to me, to your friends, and for what you have done." He had confidence, he assured her, that she would outdo both *Mrs. Wiggs* and *The Marriage Game.* He wished that he could "lift" her "over the rough places"; "even more," he wished he "never roughened them" for her.[15]

They shared an interest in the growing women's movement. Both marched in the 1915 New York women's suffrage parade. Two years later, he encouraged her to go to Washington for a national demonstration on behalf of women's suffrage. To Jean he confided his pride in her mother and told her of his great satisfaction that New York had ratified the suffrage amendment.[16] On this issue, as on support of Southern blacks, Flexner was impatient with President Wilson.

While devoted to his own family and his demanding job, he still kept a close eye on his brothers and sisters. Often he conferred with Simon about family troubles and continued to give financial help to several siblings. When his older brother Henry died in 1913—the first of the nine children to do so—he joined Simon in giving Henry's family temporary support. He worried, too, that Bernard, who was still in Louisville, had taken on the role of paterfamilias that he had himself relinquished a decade before. He suggested to Simon that they find some way of lightening Bernard's growing burden. When Jacob became ill a few years later, Abraham went to Chicago to meet Bernard, Washington, and Mary to work out a plan to provide financial help for Jacob and his family. In 1918 he journeyed to Boston, where his brother Isadore was hospitalized with a serious spinal ailment. "We are looking after him," he assured Jacob, "as best we can."[17] For the rest of his life he remained close to his brothers and sisters, often helping their children through troubles as well.

At his new post at the General Education Board he was overwhelmed by the "kindness and deference" of his associates. Not only Buttrick and Gates but the younger Rockefeller and other members of the board did him "the honor of talking with [him] about several matters of moment." He found the atmosphere at 61 Broadway, where the offices were located, very different from that of the Carnegie Foundation. Here he felt that he was surrounded by friends rather than by "a single protector" in Henry Pritchett.[18]

Although he had parted with the Carnegie Foundation, his friendship with Pritchett remained an important part of his life. Pritchett consulted him often about projects that he was considering. At Pritchett's request, Flexner gave him the names of persons who might undertake a survey of college libraries. He "wracked his brain" to find someone who could do a study of graduate schools. "Time was," he said, "when it was my highest ambition to do this myself." The graduate school could not be studied, he told Pritchett, without considering its relationship to the entire educational system. If secondary education were finally remodeled as he hoped it would be, the college could be "a good deal abbreviated," which in turn would enable graduate and professional schooling to "go on a new basis." When asked about a possible survey of schools of pharmacy, Flexner advised Pritchett that pharmacy was not worthy of so much attention, suggesting instead "a fearless investigation" of dental schools. Dentistry, he said, was "in the same primitive condition as medicine had been before the appearance of the Johns Hopkins Medical School."[19]

At the General Education Board he plunged into his new responsibilities. He divided his time at first between completing the report on prostitution and taking on new assignments. He wrote on educational topics, quickly becoming an effective propagandist for the board's work. His history of the board, completed in 1914, was widely disseminated among educators, journalists, and political leaders. The following year he wrote an article in the *Independent* about the growing number of board programs and how they affected the nation. He described the efforts to make southern agriculture more prosperous, to promote high schools and rural schools throughout the South, to strengthen private colleges and universities, and to encourage full-time teaching in schools of medicine. These were all practical programs to make education "more effective, more economical, more intelligent, [and] more liberal."[20] No decision on medical education, a subject on which he was considered the expert, was made while he was away from the office.

As he gained power and influence, the men around him—Buttrick, Gates, Rockefeller Jr., Eliot, and other members of the board—became his friends and confidantes. After only a year and a half, his chief, Wallace Buttrick, departing for China, told him that he had "a tear on [his] cheek and a lump in [his] throat" in leaving him. "You are very dear to me, my friend, and the thought of being away from you for four months and more is not pleasant." When George E. Vincent, a member of the board and president of the University of Minnesota, was asked by the younger Rockefeller to become president of the recently established Rockefeller Foundation, he consulted Flexner "in strictest confidence" for "advice and counsel." "What ought I to do?" he asked. He raised questions about the advantages and limitations of the Rockefeller post.[21] In a very short time, Flexner had won the confidence of some of the most influential figures in American education. By those closest to him, he was seen as approachable, even-handed, and thoughtful.

Among his first projects was a series of surveys of public education in the southern states. After his survey experience at the Carnegie Foundation and his work for Gates and the younger Rockefeller, he was the logical person to undertake such studies. The work began in Maryland, where the state legislature in 1914 determined to overhaul a school system that was highly politicized and controversial. The General Education Board was asked for help, and Flexner volunteered for the assignment. No longer required to do the field work himself, he hired several investigators, including Frank P. Bachman, a painstaking scholar and administrator, who had been an associate superintendent of schools in Cleveland. Bachman carried out the bulk of the work on this and future surveys, while Flexner did the overall planning, made contacts with state officials, and edited the final reports. Flexner, however, was rarely able to stay in his New York office. On a number of occasions, he joined Bachman in the field, once reaching him by taxi at a rural school some six miles outside of Baltimore.

When Bachman produced the first chapter of the Maryland report, Flexner, keenly sensitive to its intended audience, found it ponderous, academic, and far too long. "This is not an academic enterprise," he scolded his associate. "We are not writing a scientific treatise . . . for the benefit of a few high-brows." The report needed to be so short that it would be read by laypeople all over the state. Legislators needed to want to know its contents. "Every newspaper," he said, "will want to comment on it editorially."[22] Flexner rewrote all of the chapters, shortening them, simplifying language, and substituting his own blunt and hard-hitting prose.

The final report, less than two hundred pages long, called for a complete overhaul of the state's educational structure. It sharply criticized low teacher salaries, poor school attendance, weak teacher training, and political meddling. A detailed set of recommendations was laid out. The impact was unexpected. Most of the state laws on education in Maryland were repealed. A new state board of education was created and at its head was placed a powerful executive officer, as Flexner had recommended. New standards were set for superintendents, teachers, and school attendance. A minimum school year was established for black as well as white schools. Published in book form, the report became a model for educational surveys. It was widely used in classrooms of schools and teachers colleges. "We all take our hats off to Dr. Abraham Flexner," wrote the Maryland superintendent of education, "who so ably mapped out and gave direction to the work."[23]

The superintendent addressed Flexner as "doctor" because Flexner had been given an honorary degree by Western Reserve University in 1914 for his work on medical education. While he did not use the title himself, many others, including university presidents and associates, did. Simon was irritated that he and his brother were now frequently confused with each other and ascribed the problem to the use of the "doctor" title. "In this country," he told Abraham, the title had only "one meaning," that of medical doctor. Flexner replied that he was doing his best to keep people from calling him "doctor" and that nobody over whom he had "any influence" used the title.[24] But the title nevertheless stuck, and eventually, perhaps without too much regret, he gave up correcting people.

The success of the Maryland survey brought invitations from other states for similar studies. Over the next few years Flexner planned surveys in Delaware, Virginia, North Carolina, Kentucky, and Alabama. While Bachman's writing improved, it still did not meet Flexner's demand for clear, sharply focused reports that stirred readers to action. He complimented Bachman that there were fewer "to be sures" in the Delaware report but chided him: "Where in the dickens did you pick up 'modicum'? There seem to be a lot of 'modica' in Delaware that they won't have . . . when I get through with the manuscript!" The effect of the reports was clear. Delaware not only agreed to a thoroughgoing reform of its schools but increased the education budget from $453,000 to $1,744,000.[25] Other states, seeing the impact of the Flexner-Bachman reports, conducted their own surveys or hired outside experts to do the work.

Flexner sharply criticized Bachman for agreeing with segregation-minded officials in Delaware to establish separate school boards for white and black schools. "This amounts to perpetuating a distinction which is undemocratic," Flexner chastised him; every county and district board "must have an equal responsibility for white and colored schools." The Rockefeller organization, he warned, "would be in a pretty fix if [it] sponsored a position of this sort."[26]

In 1915 Flexner began his most sensitive and controversial school survey. In the steel town of Gary, Indiana, the superintendent of schools, William A. Wirt, an energetic and imaginative former student of John Dewey's, was gaining national prominence through his "platoon system" of breaking up groups of students for alternate periods of study, work, and play. Wirt saw himself as trying to realize Dewey's ideal of the school as "an embryonic community," complete with exposure to various occupations and "permeated throughout with the spirit of art, history, and science." Schools were given machine shops, laboratories, auditoriums, playgrounds, libraries, swimming pools, and gardens—all with the idea of making the school the heart of each community's social life. Open day and evening throughout the year to adults as well as children, the Gary schools were intended to be a major force in uplifting the city.[27]

By making full use of the schools, politicians realized, important economies could be realized. While some students were at play or in the auditorium, others would be in the shops and laboratories. Still others would be in the classroom. Fewer schoolrooms and thus fewer schools would be needed. By imaginative scheduling, a student could take part in a great variety of activities, including vocational training, art, music, laboratory work, health classes, field trips, and movies, as well as class-room learning. Special classes in remedial education, advanced study for gifted students, and adult education in the evening were also provided. To many educators across the country, struggling with the burdens of teaching growing numbers of students within limited school budgets, it seemed a magical way to be progressive and save money at the same time. The Gary plan, in the eyes of some, thus embodied two separate and contradictory goals. On the one hand, it represented a "drive toward effi-ciency, economy, and scientific management"; on the other, it made pos-sible "a natural and enriched schooling in which children learned by doing."[28]

When Flexner was asked by Rockefeller Jr. in 1915 to list for the board the most important educational issues of the day, he put the Gary plan at the top. With the board's approval, he wrote Wirt to ask for his coopera-tion in carrying out the study. "It seems to me," he told Wirt, "that a thor-ough scientific study of these schools from every legitimate point of view would be of very great value." By this time, the Gary plan was the most talked-about topic in education in the country. Scores of articles appeared in major newspapers; John Dewey, not surprisingly, wrote favorably of its potential; and the journalist Randolph Bourne aroused the interest of in-tellectuals with a stirring series of essays about it in the *New Republic*. For Bourne, the Wirt plan justified industrial education by demonstrating un-equivocally that "learning can come only through doing."[29]

Flexner, too, saw great possibilities in the Gary system. On starting his work with the General Education Board he had been quickly drawn into the Progressive Education Association, the most important school reform organization in New York City. He was then appointed to the board of education by the progressive young mayor, John Purroy Mitchel, on the mayor's first day in office. He became the mayor's lieutenant in all mat-ters affecting the schools. As a board member, he approved the appoint-ment of Wirt as a consultant to demonstrate his "platoon system" in New York. The Progressive Education Association, with Flexner now among its leaders, strongly supported the initial demonstrations of the Wirt pro-gram in the Bronx and Brooklyn and then their extension to other schools. Mitchel, faced with a straitened budget and an overcrowded school system, called in 1915 for the extension of the Gary system to all New York public schools. The school population had doubled over the preceding two decades; one of every eight children was schooled part-time or in double-session classes. A Progressive Education Association spokesman predicted that the plan "would enrich the children's school life, seat thousands, and save millions."[30]

But once the General Education Board began its study, Flexner was in a quandary. He was the director of an impartial scientific appraisal of the Gary school system and at the same time a member of the school board sponsoring the system's demonstration in New York. Further, he was the agent of a Rockefeller enterprise at a time when the oil tycoon was under heavy criticism for the deaths of dozens of miners in a Colorado coal field strike. At first, he tried to distance himself from the survey by approaching an independent scholar, the Stanford educator Ellwood P. Cubberley, to do the work. But after several weeks of discussion and a joint visit to Gary, he became disillusioned with Cubberley. The Stanford expert, he believed, had too many commitments, demanded too high a compensation (one thousand dollars a month), and had just released a hastily written study of the Salt Lake City schools. The last, he criticized, was "a dreary, tame, and feeble performance, poorly written and altogether deficient in detail and incisiveness."[31] Summarily, Flexner dropped Cubberley and determined to do the work himself.

Of the study's significance Flexner had no doubt. It was "of national importance," and the pressure for the Gary system's "wholesale introduction" in New York and elsewhere was "something tremendous." The study, he wrote, "ought to go a long distance toward deciding the question." He conferred with Buttrick, Rockefeller Jr., and Eliot, all of whom urged him to take on the assignment. Perhaps he had wanted to do it all along. In the winter of 1915–16 he assembled a team of eight experts, most of them university specialists in education, to study the costs, methods of teaching, curriculum, and outcomes of the Gary system as measured by performance tests.[32]

But even as the study was getting under way the Gary plan was becoming more and more controversial. In New York, opponents of the plan included not only the superintendent of schools, William H. Maxwell, and most of the system's teachers, but a steadily growing group of parents and citizens, and the Tammany-controlled Democratic party. Maxwell was convinced that the Mitchel administration was pushing for the Gary system only to save money and that it had not been sufficiently tested. After visiting one demonstration school, Maxwell told reporters that "the only thing new was some children digging up a lot." Teachers protested that the new system would add several hours weekly to their workload. Tammany leaders, seeing a sensitive political issue, pushed the formation of "mothers clubs" and "anti-Gary leagues" that warned of children being shortchanged or lost amidst the frequent changes of location each day. There was no time even to call the roll between changes, charged one flyer, "and so, many children stay out on the street or remain in the playground." Children were losing their way, no one knew where they belonged, and "in the grand rush no one ha[d] time to find out." It was false economy, the critics argued, to control school costs at the expense of the children. The plan was the work, said one parent, "of every wild-eyed, long-haired, be-whiskered demagogue" in New York.[33]

An all-out political war broke out over the Gary plan. The progressive forces lined up behind the Mitchel administration, while the growing army of opponents coalesced around the Tammany leaders. In the mayoral campaign of 1917, Mitchel stoutly defended the Gary plan, calling it "the most valuable educational contribution of the last one hundred years." Children in the platoon schools were "happier," he said, the programs offered children were richer, and schoolwork had lost its "drudgery." The rival candidate, Brooklyn judge John F. Hylan, countered with efforts to arouse parents across the city to "banish this vicious Gary system." Hylan and others saw in the Gary plan the power of "Rockefeller interests" aiming to make the public schools "an annex to the mill and factory." Flexner, in particular, was singled out as the Rockefeller agent on the school board who was trying to force "Garyized" schools onto the city's children. By the spring of 1917 violence erupted in many places across the city. Strikes, picketing, demonstrations, and heated oratory became a part of the daily routine at a number of the city schools. School windows were smashed and buildings were stoned.[34]

Flexner found himself in an increasingly uncomfortable position. The attacks mounted in ferocity. At times he seemed to regret taking on the Gary study. The Rockefeller interests, according to one handbill, were "spreading their web over the schools of the country" and Flexner was "the ruler" of the New York City school board, the person who had made the board an "instrument of politics" by endorsing the Gary plan. The aim of this Caesar was "to teach the common people to produce efficiently and docilely for their governing class," while keeping children from acquiring "Greek or Latin or anything more than the simplest mathematics."[35]

Under pressure, Flexner resigned from the school board in the spring of 1917. He let Buttrick and Rockefeller speak for the General Education Board in answering his critics. Rockefeller wrote to the leaders of one anti-Gary group that Flexner's service to the city had been "purely in his individual capacity" and that the forthcoming report of the General Education Board was unfinished so that none of them was "in position to form a judgment" on the Gary plan. Flexner had grown tired of the turmoil. "I don't want ever again to do another remote and elaborate survey," he wrote Anne; "that is work for younger men!"[36]

The overwhelming defeat of Mayor Mitchel in the November election was a debacle for the Gary movement. Hylan quickly moved to end New York's experiment with the platoon system. Local interest in it began to decline. Flexner and other progressives were deeply shaken by the return of the schools to Tammany control. In the country at large the defeat in New York was taken as a sign to slow down the Gary movement. Many looked now to the pending report of the General Education Board to learn what Flexner's team of experts would say. The significance of the study for the national debate was greater than ever. Flexner was keenly aware of the need to steer the report through the shoals of anti-Rockefeller sentiment, political partisanship, and differences of opinion among members of his own team. It was the most sensitive and demanding of all the Flexner educational surveys.

While all of his experts wrote separate monographs, seven in all, Flexner himself wrote the final report, with Bachman's help. How deeply was he influenced by the electoral defeat in New York and the public attacks on him? At the outset he had been strongly supportive of the Gary experiment. He liked Wirt personally and applauded his courage in undertaking reform in the "Godforsakenest hole [he] ever tarried in." He sent each of his experts a copy of Bourne's highly favorable essays on Gary. As the individual reports came in, he sent them to Wirt for comment, and in several cases forced changes based on Wirt's reactions. At one point, he expressed the wish that his own daughters might have had "some of the opportunities that all these children" were being given.[37]

Now he was determined to write a report that was as objective and fair to Wirt as possible. But he was undoubtedly influenced by the New York experience and the need to be seen as an impartial investigator. The result was a book that balanced the promise and the faults of the platoon system in a way unusual for Flexner. Unlike his hard-hitting, action-oriented reports on medical education and prostitution, or the surveys of state school systems, none of which left any doubt as to where Flexner stood, the Gary study could be read as either favoring or not favoring the system. The *New York Globe,* for example, which had fought the Gary plan in New York, praised the Flexner report under such headlines as "Pupils

Do Just About as They Please," while the *Boston Evening Transcript*, which favored the plan, lauded it as "a very wise, sensible, and inspiring book, good-tempered and fair." The professional reviewer for the *Journal of Education* found it "honest, intelligent, [and] inspiring."[38]

Flexner praised a number of features of the Gary system. He lauded its democratic spirit, its organization, its imaginative use of school plants, and its "progressive, modern conception" of what a school should be. Wirt's plan, he wrote, "is as large and intelligent a conception as has yet been reached in respect to the scope and bearing of public education." In its working, however, the plan had led to confusion and weakening of basic educational skills. Many of the Gary children, he noted in his account, citing a number of measurements, lagged in spelling, arithmetic, and reading. Knowledge of history, geography, and mathematics, too, was often wanting. Activities outside the classroom, furthermore, were not truly integrated into the child's learning experience. The system, in short, for all its promise, did not produce "generally good work." Enforcement of performance standards was only "spasmodically" in evidence. The effort to achieve economies had resulted in poor student performance. Despite these weaknesses, he concluded, the Gary community should be praised for its "courage, liberality, and imagination" and should be encouraged in its efforts to make "schools adequate to the needs and conditions of modern life."[39]

It was a bravura performance. He had fashioned a careful, impartial critique that rescued the Rockefeller philanthropies from charges of outright bias and a desire to control the nation's schools. At the same time, he had called attention, mostly favorable, to the Gary system. The immediate effect was to dampen enthusiasm for the Gary experiment while keeping alive the promise of Rockefeller support for further educational reform. The General Education Board, in fact, with Flexner in the lead, was already working on its own plan. Influenced in part by the Gary experience, the board hoped to create "a modern school" that would serve as a model for school reformers. Flexner had long wanted the chance to create a well-supported progressive school stressing modern studies and downplaying the ancient classics. "Always," writes one historian, Flexner sought "a model and a compelling example." Foundation money was for him a catalyst, "something to create striking interest" that would result in "a wave of emulation."[40] Unlike the schools of the Gary experiment, his school would not be accused of scrimping on money.

Soon after joining the board, he was made a member of a committee studying the effectiveness of teaching in the United States. The committee's report of 1914, largely his work, called for more experiments and demonstrations to break the lockstep of existing teaching, especially at the high school level. What he envisioned was a model or experimental school to "focus and assist" progressive tendencies in education, which he said were then "unorganized and precarious."[41]

At a plenary meeting of board members and officers in the summer of 1915 at a Maine resort, elementary and secondary education were the themes of a three-day discussion. What could the board do to improve teaching in America? Flexner, who prepared the program, hoped secretly for a decision to fund a model school. The discussion was led by Eliot, who had long agreed with Flexner's views about what American schools needed. Did the two conspire in advance to shape the outcome? Before the meeting, Eliot prodded Flexner: "You must have . . . plenty of ideas, suggested by your own experience as a teacher of boys."[42]

Eliot told the assembled group that too many schools taught only "memory studies [such as] English, Latin, American history and mathematics." They provided "no real acquaintance" with the sciences and the arts that had "revolutionized all the industries of the white race." What was needed in the curriculum was more chemistry, physics, biology, and geography, as well as music and manual training in shop work and domestic science. To those familiar with Eliot's campaign for reform in secondary education, it was a familiar recital. At the end of the talk, he remarked that past educational experience was too often lost and cited Flexner's earlier school in Louisville as "one of the most interesting and successful experiments" he knew of. As if on cue, Flexner was called upon to explain his ideas. Extemporaneously but enthusiastically, he described in detail his Louisville experience and ended with the proposal that a "modern school" be created based on Eliot's remarks.[43]

The following morning came his "real triumph" when the organizing committee recommended that a study be made of "a modern school" and that the study be publicized and widely distributed. Implicit in the recommendation was a commitment, if the report was satisfactory, to fund a model or experimental school. "It was a great moment, Sweetheart," he told Anne, "and I was happy, if ever man was happy." Rockefeller, as expected, assigned the task of writing the report to him, saying: "Your work will blossom and we shall have good fun in this hard old world before we are turned out to graze." Buttrick drew a sketch of him entitled "In the Hour of Victory" and slid it across the table. Eliot ended the meeting by adding to Flexner's accolades: "I have long wanted some such experiment, now I confess I should regard it as a calamity, if we, having in our service the one man best fitted in the entire country to organize and conduct such a school, should fail to give him and the country the chance." The ebullient Flexner saw the board becoming "a dynamic force" in modern education."[44]

Gates was skeptical. The chairman wrote Rockefeller Jr. that the real question was not the weakness of the schools, which was generally acknowledged, but whether a model program could "correct the evils and do it on any considerable scale." Not one teacher in fifty, he said, was capable of making a difference in students' lives. The student who could bring "life and power" to studies was likewise rare and would succeed regardless of school arrangements. "No man was yet ever made," said the crusty individualist, "that was not self-made," and few teachers were skilled enough to be of much help. "If all teachers were big Flexners and all students little Flexners all would be easy." But education could not be conferred "even by the genius of a Flexner." Any effort to establish an experimental school, he concluded, would need to be undertaken very cautiously and only after thorough study and after subjecting the plan to "the criticism of experienced educators in great numbers."[45]

Flexner worked on the plan in the late summer and fall while still involved in the state school surveys and the Gary schools project. It was a labor of love. For a quarter-century he had been preaching the gospel of progressive learning: learning by doing, discarding the classics, putting emphasis on science and modern studies, treating the child as an individual, and abolishing the theory of mental discipline. The mind of a child was disciplined, he wrote, in the only way it could be disciplined—"by energizing it through the doing of real tasks."

By the time of the board meeting in January 1916, he had finished a draft of his ideas that was accepted as the working outline for the creation of a "modern school." Rockefeller's and Eliot's enthusiasm carried all before them. "It seems as though the dawn has really come," Rockefeller told the board. "If I only had had such an education as is here outlined." Gates, however, remained opposed to creating a school with board funds.[46] So strong was the board's support, however, that he kept his silence as the school project unfolded.

The Flexner plan contained little that was new, but it was written in now-characteristic Flexner style: blunt, assertive, colorful, demanding action. When published in the *American Review of Reviews* that fall, it evoked a storm of criticism, especially from defenders of the classics.[47]

The classics, he charged in his report, had outlived their usefulness and had no value for the average student. Even those who studied Latin throughout high school and college were unable to understand or make use of a simple Latin document. "Stumbling and blundering through a few patches of Latin" did not lead to intellectual discipline or a knowledge of Roman culture. Mental discipline, moreover, was an archaic concept that flew in the face of modern theories of learning. The schools were altogether "too much under the shadow of the past." Rote teaching of grammar, accumulation of "useless historical facts," memorization of mathematical formulas, reading "obsolete" works of literature—all without social context or concern for the individual student—were relics of a hidebound tradition. Even the existing progressive schools did not go far enough in shedding the old patterns. A modern school, he asserted emphatically, must start from scratch; its curriculum should embrace "*nothing for which an effective case cannot now be made out.*"[48] The interests of the child, as he had taught many years before in Louisville, were foremost, and the teacher's job was to find and use those interests in encouraging learning.

The new Flexner school, as he described it, would be built around the quadrivium of science, industry, aesthetics, and civics. Modern languages would take the place of Greek and Latin. Much of traditional mathematics would disappear. Science would be given a central place in the curriculum and be taught, so far as possible, by experiment and by observing such natural objects as rocks, animals, and trees. Industry, too, was best understood through hands-on experience in such skills as shop work, woodworking, printing, and dressmaking. Here he cited the experience of the Gary schools.

In the humanities or "aesthetics" he wanted to stimulate interest in the arts and especially in reading. What students actually read or painted or sung was less important than that they carried away an interest in these activities. Finally, the study of civics or social studies, crucial in a democratic society, needed to concentrate on a broader understanding of history and on current events. Flexner acknowledged his debt to the contemporary historian James Harvey Robinson, who was preaching a "new history" that pushed beyond wars and politics to include the lives of ordinary men and women. At the "New School" in New York, Robinson and his colleagues were doing away with the old formal lectures on Aristotle and Grotius, he said, and asking instead "what this old world is doing and suffering."[49]

None of these divisions among proposed subjects was sacrosanct. On the contrary, wrote Flexner, teachers must take a holistic view of their responsibilities and ignore traditional boundaries. Every exercise should be a lesson in spelling; the study of science, industry, and mathematics could not be separated; science, industry, history, civics, literature, and geography would "to some extent" use the same material."[50] An intensive effort must be made, he stated, to break down the rigid separation among school subjects.

In December 1916, the board made public its plans to build a school in New York. The school—to be called the Lincoln School, after the Civil War president—would be built in cooperation with the faculty at Teachers College of Columbia University. Flexner had urged the board to create a completely independent school but was overridden. According to the agreement, the school was to be "a laboratory for the working out of an elementary and secondary curriculum which shall eliminate obsolete material and [be] adapted to the needs of modern life."[51] Flexner, as expected, played the dominant role in launching the school; he was a member of a joint administrative board set up to oversee the project. The curriculum that grew out of the planning group reflected closely the ideas in *A Modern School.* Familiar subjects were divided and realigned around "units of work" or "core projects" that combined reading about subjects with direct experience in real life. First and second graders would learn about civic life while building a play city; a celebrated third-grade project focused on the history, construction, and commercial uses of boats as a way of interesting students in history, engineering, economics, and science; eighth graders visited factories and farms while studying the "power age" and its influence on culture and environment; graduating seniors learned about "living in contemporary America" though trips to slums and middle-class neighborhoods as they read textbooks on social problems.

Behind the scenes, Flexner did his best to shape the outcome. A close friend, Otis W. Caldwell of the University of Chicago, who had worked on the Gary project, was hired to direct the school. Flexner helped select the site for the new building. Prospective teachers ran the gauntlet of long interviews with him. One woman, about to be hired to teach foreign languages, was rejected when he learned that she had never been abroad. "She is quite out of the question," he informed Caldwell, "in a high grade school." His standard was men and women teachers whose ideas were highly original, who brimmed with energy and enthusiasm, and whose methods would set a standard for other schools.[52] In the back of his mind, surely, was his own experience at his school in Louisville.

"I did not visit a single class," said Eliot of the new school in 1918, "which failed to call upon the children for active participation." The class in elementary mathematics was the best that he had "ever seen." Pupils in advanced English were inspired with a strong desire to read, he said. All manner of opportunities beyond the classroom surrounded the Lincoln student—industrial shops, scientific laboratories, a gymnasium, a music room, home economics, laboratories, a strong library, and a first-rate testing and guidance program. The Lincoln School, carefully planned, lavishly supported, and well organized, became the high point of the progressive school movement in America. It was a demonstration of what was possible if all the needed resources were provided. Its influence radiated out to school systems across the country. No other school, in the opinion of a leading historian of American schools, exerted "greater or more lasting influence" on American education."[53]

In what ways did the Lincoln School affect the course of American education? In the years during and after the First World War, the experiment was followed closely by hundreds of educators. Visitors from every state trooped through its classrooms until a limit was finally established. A number of its innovations were directly copied in public school systems. Such cities as Cleveland, St. Louis, Denver, and Chicago asked for help in setting up their own experimental programs. Its faculty was hired by dozens of teachers colleges to spread the new gospel. Particularly influential were the idea of the core curriculum, the joining of history with geography and civics in classes in "social science," the merging of theory and practice in science teaching, and the strong emphasis on vocational education.[54] It was through such ideas, as mentioned in the introduction, that Flexner's influence came to the public schools of Rochester, New York. While all of these departures had been tried elsewhere, it was the well-publicized curriculum of the Lincoln School and its energetic leadership that captured the nation's attention.

Some of the school's innovations, such as allowing students to learn at their own pace and doing away with traditional classroom punishments—which had been characteristic of Flexner's school in Louisville—clearly worked best in an environment of wealth, small classes, and a highly selected student body. Only a fraction of the many who applied to the Lincoln School were accepted, although a number of poor and some black students were given scholarships in order to include children "of varied social antecedents." About a third of the students in the first class paid no tuition.[55]

Among the first students to enroll in the Lincoln School were Rockefeller Jr.'s children, Simon Flexner's sons, and Abraham's daughter Eleanor. "The Rockefeller boys," according to one account, "walked or roller-skated up Fifth Avenue until they tired, at which point they would get into the back seat of the limousine [their father] had ordered to crawl along beside them." The Rockefellers remained loyal to the school throughout the children's school years. Simon's son, the historian James Thomas Flexner, said that on reaching Harvard he found the teachers there less exciting than those at the Lincoln School. Eleanor Flexner, who became a well-known feminist, told an interviewer that she had been "very happy" at the school and that "there literally was not one thing that the boys had that the girls didn't also have, sports, shop work, industrial arts, domestic arts, everything was similar for boys and girls." She was very embarrassed, however, when her father came to visit. "He had a ghastly habit of standing behind me in class," she remembered, "and patting me on the head until I finally blew off."[56]

The achievements of Lincoln students were legendary. They published prose and poetry while still in school, composed a symphony and played it on instruments they made, scored well above average on college entrance examinations, and did superior work in college. All but three of the school's first seventy-eight graduates completed college. Their precocity was celebrated in *New Yorker* cartoons. The president of the Progressive Education Association, Charles P. Howland, came away from a mathematical demonstration by pupils eleven to sixteen years old so impressed that he called it "revolutionary in character." The students were "two years ahead of anything" he had ever seen; they "knew the principles underlying well made graphs" of city budgets and the effects of daylight savings laws; they could explain "in simple and correct language, not memorized, exactly what they [we]re doing." One girl gave "a simple and fluent explanation of logarithms" that "made me gasp." The proud Flexner told Rockefeller that the achievements of the pupils were "astonishing."[57]

The critics of the "modern school," however, were loud in their denunciations of both Flexner's ideas and the attention given to the Lincoln School. Traditionalists, not without cause, saw the school as an all-out attack, heavily financed by Rockefeller money, on the classical high school. Flexner's abandonment of the classics, said the *New York Times,* carried the idea of a practical education to a dangerous extreme. An officer of the

American Academy of Arts and Letters called Flexner's ideas "frankly util-itarian to the verge of materialism." Flexner was vigorously criticized by the Princeton dean Andrew F. West for discarding the idea of mental dis-cipline. More importantly, West charged Flexner with a selective use of statistics to show that high school students did poorly in Latin. The pres-ident of the Massachusetts Teachers Association, agreeing, said flatly that Flexner had "misused statistics in a way to utterly deceive and mislead his readers" and demanded that he retract his statements. Even George Vin-cent, president of the Rockefeller Foundation, urged him to "admit in the most unequivocal way that a mistake was made."[58]

Although he did remove the offending passages in later editions of *A Modern School,* he refused to admit error and continued to assail Latin study on other grounds. Throughout his life he found it difficult to pub-licly reverse a position once taken—though privately he often changed his mind. In his new position of public prominence, his unyielding stance on classical learning brought charges of being "opinionated," "stubborn," and "close-minded." Understandably, he became the bête noir of classi-cists and defenders of the old order. When the preeminent classicist Gilbert Murray was introduced to Simon Flexner, he asked whether he was the "good" or the "bad" Flexner.[59]

But history was on Flexner's side in the debate over the classics. Most of the publicity surrounding his work on the Lincoln School was favor-able. Educators generally hailed his achievement as a landmark in Amer-ican education. Forty thousand copies of *A Modern School* were distrib-uted across the country. Without question, the Lincoln School project was close to Flexner's heart. The medical studies had come to him un-bidden and were at first entirely strange to him. His work on prostitution had no connection to his previous education or experience and was an un-welcome intrusion. But the reform of America's schools had been a pas-sionate commitment since his schoolmaster days in Louisville. In a score of letters he had voiced the hope that he would one day have a chance "to make a difference" in American education.

Now he believed he was beginning to have an impact, though he wor-ried—justifiably, as it turned out—about the regressive effect of the First World War on the reform movement. The "standpatters," he told Simon in November 1918, lived in the hope that the revolution in education would "go backwards when the war" ended. But the need for a school that "would "provide children with mastery of the tools they need to live *this* life in *this* world," he said, would be greater than ever. "One day," he sighed, "men will marvel that education was ever regarded as anything else than a training for doing jobs and being useful in the world one is to live in."[60] His views on education at age 52 were among the most radically utilitarian of his contemporaries.

For all his involvement with the Lincoln School and the school surveys in the first half-dozen years at the General Education Board, Flexner was indefatigable in his search for still other ways to affect the course of American learning. Always impatient, he was not satisfied that he had done all he could to effect change. To gain more attention for his ideas, he wrote a series of articles on education for such journals as the *Atlantic Monthly*, the *Independent*, and *School and Society*. In "Parents and Schools," he urged parents to be well informed about their children's schools and to cooperate with teachers but not to interfere with curriculum planning or teaching in the classroom. "Running a school or a class is a technical or expert job," he warned, "and untrained people, seeking to break in, are likely to do more harm than good." What parents could and should do was to raise questions. They should make school officials "tell *why,* make them show *why*" they were teaching certain subjects. No longer was the schoolmaster able "to pursue his own sweet way," for parents were going to inspect him as they inspected every other factor in the child's life.[61]

In another *Atlantic Monthly* article he argued, more emphatically than ever before, that the study of "time-honored subjects" to inculcate such mental processes as reason, memory, imagination, or observation was futile. Further, it was contrary to modern understanding of how children learn. Yet the disciplinary theory of learning still ruled in the secondary school. Any deviation from it was virtually impossible because of the college's demand for particular subjects as a condition of admission. As a result, American students did not study languages "as a way of getting at and conveying ideas"; they did not study history "as a way of arousing and satisfying social curiosity"; they did not study science "because they wonder at the world about them"—no, they studied them all "for the purpose of disciplining faculties that do not exist." When the article appeared, Gates called him up to say—"in a breathless series of superlatives"—that it was the best thing he had ever written.[62]

In a letter to President A. Lawrence Lowell of Harvard, Flexner pleaded for a modus vivendi between the college and the high school, denouncing the college entrance examinations as "practically destroy[ing] the possibility of scientific educational experiment in the secondary field."[63] For Flexner, domination of the high school curriculum by the college was a great evil that must give way to greater flexibility for the high school in meeting the needs of its students.

Flexner's energy found other outlets. At 61 Broadway, he joined with other reform-minded officers and board members to try to shape the course of the Rockefeller philanthropies. When the Rockefeller Foundation was created in 1913, sharing offices with the General Education Board, he teamed with the dynamic attorney Raymond Fosdick (later president of the Foundation) to urge that it deal with such controversial issues as crime, the use of drugs and alcohol, venereal disease, and juvenile delinquency. In the summer of 1916, he conceived a plan to give support to young scientists to increase the number of university teachers with active research interests. He likewise championed a program of medical fellowships to raise the quality of teaching in medical schools. In 1918 he began a study of business schools, asking President Lowell for an accounting of the expense of running the Harvard Graduate School of Business Administration. He developed, too, a program costing nearly a million dollars to improve the taste of industrial and commercial designers. At Harvard, he led efforts to appropriate five hundred thousand dollars to begin a graduate school of education.[64]

Outside the Rockefeller organization, he spoke publicly, addressed meetings of educators, and undertook private commissions to study particular schools. In one instance, he boldly told a national organization of social workers that their work did not constitute a profession in the same sense as medicine or engineering. What were the criteria of a profession? Flexner listed a number of "objective standards"—it must be intellectual in character, be rooted in the learned disciplines, involve a large degree of personal responsibility, have a limited and direct practical role, set uniform and high standards for practice, and be dedicated to public service. By these tests, social work was not yet a profession but more a kind of mediation among physicians, legislators, the schools, and organized charities. It was "in touch with many professions rather than a profession in and of itself."[65]

At the request of the trustees, he undertook a survey of the famous Groton School, which was run by the redoubtable Endicott Peabody, perhaps the most famous schoolmaster in America. Some of the school's alumni, trustees, and parents were dissatisfied with the rigid, traditional curriculum and Peabody's paternalistic, strongly Christian style. For Flexner, the product of a Jewish immigrant family, the chance to examine such a bastion of educational privilege must have been irresistible.

His report, though deferential to Peabody, was a merciless attack on Groton's purpose, courses, and teaching. The whole purpose of Groton, he told the trustees, was limited to preparing boys for the college entrance examination rather than "awakening and disciplining" their intellectual capacities. The time given to Greek and Latin should be shortened if not eliminated; new course options, including science and vocational studies, should be introduced; and the focus of teaching should be shifted to the varied interests of the students. "A boy is an animal living largely in the present," he wrote, "if he is effectively to be led higher, his guide must begin by meeting him on his level." Teaching at the Groton School, he found, was rigid and mechanical, ranging in quality from "poor" to "very poor." The minute regulation of the boys' lives he criticized as not permitting individuality or allowing learners to proceed at their own pace. Although the trustees received these criticisms for the most part sympathetically, implementing his suggestions for improvement had to await Peabody's retirement.[66]

All in all, it was an auspicious beginning of a national career in shaping the forms and practices of American learning. By the end of the decade he was firmly entrenched as the most effective officer in the Rockefeller philanthropies. Frequently he dined with the Rockefellers and the Eliots, who became his close allies. He was close to Buttrick and Raymond Fosdick, the rising star in the Rockefeller organization. After one dinner with the Fosdicks and Raymond's renowned brother, the minister Harry Emerson Fosdick, he described a "bully time" discussing the place of religion in "this mess of a universe." When Harry Fosdick contended that religion was a way to bring meaning to "the chaos of good and bad," Flexner responded that religion was "organized human cowardice, a spiritual cocktail analogous to the drink a tired and harassed business man takes before dinner to mellow himself."[67]

Buttrick grew ever fonder of him. "You have grown into my very life as a brother beloved," he told him as Flexner set sail on one of his frequent trips to Europe. The younger Rockefeller, too, wrote him that he was loved by his many friends for his qualities of "sweetness, gentleness, [and] forbearance." Even the gruff Gates, who harbored ill feelings toward many of his Jewish contemporaries, told him that in his entire life he had known only three Jews of "inflexible courage" and proceeded to name him and Simon Flexner as two of them.[68] Small wonder that Flexner felt secure in his position at the board.

Among his fellow workers at 61 Broadway he gained a reputation for brilliance, hard work, solitude, obstinacy, and innovative ideas. Few thought that they knew him well. He was often reclusive as he mulled over ideas in his office or worked on one of his reports. As his power and influence grew, he became ever more confident of his position and the soundness of his ideas. He continued to welcome intellectual combat and fierce argument but had little tolerance for those without keen intelligence or rhetorical skills. Raymond Fosdick praised his "indefatigable curiosity" but noted that "his passage through life was never slowed by hesitation or lethargy." A younger colleague, Alan Gregg, who was fond of him, remembered him as "extraordinarily bold and usually correct when it came to appraising and evaluating a system of education." As a man trained in the classics, he "knew what good teaching was . . . how to get it and how to give it." But he was "terribly restless" with routine office duties and could be "virtually inaccessible" for days or weeks at a time. He had little time for gossip or idle conversation. While others were talking and meeting visitors, "Abe was writing books and putting things together in a way that was extremely effective." Gregg recalled a luncheon of board officers where Flexner "went right down the table [explaining] how completely unfitted for his position every man at the table was. He left us all gasping. There was no mercy, nothing spared."[69]

Yet the warm-hearted Buttrick, who was described as having an "uncanny comprehension of human nature," could tell Eliot that he thought Flexner was "lovable" and essentially a "timid" person. By this he said he meant that Flexner's "self-assertion," which sometime looked like arrogance or conceit, was often the defense that timidity put up. In most respects Flexner was not timid, he told Eliot, but "in certain real respects" he was. In any case, "he is growing all the time and . . . he does change his mind and thus exhibits rare courage." In all their years together, said Buttrick, Flexner had impressed him more and more with his "loyalty, affection, and moral earnestness."[70] Perhaps, unacknowledged, Flexner suffered from the discreet anti-Semitism in the circles around him and felt he needed continually to prove himself. Friends and foes alike found him in action a courageous, knowledgeable, and impressively quick-witted figure. The object of endless speculation, he never acknowledged the interest of others in his personal life.

His energy and drive seemed not to falter as he approached and then passed his fiftieth birthday. He had begun a program of vigorous exercise, regular visits to the gymnasium, and frequent tennis. "I have not in years had the feeling of physical well-being," he told Anne, "that I mark with the morning following an hour's tennis." At noon each day he walked some thirty blocks to his apartment.[71] All through his early years at the board he remained physically active and was rarely sick or missing from work. In January 1918, however, he slipped and fell on an icy pavement and broke his leg. It was set by a New York surgeon, but the cast slipped out of place before healing and the leg had to be rebroken and reset. This time the leg was placed in a very heavy cast that was not sufficiently cushioned where it rested on the instep. It was excruciatingly painful, and when the cast was removed it left a blackened blister that refused to heal.

For more than a year he was in and out of hospitals, especially the Rockefeller Institute Hospital in New York and later the Johns Hopkins Hospital. At Johns Hopkins, the eminent surgeon William S. Halsted tried a number of procedures that all ended in failure. At one examination Halsted was joined by surgeons John T. Finney and Walter Dandy in examining him. As the three men bent over the small hole in his foot, Flexner said he thought the three balding heads "looked like the three balls of a pawnbroker's sign." For a time it looked as if the foot might have to be amputated. "I am weary—oh, so weary—of hope deferred," he wrote in December, "of hospital sights and sounds . . . weary of this eternal sitting—and perhaps all to no end." Finally, the surgeons were able to close the open wound with a thin membrane that held but remained vulnerable for the rest of his life.[72]

His long stay in Baltimore was not without its benefits. He was joined by his secretary, Esther S. Bailey, who was fiercely loyal and protective. In constant touch with the New York office and undisturbed by business callers and other distractions, he worked in his hospital room on articles, on memoranda for the General Education Board, and on ideas for the future. He spent a good deal of time talking about medical education with the many doctors who came to see him. His daughter Jean was convinced that this time was "one of the most fruitful of his life" as he began to shift his thinking more and more to the reorganization of medical education.[73]

Until then, his time at the board had been spent largely on projects in primary and especially secondary education—the state surveys, the Gary schools, the "modern school" paper, the Lincoln School, programs to aid black and white schools in the South, articles on education—as well as encouraging, so far as possible, full-time clinical teaching in schools of medicine. In a series of memoranda he now began to lay out the case for a special program to promote more vigorously the reform of medical education around a core of high-quality, regionally dispersed schools. On his release from hospital treatment in 1919, he took up the campaign more actively and secured a meeting with Gates to propose a program.

Fortunately for Flexner, scientific medicine had long been a favorite topic of Gates's, and he was predisposed to look favorably on Flexner's overture. His only question, in Flexner's memory, was "How much will it cost?" It would take several hundred million dollars, he told Gates, but if the senior Rockefeller would give fifty million as an incentive he believed that he could raise the rest from private and local sources. On September 20, 1919, the senior Rockefeller notified the board that he would give twenty million for the purpose; in the next few years he added more gifts, making a total of fifty million for the enterprise.[74]

These gifts enabled Flexner, over the next decade, to exert a decisive influence on the course of medical training and to leave an enduring mark on some of the nation's most renowned schools of medicine. He would create a national system of regional hierarchies in medical education that would have a lasting effect. In carrying out this program he would reach the pinnacle of his power.

8

At the Pinnacle

The munificent gift of John D. Rockefeller was without precedent. It changed dramatically the place of medical training in the nation's priorities. It made clear that the much-heralded exposé of conditions in the medical schools of 1910 was not forgotten. It gave implicit recognition to what many had come to believe—that Abraham Flexner was uniquely qualified to undertake a restructuring of the nation's medical schools.

No one else, it seemed, had the understanding of education, the knowledge of medical schools, the ability to organize, and the capacity to move easily in the separate worlds of academia, government, and philanthropy. The Rockefeller gifts, which eventually reached more than eighty million dollars from the General Education Board alone (more came from the Rockefeller Foundation), rested at bottom on the confidence that the Rockefellers and their associates had in Flexner's judgment and capacity. These huge sums were augmented by grants from Flexner's friend Henry Pritchett at the Carnegie Foundation and sometimes from other philanthropies. More money came from the schools themselves, which were required to raise sums to match or exceed these gifts.

Some measure of the immensity of these new sums—estimated by Flexner at not less than six hundred million dollars (perhaps six billion dollars in today's currency)—can be seen by comparing them with the total outlay for medical schools in 1910. In his Carnegie report of that year, Flexner stated that all 148 American medical schools together spent just over four million dollars on educating students. About 70 percent of this amount came from student fees. By 1920 the expenditure had reached perhaps twelve million dollars.[1] It was a new era for the training of doctors, and Flexner was at its center.

In winning so large a vote of confidence, Flexner realized the hope he had voiced a half-dozen years before: that the General Education Board would play in America the role, at least to a considerable degree, that governments did in Europe. From his earliest visits to American schools,

Flexner had been struck by what he saw as the disorder and commercialism of American medical training. While making the 1910 survey, he had begun to take steps to promote consolidation, assert priorities, and suggest new directions. Reform in America, he was convinced, would come not from governmental direction or planning but through major financial incentives. Philanthropy, not tax monies, was the means of elevating the training of doctors.

Flexner's confidence in his ability to manage such huge sums almost single-handedly is staggering. The nation's system of medical training, after all, was huge, disparate, complex, and subject to immense local variations, as disorganized as any in the world. "It seems queer—doesn't it?" he wrote, "to be a factor in these huge enterprises. The money part of it amuses me . . . it doesn't thrill or excite me any more than eating or drinking. My thrill comes in the creative sense I get at times from participation in adventures that promise to add something to the joy or take something away from the tragedy or pathos of life."[2]

His ideas about the right course for American medical education were far advanced. In the Carnegie report he had outlined a series of mergers and eliminations that would reduce the number of medical schools to thirty-one, all closely allied to universities, most in large cities, and all with adequate facilities for clinical teaching. Only in the South did he see the need to tolerate "greater unevenness" because of the South's educational backwardness.[3]

He had hinted, too, that full-time teaching in the clinical branches as well as the foundation sciences of medicine would in time become necessary. The survey of European medical schools and his mission to the Johns Hopkins School of Medicine strengthened his belief that commercial incentives for clinical teaching were damaging to American medicine and had to be suppressed; only hiring university-paid teachers in full-time service would enable clinical research to prosper and promote the science of medicine in America. The new type of clinician would be an investigator, as in Germany, rather than a traditional consultant. Although Frederick T. Gates provided the initiative for the full-time plan, it was Flexner, more and more, who came to explain and promote the plan at Johns Hopkins and other schools.

After joining the board, he began promoting the idea of full-time teaching in medicine, identifying those schools most likely to implement it, and then encouraging fund-raising efforts to match the Rockefeller grants. At a board meeting in October 1913, a policy of offering help to only those schools willing to make the commitment to full-time teaching was made explicit. Although not yet a board member, Flexner was called in by Gates to make the case for full-time teaching. He spoke for twenty minutes. Charles W. Eliot then said he would vote "with enthusiasm" for the plan and that it was "the most important action the Board [had] ever taken." One by one, the other board members concurred. Flexner was jubilant: "I had not only drafted the . . . Report of our Committee [but] the resolution carrying it out and all carried unanimously." At the lunch following the meeting, Eliot told Flexner that he was "the only person" who seemed "to know exactly how to do it."[4]

For the next fifteen years, until he left the board in 1928, Flexner alone carried out the scores of negotiations with medical schools. He came to know virtually every dean and university president in the country; he was called upon to name persons for key medical appointments; he committed millions of dollars of Rockefeller money; and he easily carried the board with him on all policy matters. Detailed proposals for the reconstruction or modification of at least twenty schools of medicine came from his pen. Other schools turned to him for advice as well. His influence over grants in medicine extended to the Rockefeller Foundation (created in 1913 and sharing offices and staff at 61 Broadway), to the benefactions of the Commonwealth Fund (which was also interested in medicine), and even to Rockefeller gifts to medical schools in Europe. He tried to educate the public about the training of doctors. He wrote popular articles—"The German Side of Medical Education" and "The English Side of Medical Education"—that extolled the cause of reform. University teachers of clinical medicine in Germany were held up as examples, and he lamented that they "hardly exist[ed] as yet in America."[5]

During all this time, he had no assistant for medical affairs and took few people into his confidence. He did not even have a secretary until 1915. Nevertheless, he carried out the extensive projects—state educational surveys, the Gary School study, the Lincoln School—described in the last chapter. When he left the board in 1928 it took more than a year for his fellow officers to sort out all the commitments, discussions, and promises he had been a part of for fifteen years.

His first great project was to identify those few schools ready to undertake major change with the monies then available to the General Education Board. Between 1913 and 1919–20, when there were large gifts, he concluded agreements with Washington, Johns Hopkins, Yale, Chicago, Columbia, and Vanderbilt universities. About eight million dollars was spent on this handful of schools. All these early grants involved an effort to replace local teachers of clinical medicine with a network of well-trained clinical scientists who were teachers and investigators. His aim was to create a science of clinical medicine and to make medicine a profession where only excellence was acceptable. More than any of his contemporaries, with his "agile command of resonant symbols and ideals," Flexner was becoming a master of new ways to organize knowledge in medicine.[6]

More than a quarter of the early grants went to William Henry Welch and his colleagues at Johns Hopkins. The long and bitter negotiations with the clinical faculty had dragged on for two years following Flexner's initial mission in 1911. In the final phase of deliberations, with Welch moving slowly but surely, Flexner became increasingly impatient. He wrote to Dean J. Whitridge Williams in 1913 that Welch and his supporters were "much too tender" on the clinical holdouts who had made enormous profits from their Hopkins connections. Finally, in October, agreements were reached to reorganize the departments of medicine, surgery, and pediatrics on the "full-time or university basis." The professors of surgery and pediatrics, William Halsted and John Howland, gave up their private income, but Lewellys Barker, an early champion of full-time teaching, found he could not do so; the appointment in medicine went to Theodore C. Janeway of New York. Welch warned that any expansion of the plan would require further support.[7]

The public spotlight on the Hopkins grant brought a flood of applications for similar support. All were politely turned aside. Flexner did visit some of the schools and advised others. Some were resolutely persistent. The Albany Medical College, which had a loose affiliation with Union College and several other professional schools, importuned Flexner repeatedly to examine its promise as a leading medical center. A dean would be recruited from outside, the authorities promised, and the faculty would be asked to resign so that the new dean would have a free hand. A full plan of reorganization was laid before the General Education Board. But Flexner was blunt. "The future of the Albany school," he wrote, "is so doubtful that a good man may feel some hesitation in accepting the post."[8]

Flexner had already picked his next targets. Yale and Washington University were to join Johns Hopkins in reorganizing clinical teaching on the full-time plan. He was much impressed by two men, Professor Milton C. Winternitz at Yale, a Johns Hopkins–trained pathologist; and Robert S. Brookings, a powerful leader of the Washington University board of trustees, with whom he had developed a close friendship since his visit of 1909. The reorganization at Washington University had, in fact, already begun before Flexner came to the General Education Board. After his sharp criticisms following the first visit, he had advised Brookings to abolish the school, form a new faculty, raise an endowment, and restructure the entire clinical facilities from top to bottom. Of the dozen schools of medicine in Missouri, only Brookings's school, he advised, had any chance of becoming a first-rate educational center. The faculty had agreed to Flexner's radical plan, and he now saw a "manifest destiny" to create in St. Louis a center of scientific medicine for the entire Southwest. Brookings was sent to visit Johns Hopkins; he then traveled to Europe to study medical schools. On his return he took control of the planning and fund-raising for the new school.[9] Constantly he looked to Flexner for support and encouragement.

As the first and most important appointment in the new enterprise, he sought at Flexner's and Pritchett's suggestion to recruit as dean the forty-year-old David Edsall, a nationally respected figure in preventive medicine at the University of Pennsylvania and a future powerful dean of the Harvard Medical School. Edsall, after a brief survey, proposed the establishment of seven major chairs to be filled by the best-qualified men in the country. Brookings tried also to recruit Halsted's preeminent student in surgery, Harvey Cushing, who also visited St. Louis. In the meantime, the university was able to make final strong teaching arrangements with both the Barnes Hospital and the St. Louis Children's Hospital.

Although Edsall and Cushing declined their offers of appointment, Brookings and his colleagues were nevertheless able to bring aboard some of the most talented and promising of America's leaders in medicine: the pathologist Eugene L. Opie from Simon Flexner's Institute in New York; John Howland, who spent a year in St. Louis before going to Johns Hopkins; the Hopkins-trained physiologist Joseph Erlanger; the biological chemist Philip A. Shaffer from Cornell; Robert J. Terry, an outstanding anatomist from the old Washington University faculty; and George Dock, a Pennsylvania graduate and leader in developing the clinical clerkship in America, who became dean. Flexner was closely involved in all these appointments. In the case of one search, he warned authorities in St. Louis "to make no offer to anyone" until he had approved it.[10] It was an impressive achievement. As with Welch in Baltimore, Flexner built his trust around a single strong figure in Brookings and would follow this practice in each of his major restructurings.

When the full-time idea was approved by the General Education Board in 1913 and Johns Hopkins was given its endowment, there was no question in Flexner's mind which school would be next. The application from Washington University followed by less than a month the request from Baltimore. Brookings told Flexner that he was convinced of the rightness of the full-time plan. He was not impressed, he said, by the criticisms from organized medicine and clinicians generally. To achieve greatness, he wrote, the American system had to "eliminate entirely the money microbe." "I want you to know that the full time plan has taken full possession of me."[11] With very little discussion, the General Education Board voted a grant of $750,000, later raised to $1 million, to enable Washington University to follow Johns Hopkins in placing the chairmen of medicine, surgery, and pediatrics on full-time salary. The university was required to match the gift.

In his remarks at the rededication of the school in 1916, William Henry Welch called the St. Louis reforms "the second epoch in medical education" following Johns Hopkins. The school, he declared, would be "an example and stimulus" for the entire country.[12] In the St. Louis newspapers, the reorganized school was hailed as "the Johns Hopkins of the West."

Yale was next. In his 1910 report Flexner had praised the quality of the small medical school in New Haven but warned of its need for endowment and control over the teaching beds at the New Haven hospitals. The grants to Johns Hopkins and Washington University were followed by an application from Yale. Flexner was persuaded to go to visit the medical school in New Haven and the New Haven Hospital. The key to the rejuvenation of clinical teaching, Flexner saw, was the hospital, which badly needed new facilities, especially laboratories, and had to be brought under control of the Yale medical faculty. Flexner moved aggressively. He succeeded in persuading the hospital chairman to surrender control over teaching in the hospital. In return, the university would build the needed facilities and staff them with well-qualified faculty members. Flexner committed five hundred thousand dollars from the General Education Board, and the university was to raise the rest. Over the next four and a half years, Yale brought in nearly a million and a half dollars, surpassing the General Education Board gift. The university promptly agreed to introduce the full-time principle into the main clinical departments.[13]

Arriving at Yale, Winternitz quickly impressed Flexner with his energy and ideas. Unlike many of his contemporaries, Winternitz wanted the medical school to be very closely integrated into the university. The two men became lifelong friends, and in later years Winternitz would refer to him as his "Uncle Abe." The only resistance to Flexner's initiatives at Yale came from Gates, who fought the Yale Medical School grant on the grounds that a medical school could not be developed in "a small town so close to New York."[14]

The quick initiatives at Johns Hopkins, Washington, and Yale universities set the stage for the reorganizations to come. Full-time teaching was now not hypothesis but reality. Flexner was convinced, as were his colleagues at the General Education Board, that full-time clinical teaching was on the way to replacing the part-time teaching of practitioners, especially at the chairmanship level. Each clinical department would have a full-time professor to direct teaching and research. The part-timers would go the way of the part-time preclinical teachers a generation before.

Opposition to the full-time idea, however, was heated and widespread. As the movement began to gain momentum, hostility to Flexner and his grants was more open and pronounced. The opinion of the nation's medical journals, by and large, ranged from skepticism to outright condemnation. The American Medical Association's Council on Medical Education, led by the highly critical Arthur Dean Bevan, waged an unceasing campaign against the strictness of Flexner's plan and his unwillingness to make compromises. The Johns Hopkins plan, said Bevan, was "absurd" and "grotesque," the clumsy work of a layman.[15] Virtually all clinicians across the country opposed the advance of full-time clinical teaching.

Tension between Flexner and Bevan over full-time teaching mounted when the American Medical Association began to pressure the severely lagging southern medical schools to raise standards. These schools, including the black schools of Meharry and Howard University, were required to meet the same high standards as all "Class A" medical schools. Flexner was deeply concerned. "Bevan is doing a great deal of harm in the South," he warned Pritchett.[16] Flexner decided to intervene directly, writing the Council on Medical Education in 1914 that while he was interested in promoting the best medical schools in the South and in getting rid of inferior schools, he took sharp issue with the timing and methods of the council. "As far as I know," he acidly observed, "no well-informed educational authority endorses the position now occupied by the Council."

He cited the efforts of the General Education Board to create high schools in the impoverished South, explaining that the senior classes in these schools were as yet very small. Most of their graduates, moreover, had been prepared not for college but for occupational and vocational pursuits. To follow the American Medical Association's requirement of one year of college science as a condition of entering medical school would put the association, in Flexner's words, "on the side of unreality, insincerity, and educational humbug."[17]

Flexner even threatened to organize a revolt to "detach the south" from the American Medical Association's area of influence. Tactful interference by Pritchett, however, temporarily calmed the feud. Flexner admitted that his challenge to Bevan "was unwisely heated in tone and language."[18]

If Flexner made enemies over the full-time plan in the American Medical Association, he made still more at Harvard. From the beginning it was expected that the Harvard Medical School would be a major beneficiary of any money given to medical education by the General Education Board. Former president Eliot was a powerful member of the board and Flexner's ally, and Eliot's energetic former assistant Jerome Greene was an active board member. Flexner himself had described the Harvard laboratories in 1910 as "unexcelled" and the clinical material "abundant," warning only of the faculty's lack of control over appointments and teaching beds in the Boston hospitals.[19]

Even before the Johns Hopkins gift was made final, a Harvard committee made up of Henry Christian, chief of medicine, and Harvey Cushing, chief of surgery, at the new Peter Bent Brigham Hospital, and David Edsall, chief of service at the Massachusetts General Hospital, was formed to request a grant. They asked for fifty-one thousand dollars a year for five years in order to hire fifteen full-time assistants to put several departments "on a satisfactory university basis."

The committee members were all trained in other schools, a break with Harvard tradition, and were spending a large part of their time on teaching and research. If change were to come in clinical teaching at Harvard, it would come from these men. The hiring of assistants, they argued, would enable them (and others) to spend more time on university responsibilities. Should there be limitations on the practice of a clinical professor? they asked in their report. "Yes" was the response, "because his primary interest and his main work should be hospital services and teaching." Should he be allowed a consultation practice at the hospital, for pay? Yes, a limited amount, said the committee, because it was the only way a teacher could see cases repeatedly during his teaching career.[20] Here, unknowingly, the committee drew a line that would keep Harvard from getting a grant like that of Johns Hopkins or Washington University.

Two months later Wallace Buttrick reported to Christian that the General Education Board was studying the question of clinical instruction and would send Flexner to Harvard for a thorough review. In June, Flexner met with Christian and made a series of detailed requests, including a request for a clear statement of the relationship between the medical school and the hospitals it used for teaching.[21] Four months later, he met with the committee and toured the school's facilities. He wanted to defer any action on the Harvard proposal until the full-time arrangements with Johns Hopkins were firmly in place. The Baltimore school was going to be the model for support of clinical teaching.

Slowly, it dawned on the Harvard authorities that their March proposal was not going to be approved; full-time appointments in clinical medicine were now the sine qua non for a major gift. This was made official at the October meeting of the General Education Board, and Harvard was notified that its proposal had been rejected.

Shock and recrimination followed. Why had Christian, the chairman, not seen the direction of General Education Board planning and thought? Had his own dislike of the strict full-time idea caused Harvard to lose a chance for major improvement? Was Harvard being treated unfairly? "There is some feeling here," wrote President A. Lawrence Lowell, "that we were scarcely treated quite fairly . . . because we did not know what was going on." Lowell complained that Flexner had never consulted him while in Cambridge. But the pathologist William T. Councilman blamed Christian and the committee for not keeping the faculty informed and imagining that the committee members alone were interested in the outcome.[22]

Christian defended himself to Eliot, complaining that the issue had come down to "personal considerations" where the salaries of prospective full-time professors were concerned. Jerome Greene, who described himself as disappointed and mortified, defended Flexner and warned Lowell that the General Education Board had gotten the impression that Harvard was "unwilling to go in heart and soul for a program leading to full-time service to the total exclusion of income from private patients." The unhappy outcome, he told Lowell, was the result of Christian's attitude. The full-time plan, he added, was the goal toward which "the best schools of medicine" were moving.[23]

President Lowell now took charge of negotiations. He proposed a plan for full-time appointments at the Brigham Hospital that would meet General Education Board requirements. The previous discussions, he told

Greene, were the result of misunderstanding. He had in mind the appointment of three full-time professors, as at Johns Hopkins, who would receive no pay from private practice.[24]

But Lowell encountered problems that proved insurmountable. The Brigham Hospital was not fully integrated into the Harvard teaching program, and efforts to change the arrangement failed. More importantly, the medical and surgical chiefs at Brigham, Christian and Cushing, were skeptical of the full-time plan. Cushing told Lowell that the Hopkins experiment was a desperate measure taken only because the school was in a rut. Harvard needed no such extreme action. He did not believe that the Brigham trustees would accept Flexner's "radical experiment"; he was willing to step aside, however, if the other parties wanted to follow that route.[25]

The Brigham trustees, as expected, did not want a new chief surgeon, even if Cushing were to remain on its staff. The frustrated Lowell wrote Flexner in January 1914 that his proposal was not ready but that he had been working on it for only three months; Johns Hopkins had taken much longer to write its proposal, Lowell pointed out. Finally, in April, he advised Flexner that he had found it impossible to complete the Brigham proposal. He did say that Edsall at the Massachusetts General Hospital had signaled his willingness to accept the full-time principle but doubted that this would be acceptable to Flexner. This proved to be the case. Flexner dismissed Edsall's plan because it lacked the "sine qua non" of university control over hospital appointments in full-time departments. The situation in Boston was "impossible," he said, "being too tenuous, complicated and impermanent."[26]

The now-embittered relations with Harvard were worsened by another General Education Board decision to award money for an institute of hygiene—intended to be a model for public health teaching and research— to Johns Hopkins University. Again, it was Flexner who played the dominant role in choosing the site. Although Harvard had pioneered public health education, it was passed over once more because of its failure to commit to full-time teaching. A committee that included Flexner visited Harvard, Columbia, Pennsylvania, and Johns Hopkins, but the outcome, in the view of the Harvard participants, was a foregone conclusion. On the visit to Harvard, Flexner had again criticized the loose relationship between the university and the Massachusetts General Hospital. Although Harvard had several outstanding men, he said, it lacked leadership and the situation in the medical school was "chaotic." Now even Eliot was angry. Johns Hopkins, Eliot told Flexner, was "a small and weak university" in "a provincial community" that could not compete with Harvard or Columbia in its resources for a school of public health.[27]

Eliot himself now determined to place a full-time proposal before the General Education Board that it would not reject. President Lowell willingly surrendered the leadership of the negotiations to him. The former president recruited a distinguished committee that included Edsall and William S. Thayer, a Harvard graduate now at the Johns Hopkins Hospital.

It was Thayer's task as an outsider to conduct a thorough survey of Harvard's medical school in the light of current trends in medical education. Thayer was blunt. While Harvard's medical school had been a leader in the past, with its research resources and potential, it "ought to be *the* leader." Individual clinicians had made some contributions to research, but the clinical departments as a whole were not coordinated and had not been properly led. The lack of control over key hospital appointments, moreover, kept the medical school from seeking the best available person for each position. "Clinically speaking," wrote Thayer, "Harvard has been generally regarded as a local institution." Cushing and Edsall were the exceptions. He recommended that Harvard, in addition to Brigham, seek control over the major clinical departments at the Massachusetts General Hospital. To be successful in its approach to the General Education Board, advised Thayer, Eliot's committee needed to be especially sensitive to the importance of barring clinical professors and their assistants from seeing private patients for pay. To be at the "beck and call" of private patients, he warned, would make it impossible for the chief of a department to direct effectively the teaching and research of his group.[28]

The tentative proposal submitted by Eliot in December (it was agreed that to avoid further embarrassment no formal application would be made) went a considerable distance toward satisfying the General Education Board policies. Eliot and Flexner had been in close touch as the committee had worked on the proposal. The proposal committed Harvard, in principle, to establish full-time professorships in medicine, surgery, pediatrics, obstetrics, and nervous diseases as quickly as suitable relationships could be worked out with hospitals and new income found. This might take some time, perhaps a number of years, because of the difficulty in finding qualified full-time clinical professors. Those few who were now qualified had made financial sacrifices, expecting a larger future income from private practice, and were not likely to be candidates. In the meantime, the committee agreed, a number of part-time clinicians would continue to carry on the teaching and research. The plan thus combined a commitment to full-time appointments in the future with a continuation of part-time teaching in the clinics. Implicit in the plan was a "whiggish expectation," writes historian Steven Wheatley, that everything would work itself out as new appointments were made.[29]

It was not enough. Buttrick, to whom the proposal was sent, responded immediately that he did not think it adequate to fulfill the board's policy of helping only schools with strict full-time teaching policies. In a memorandum to Buttrick, Flexner reminded him that the very purpose of full-time teaching was "the *suppression* of the part-time departments." Eliot's proposal, Flexner wrote, "continues the old order and simply adds the new order." It would not change the character of the medical school, as had happened in Baltimore and St. Louis. If the Harvard proposition were approved, the board would be deluged with similar halfhearted applications from other schools.[30]

Discussions dragged on until April 1917, when the project was abandoned. Eliot made it clear that while he thought the full-time policy a clear improvement in clinical teaching, Harvard was not willing to make it the exclusive policy of the school. No wholesale transformation of the Harvard Medical School, as Flexner had demanded, was needed. The negotiations closed on a sour note. Eliot accused the board of departing from its firm policy of not interfering with the local management of an institution. Lowell saw "a prejudice which I do not fully understand." One angry faculty member told Henry Pritchett: "There are circumcised [sic] folk in NY, circumcised alike in pecker and intellect, who can see nothing good in the Harvard Medical School . . . Every now and again the savor of their skunkhood comes my way."[31]

Flexner had prevailed. Buttrick's response and the silence of the board made it clear that no one was going to challenge his program. Even Eliot acquiesced in the board's final denial. The power of Flexner's logic and the strength of his personality were now unmatched in the counsels at 61 Broadway. He seemed unshakeable in his self-confidence, unafraid of criticism, and mulishly stubborn in defending his position. Most important, his record of success in carrying out a large number of delicate projects silenced any serious criticism. Over and over he painted for the board a picture of American leadership in medical education once the commercial spirit was crushed. His mission, as he saw it, was making medical schools, rebuilt or newly created, that were integral parts of universities in control of first-rate teaching hospitals and were free of money-making concerns.

He saw himself as fighting for high ideals and against avarice. He dismissed criticism that he was selfish and short-sighted. By the end of the Harvard negotiations, he believed he was succeeding in his mission.

While the discussions with Harvard were grinding to a halt, Flexner was turning his attention to Chicago and New York. Neither of these great cities, in his view, possessed a modern medical school or one that promised much for the future. He now determined to create full-fledged schools based on his ideas at the University of Chicago and at Columbia University. The initiatives he took with regard to these schools proved to be as difficult to enact as those at Harvard, but his success was greater. In Chicago he faced once again the hostility of Arthur Dean Bevan, who was the leading surgeon of the Rush Medical School, an independent school with a loose relationship with the University of Chicago, while at Columbia he would have to deal with his old nemesis Nicholas Murray Butler.

The University of Chicago owed its very existence and prominence to the early benevolence of the elder Rockefeller. But William Rainey Harper, the first president, had alienated Rockefeller and Gates in the early 1890s by refusing to create a separate medical school stressing scientific medicine on the university campus. Gates had convinced Rockefeller to follow the Johns Hopkins example. When Harper moved to absorb the distant Rush Medical School, dominated as it was by practitioners, as the university's school of medicine, while offering only the preclinical subjects on the university campus, Rockefeller and Gates cut off any further aid to the medical school. Harper's action left a bitter residue in relations between the university and the Rockefeller philanthropies. The university had made a fatal mistake, wrote Gates, in turning over "to all intents and purposes . . . the whole thing to Rush Medical College."[32]

In 1916, after two decades of hostility, Flexner took up the cause again. He was able to persuade Gates, Buttrick, John D. Rockefeller Jr., and other board members that the time had come to bury the hatchet and to try once more to build a full medical school at the University of Chicago. Harper's successor, Harry Pratt Judson, told Flexner that he was interested but "alarmed" by Bevan's position as a bitter opponent of the full-time plan.[33]

Flexner came to Chicago to talk to Judson and to his close friend, philanthropist Julius Rosenwald, head of Sears, Roebuck and Company and a trustee of the university. In July 1916, Flexner prepared a plan that praised the opportunity open to the university to create a national medical center. Unlike Boston, New York, and Philadelphia, which were hampered by their old-fashioned medical schools, Chicago was free to build a new school on its merits "without compromise or embarrassment." Not only did Chicago have a university of the first rank, it possessed in Frank Billings, the most powerful figure in Chicago medicine, a strong supporter of building a full clinical program at the university. Billings, Flexner wrote, was a leader like William Henry Welch: "wise, clear-headed, and absolutely unselfish."

Flexner strongly recommended building a full medical school modeled on Johns Hopkins and located on the university campus. It would require the building of a university hospital at a cost of two and a half million dollars. The Rush Medical School, under his plan, would become a postgraduate school for missionary training and for practitioners needing advanced education.[34] Judson agreed, Rosenwald offered a half-million dollars to begin the campaign, Billings signaled his willingness to lead a fund drive, and Flexner committed one million dollars each from the General Education Board and the Rockefeller Foundation toward the start-up costs of five million dollars.

Nothing could have been better calculated to bring Bevan to full boil than this direct intrusion into Bevan's backyard. Bevan was a Rush graduate and since 1902 a mainstay of the Rush faculty. Judson told Flexner that Bevan was "very bitter" and "much alarmed" about the university's decision to build its own clinical school and hospital. Bevan, he said, had done all he could in the meantime to secure a union between Rush and the state university at Champaign–Urbana. But Bevan did not know that the University of Illinois had also approached Flexner, albeit without success, to fund a full-time system at the College of Physicians, with which the university had an affiliation.

Against strong opposition from Bevan, the Rush faculty, the alumni, and many Chicago physicians, negotiations moved forward over the next several years. In an address to the American Medical Association, Bevan attacked lay interference with physician training. He denounced the full-time teaching experiment as a failure and attacked the foundations—meaning Flexner—for using their millions to "bribe" universities to do something in which they did not really believe.[35]

Flexner's response was scathing. Medical education was preeminently education, not "only medicine," and doctors were simply "not competent" to manage the subject. No quarrel existed with the laboratory scientists, Flexner said; it was only the "old-time type of physician and surgeon" being pushed off the stage who was fighting a rearguard action.[36] One can imagine the effect on Bevan's blood pressure on hearing this! The two men were about the same age.

As the plans for rebuilding medical teaching in Chicago dragged on, Flexner was busy elsewhere with a dozen other initiatives, especially the effort to reconstruct Columbia's school of medicine. The triumph in Chicago encouraged his belief that he could bring order out of the tangled situation in New York. But the situation in New York was even more complex than that in Chicago. While both Columbia University and the Presbyterian Hospital saw the advantages of combining their resources into a single medical center, the clash of traditions, strong personalities, and bitter quarrels over the site of a new medical school and hospital made agreement seem impossible. The philanthropist Edward Harkness, son of a John D. Rockefeller ally in the oil business and a Presbyterian trustee, had signaled his willingness to fund a new hospital, to be used as the teaching hospital of the medical school. It would be a center for scientific investigation.

But contrary to Harkness's understanding, President Butler of Columbia failed to carry out his part to raise the money to move and reorganize the medical school. The dean of the school, Samuel Lambert, had long wanted a geographical union and urged that the faculty be brought into the negotiations.[37] The deadlock in the discussions brought a suggestion to Harkness from John D. Rockefeller Jr. that Flexner be asked to form an "ideal plan" for medical education in New York.[38] Harkness agreed immediately, and President Butler, doubtless with some reluctance, concurred.

Throughout the summer and fall of 1917 Flexner conferred with Presbyterian and medical school officials. He met several times with Butler, asked for vast amounts of data, and then submitted his report in November. It was vintage Flexner: the medical school and hospital would be reconstructed on a single site; Presbyterian would be the university's sole teaching hospital, with its appointments controlled by the university; and the clinical faculty members would surrender their claim to private fees and become full-time university teachers.[39] To implement the plan, the General Education Board, the Rockefeller Foundation, and the Carnegie Foundation (Pritchett had joined the discussions) would each give a million dollars, and the university and hospital would raise the rest.

At first, the response from all parties seemed favorable. Gradually, however, it became clear that Butler did not accept several key parts of the Flexner plan, especially the full-time system and the dropping of

Columbia's teaching affiliations with other hospitals. Pritchett, too, was becoming impatient with what he described as Flexner's "absolutism" on the full-time arrangement.[40]

But Flexner was firm. He had no confidence in Butler's judgment or capacity to lead. He likened the Columbia president to the wartime Kaiser Wilhelm II, both of whom, he said, had to go before there could be peace. Pritchett's impatience, too, he gently set aside, reminding him that the General Education Board had had a policy on full-time teaching since 1913. At this stage in the development of clinical teaching, he was doubtless right that any deviation from the full-time principle might crush the movement to end the commercial impulse in academic medicine. With the full support of his board, Flexner held all the high cards, and the parties were forced to accept his terms. The Presbyterian trustees, led by Harkness and exasperated by Butler's intransigence and evasiveness, demanded at a joint meeting with university representatives, that Butler be eliminated from the negotiations.[41] Harkness then went directly to the Columbia board of trustees and succeeded in having Butler replaced by the board chairman in the negotiations.

Flexner had won. A memorandum was approved by both Columbia and Presbyterian that met all of Flexner's terms. Although the details of the reorganization took a number of years to complete—and further dissension reared its head—the Flexner plan was substantially implemented in the 1920s.

His success in New York and Chicago, added to the reorganizations in Baltimore, St. Louis, and New Haven, led him to believe that the "experimental" period of full-time clinical teaching was drawing to a close. He was now certain that the full-time university teacher was the model for the future, even if the model was modified at times by allowing a small amount of private practice. Competition for academic honors in the university and recognition of research, he believed, were rapidly replacing income as the primary goals of clinician-teachers. While still pressing for a strict definition of full-time teaching, he was becoming more flexible in his negotiations with other universities, especially those he regarded as in the "second tier" of schools.

He was doubtless influenced, too, by criticism of his unyielding resistance to deviation from the full-time plan. Pritchett continued to press him for a plan that provided for a clinical teacher to give his time primarily to teaching and research but allowed some private practice. "I think your tendency," he told Flexner, "is to go a little too far in laying down the rules." At Johns Hopkins, Theodore Janeway, the first full-time professor of medicine, spoke openly of his reservations about the Hopkins plan and the need of clinicians to have opportunities "to obtain mastery of the practical art." Privately, Janeway lamented the fact that his fees for private practice all went to the university.[42]

At Harvard, Edsall, who favored full-time in principle and became dean in 1918, was forcefully advancing what he called the "Harvard system" of full-time (also known as "geographic full-time"). He called for full-time university appointments but allowed clinicians to be paid for seeing some private patients in university hospitals. "It is distasteful," he wrote Flexner, for universities "to lay down laws regarding men's fees and activities." Medical scientists, whether anatomists or surgeons, "do not care anything about the fees except that they are not exorbitant."[43] Continually he bombarded Flexner with long letters urging him to modify his position.

Most of the leading medical schools were thus by 1919 moving toward clinical appointments that required either strict full-time service or an arrangement that approached it. Without Flexner's vigorous initiatives and the monies he commanded, it is unlikely that so strong a movement could have gained so much momentum. The Johns Hopkins historian and clinician A. McGehee Harvey summed up the changes of these years: "No single event has had a more profound effect on medical education and medical practice than the movement to full-time positions in clinical departments."[44]

When the elder Rockefeller made the first of his large gifts to medical education in 1919, Flexner made it clear that it would be used for improvement of certain schools and not for standardization of all schools. To put medical education on "a modern basis" everywhere in the country would require at least two hundred million dollars. With the smaller amounts available, it was important to invest the money wisely to achieve the largest possible return. Some of it would of necessity be given to schools that did not meet Flexner's criteria, including the full-time plan. The objective was to create a national plan for educating doctors that was as complete as possible amidst the complex and uneven conditions that existed. A uniform policy was simply not possible. A suggestion from the American Medical Association that the money be spent on reeducating the thousands of doctors trained in "old time medical schools" was turned aside. In the eastern states, Flexner advised, it was possible to concentrate on the further improvement of "the highest-type medical school," but in the South they needed "to be satisfied" with doing "the best that the situation" permitted.

Only the medical school at Vanderbilt University in Nashville gave promise of reaching "the modern ideal" in that part of the country.[45]

In the West, where professional education was almost wholly in the hands of state universities, it would be necessary to cooperate with state authorities. He told the senior Rockefeller in 1919 that a national system of medical education need include no more than thirty-one schools, ranging from Baltimore, Philadelphia, New York, New Haven, and Boston in the East to Nashville, New Orleans, and Galveston in the South (and perhaps the universities of Virginia and Georgia) to Chicago, Iowa City, Cincinnati, and St. Louis in the middle West, and Salt Lake City, San Francisco, and Seattle in the far West. The resources of the General Education Board, he advised the donor, should be concentrated on the schools where there was a real chance to make a difference.[46]

In the years following, armed with vast new monies, he set about planning a national restructuring of medical education. He made lengthy tours of each section of the country, held conferences of leading medical educators, and corresponded with scores of medical schools. He was traveling constantly, staying at home for only a day or two before starting off again on another trip.[47] After a tour of the South in 1920, he warned once more that a uniform policy in that region was not possible. Too swift a change, he maintained, might prove too much for public sentiment. The public, whatever the board did, was going to have doctors: "good doctors, if they are to be had, but doctors in any event."

Everywhere in the South he found schools unprepared to make the leap to first-class status—the Baylor University School of Medicine in Dallas was "a weak affair"; the University of Texas in Galveston medical department was "not rich enough in clinical material"; the Tulane University medical school was "unfortunately divided" between its scientific and clinical departments; the Emory University medical program had serious problems but might ultimately be acceptable; the University of Georgia medical school was making slow progress "in the face of difficult conditions"; the University of Tennessee at Memphis medical department was undergoing a transition to state control; and the District of Columbia's three medical schools were eking out "a bare subsistence."

Yet, in contrast to his approach at Yale or Washington University or Chicago, he sought to make improvement without wholesale reorganization. After his visit to Dallas, he sent the president and two members of the Baylor board of trustees to the Johns Hopkins School of Medicine for a week and promised further discussions. In Galveston, he recommended

General Education Board participation in a campaign to build a new laboratory building and small annual grants to enable the medical school to start a program of residencies. At Tulane he urged board aid "as liberally as possible," depending on a canvass of local financial support. The Emory University school, he reported, urgently needed an endowment of five hundred thousand to one million dollars, and he recommended that the board supply one-third of the amount. The University of Georgia medical school should be considered for grants of one-third of the cost of a new laboratory and dispensary building, and an additional amount of $25,000 for five years to increase its budget. The school at Howard University, one of two remaining medical schools for African Americans, "must not be permitted to disappear" and merited an immediate contribution of $250,000 toward a $500,000 endowment for teaching and equipment. The other school primarily for blacks, Meharry Medical College in Nashville, was also given support of $345,000 over the next few years. Medical education in the South, concluded his report, was "trembling on the verge of extinction," but these initial steps would put it on the road to greater stability.[48]

Two of the other southern schools he visited were marked for special treatment. Vanderbilt University in Nashville and the University of Cincinnati, across the Ohio River from Kentucky, were, of all the southern schools he visited, the only candidates, he believed, that could become leading centers of medical teaching. Both had some endowment, strong leadership, a commitment to make the medical school an integral part of the university, and a willingness to begin full-time clinical appointments. These schools were important to his overall plan because they could serve as models for other schools and produce the teachers and researchers to "colonize" and uplift them. The negotiations already in progress at Vanderbilt, he wrote in his report, had "acted like a depth bomb" across the South; every school expecting to survive now had to exert itself.[49] The German principle of emulation among medical schools, he predicted, would take hold in America as well. Help one school to excel, he believed, and its rivals would exert themselves to become more competitive.

Flexner had become close friends with James H. Kirkland, the dynamic chancellor of Vanderbilt University, following his first visit to Nashville in 1909. His summer residence at Lake Ahmic in Canada adjoined that of Kirkland. He applauded Kirkland's determination, despite overwhelming obstacles, to create "a real university" in the South. Such a development, Kirkland asserted, would be "the greatest service that could be rendered this people and this section." Himself a southerner, trained in Germany, with a Ph.D. in classics from Leipzig, Kirkland had begun the Vanderbilt transformation in the 1890s to a place of high standards, modern curricula, and advanced study. He led a long, bitter fight to divorce the university from the control of the Methodist Church. In 1913, after Flexner had described the Vanderbilt medical school as the only medical institution in Tennessee worth saving, Kirkland appealed successfully to Andrew Carnegie for a million dollars to upgrade the school. It was the largest gift the university had ever received. He then shrewdly invited Buttrick and Flexner, now with the General Education Board, to survey the needs of the whole university. Not surprisingly, the two visitors singled out the medical school and the college of liberal arts as requiring large support.[50] The General Education Board subsequently pledged three hundred thousand dollars toward a million-dollar drive to support the college of liberal arts. The close contact between Kirkland and Flexner continued during the years when Flexner was waging his campaign for full-time medical teaching.

By 1918 Flexner was persuaded that Vanderbilt should become the first-class medical school that was desperately needed in the South. The hope for Vanderbilt, he told Kirkland, "lies very close to our hearts." More visits and correspondence followed. At a discussion of medical education in the southern states in February 1919, before the large gift in the fall, the board approved a Flexner resolution that a plan be drawn to reorganize the medical school at Vanderbilt. No other school in the South, Flexner advised, could provide the medical training, research, and work in public hygiene needed to deal with such indigenous medical problems as malaria, pellagra, and hookworm disease. Kirkland was the key, he believed, for he possessed the vision and energy to transform the present school. In July, the board approved a grant of four million dollars, the largest yet made, to create a medical school "of the most advanced modern type."[51] It was, in effect, a blank check, since no firm plans for the reorganization and rebuilding were yet in place.

In the days that followed, Flexner found himself deeply involved in the details of restructuring the Vanderbilt school, reviewing curricular plans, architectural sketches, the hiring of personnel, relations with hospitals. "As you are well aware," Kirkland told him, "we have regarded your suggestions as having practically the force of orders." According to the university's historian, Flexner was more deeply involved in the planning than Kirkland. The old faculty was forced to resign, and a new, full-time corps of instructors was to take its place. A new dean was urgently sought to plan the new facilities and to guide the recruitment of faculty. Flexner, again, played a critical role, consulting with Welch, his brother, and others before recommending G. Canby Robinson, the vigorous, portly dean of the recently reorganized school at Washington University. "In a sense," writes the school's historian, "Flexner picked the dean."[52]

The ambitious Robinson, a student of William Osler and resident physician at Simon Flexner's research hospital in New York, used his experience to demand far more from Kirkland and Flexner than they were prepared to give. He insisted that a model medical center required a unified school and hospital on the main campus of the university. A tense relationship developed between Kirkland and Robinson as the latter pressed his demands. Flexner and Buttrick were frequently called upon to act as referees. Robinson came close to resigning several times, claiming that the General Education Board was "morally bound" to furnish everything he needed for a first-class school and that Kirkland should join him in pushing harder for more money. Flexner was able to mollify him with promises of future aid and by reminding him that even Welch had not started in Baltimore with everything in place.[53]

Finally, in 1921, Flexner reported that Pritchett would contribute another $1,500,000 of Carnegie money to match a similar amount from the General Education Board to make possible the plans for the new school and hospital that Robinson demanded. Four years later the first students were welcomed into a school and hospital where for the first time they found "under one roof" everything needed for laboratory and clinical training and for faculty research. Robinson, with Flexner's sometimes-reluctant support, had prevailed. In 1927, Flexner's brother Bernard, now a highly successful New York lawyer, established the Abraham Flexner Lectureship at Vanderbilt to perpetuate his brother's association with the reorganization of the medical school.[54]

The crucial alliance between Flexner and Kirkland was duplicated in Cincinnati with the progressive president of the University of Cincinnati, Charles W. Dabney. Dabney had brought a flurry of reforms to the university since his arrival in 1904 from the University of Tennessee. The aim of an urban school like Cincinnati, Dabney proclaimed, must be to serve the entire community. The university he headed, he declared in a widely quoted statement, must be not only "a university *in* the city but a university *of* the city." What impressed Flexner most was Dabney's skill in uniting the two rival medical schools in the city and his ambition to build a scientific school of medicine. As early as 1913 he told Flexner, "I desire very much to put paid whole time men in charge of the medical and other chief clinical professorships."[55]

For the next seven years Flexner followed closely the changes being made in Cincinnati. The city, he perceived, was in a unique position as the owner not only of a university and medical college but also of a large municipal hospital. Cincinnati, if successful, could well become an example for other cities. Many of its students came from south of the Mason-Dixon line. In 1919 the university appealed to the General Education Board for support in creating full-time positions in surgery and obstetrics. Flexner, anticipating the new gifts for medical education from the senior Rockefeller, replied that he hoped to be able to help. The following year the General Education Board committed seven hundred thousand dollars to the restructuring of the school, and Henry Pritchett agreed to add two hundred thousand dollars of Carnegie money. The university was to raise the remainder in a two-million-dollar campaign. Flexner then helped recruit a promising surgeon, George Heuer of the Johns Hopkins School of Medicine, to head the department of surgery. In a significant shift, he agreed to give Heuer the right to see some private patients for pay in a ward set aside for him at the city hospital. A few years later, a separate hospital for faculty practice was built with Flexner's aid and encouragement.[56] More and more, he came to accept such "geographic full-time" arrangements while still protesting the commercialism that made them necessary.

Elsewhere in the country Flexner carried out simultaneous negotiations with other schools of medicine. In two bold departures from earlier ventures, he engineered agreements to build a completely new school of medicine at the University of Rochester and to restructure the state medical school at the University of Iowa. In both cases, he relied as before on powerful local leaders. Both ventures brought him opposition, in the Iowa case particularly. But for the rest of his life he took special pride in these two schools, believing that they were his own creation and that without him they would never have attained their prominent status.

The rationale for creating the Rochester school was the failure of the New York City schools to move more rapidly in creating the kind of full-time, university-integrated school in full control of a teaching hospital that he favored. The agreement with Columbia was moving forward only slowly, and resistance to beginning the full-time plan was strong. A parallel effort to bring the Cornell University school of medicine into close relationship with the New York Hospital was likewise encountering formidable obstacles.[57] The appeal of Rochester was that it had no medical school but did have a strong, ambitious president, Rush Rhees, and was the home of the philanthropist and Kodak giant George Eastman.

Creating a medical school *de novo* meant having an unprecedented opportunity to shape its program. When the idea formed in his mind in 1920, he knew neither Rhees nor Eastman. But Gates, a Rochester alumnus, and Buttrick, who had been a Rochester trustee, were well acquainted with Rhees and were intrigued by Flexner's idea. A surprised Rhees was approached by Flexner and signaled his interest, but only if the proposed school was "unquestionably of the first class." He declined to approach Eastman himself but did arrange an interview for Flexner.

On February 5, 1920, Flexner spent the day with George Eastman in Rochester. He told Anne that it was a novel experience. As they ate breakfast in a spacious room full of flowers, they listened to the tones of a private organ, a ritual observed every morning in the Eastman mansion. Eastman himself was a "sweet-faced, gentle man with thin white hair covered by a skull cap, who puffed continually on a cigarette." After the breakfast concert, Flexner was led to a comfortable study where the two men talked from nine-thirty in the morning to four in the afternoon. At the conclusion, Eastman, who had asked few questions, told Flexner that he had made his proposal "crystal clear" and that he was deeply interested. He was invited to return for dinner at seven in the evening, where a string quartet played until their discussions resumed. Later that evening, as Flexner remembered it, Eastman offered $2,500,000 toward an estimated cost of $10,000,000 for a school of medicine. Flexner's reply, perhaps apocryphal, was that it was not enough and he would wait until Eastman sold more Kodaks. The size of the gift was then raised to $3,500,000, but Flexner declined the offer again.[58]

A few weeks later, Eastman agreed to a contribution of more than $5,000,000, including the value of a pioneering dental clinic that he had founded in Rochester. The clinic would be part of the new school, which, uniquely, was to include the study of dentistry. Flexner confidently agreed to match the total, although he had as yet no authority from his board to do so. On March 15 agreement was reached and the proposal was signed to create a school of medicine and dentistry at the University of Rochester.[59]

Three months later, the plans were announced at a gala dinner with Eastman, Rhees, and Flexner as the featured speakers. Flexner, who was given "a tumultuous greeting," heaped praise on the donor and the president. The city was fortunate, he said, "in the conjunction of these two planets." Rochester would follow Baltimore, St. Louis, and New Haven in introducing the full-time plan of clinical teaching. Clinical teachers, to be sure, would make less money than formerly, but teaching, like the ministry, was "an unworldly occupation," whose rewards come from spiritual satisfactions beyond all price. He appealed to the local medical profession to support the new endeavor. Finally, he reminded his listeners that the new school would be different from any other because it would include instruction in dentistry, thus placing dentistry on the same level as medicine and surgery. It had been his idea to combine dental students' and medical students' first two years of instruction.[60]

Flexner showed pride as well as a proprietary interest in his creation. He was in steady contact with Rhees, advising him on appointments and on where the newly hired might get the best advanced training. He took a keen interest in the plans for a new municipal hospital adjoining the medical school, the organization of the medical departments, the building of a library, and the salaries for faculty. When his favored choice for dean, George H. Whipple, a student of Welch's at Johns Hopkins and now dean at the University of California Medical School, declined a visit to Rochester, he urged Rhees to board a train for California to convince him. Whipple credited Flexner with his decision to come to Rochester.[61]

Even after Whipple's arrival, he and Rhees journeyed often to New York to confer with Flexner. In October 1922, Rhees wrote that he and Whipple were coming to see him because they needed to talk over a number of candidates for clinical appointments. Later, after the faculty was fully staffed, he urged Flexner to join the discussions on curriculum before they reached "the time when some decisions ha[d] to be made." Before the first catalogs were sent out, Flexner suggested extensive revisions that better reflected his point of view. Rhees asked also for advance proofs of Flexner's forthcoming book on comparative medical education. For the rest of their lives, Rhees and Eastman remained close to Flexner. In 1929, after he had left the General Education Board, Flexner persuaded Eastman to endow a professorship of American Studies (including a George Eastman House for the professor) at Oxford University.[62]

Not everyone applauded Flexner's creation in Rochester. Critics, especially in New York, questioned the need for another medical school in the Northeast. Other petitioners for aid found fault with so large an expenditure for a wholly new school. Pritchett, while congratulating him, questioned so large a sum being given in a region full of medical schools when there was such urgent need in the South. To Buttrick he wrote that the Rochester venture seemed "like going against all the things for which the General Education Board has stood." Flexner might argue that the board had gotten five million dollars out of Eastman, but "the reply to that" would be "that Eastman got five million out of" Flexner.[63]

The venture in Iowa raised a very different controversy. From the beginning, Gates's policy of giving aid to only selected private colleges and universities had gone largely uncontested. He could see no reason to give money to a tax-supported school. Private aid to tax-supported schools would only make it easier for the public to avoid its responsibilities. To give to one such school, he argued, would open the door to further such gifts and dilute the effort to strengthen the better schools, which were almost entirely private.

Flexner knew that the plans he had outlined to the elder Rockefeller, which included developing schools in regions not served by private schools, would meet with strong opposition from Gates. He was able to persuade Gates to go along with limited aid to several of the southern state schools and to the University of Cincinnati, a historically private institution now receiving city support. But he was strongly convinced that to bring about a national revolution in medical education he would have to find a way to build a modern school in the western states, especially in the growing states beyond the Mississippi basin. Without a change in policy, he was persuaded, the General Education Board would have no influence in "the vast territory" west of the Mississippi.[64]

The school he picked was Iowa, and the key local ally was William R. Boyd, chairman of the finance committee of the state board of education. Flexner had met Boyd at the time of the Carnegie survey in 1909 and had stayed in touch with him during his career at the General Education Board. Like Rhees, Eastman, Kirkland, Brookings, and others, Boyd became Flexner's lifelong friend.

In December 1920, Flexner returned to Iowa City to see for himself what promise the medical school held. He found that politics had been removed from the board, that capable teachers had been recruited in the medical departments, and that a complete reconstruction of the school's facilities was being considered. The reconstruction, he was told, would take eight to ten years because of the large sums of money involved. Flexner asked Boyd whether a contribution from the General Education Board could be matched by the state to make possible a speedier reconstruction. Boyd replied that it could. Other considerations were favorable. The president of the university, Walter Jessup, was "a perfectly corking good fellow" who was interested in medical education. There was great advantage, Flexner concluded his report, in dealing with tax-supported institutions. No question would arise about maintenance or development, and they were "in a strategic position in reference to public health."[65]

Flexner obtained agreement from Buttrick and the president of the Rockefeller Foundation, George E. Vincent, a former president of the University of Minnesota, that the two Rockefeller boards would contribute half of the estimated $4,500,000 cost of rebuilding. But Gates, now retired but still a formidable member of the General Education Board, was adamantly opposed. Over the next eighteen months Flexner built his case, quietly lobbying the other members of the board. Unlike the previous large grants, the Iowa gift did not require a commitment to full-time clinical medicine. Flexner did ask the dean, however, to talk to his clinical heads about their income from private practice and to prepare a memorandum that he could use if necessary. "We know, of course," he told the dean in a remarkably frank statement, "that the country needs to have and must pay for services of competent medical men, but we feel that this is the business of the patient and his family, and not of such organizations as the General Education Board."[66]

Action by the General Education Board was continually postponed while Flexner prepared the way. Pritchett, who had been approached to help in the Iowa project, made it known that the Carnegie Foundation would not participate in a grant to a tax-supported institution. Great medical schools, said Pritchett, were not developed in "little towns" like Iowa City. But Flexner responded that Germany, Holland, and Sweden contained numerous examples to the contrary. The long delay caused deep misgivings in Iowa, which was going through a severe farm depression. "If this College of Medicine ever needed help, it needs it now," Boyd wrote Flexner.[67] Rockefeller Jr. was kept advised of Flexner's efforts to woo Gates and to overcome his objections. Gates, meanwhile, collected materials, including specially prepared charts and statistics, to argue his case against Flexner.

The showdown came at the Gedney Farms Hotel in White Plains, New York, where the General Education Board held its October 1922 meeting. Gates had personally asked all board members—some of whom wanted to avoid the confrontation—to attend his "swan song" as trustee. The Iowa grant was at the center of the meeting. Raymond Fosdick, a future president of the Rockefeller Foundation and historian of the General Education Board, called it one of the most interesting debates he had ever heard.[68]

The atmosphere was electric as Gates took the floor. His white hair flying, he spoke for three hours, while Flexner spoke for less than half an hour. The speech of the former minister, an injured lion at bay, was by turns eloquent, sermonic, historical, sarcastic, and dismissive of Flexner's case. His flair for the dramatic, said Fosdick, might have led him to the stage. Gifts to state universities, Gates argued, were "needless and gratuitous." The urgent need was for more trained medical scientists who could be produced in only first-rate medical schools. It was these research scientists who were making a revolution in medicine. "Schools of the second class," Gates said, "*will take care of themselves without our aid.*" The school at Iowa City was only a well-equipped state school for the production of Iowa doctors. To describe it as a national school like Johns Hopkins or Vanderbilt or Rochester, even to speculate that it could become one, "is to take a gambler's chance with our money." Furthermore, Iowa was a wealthy state, one of five "without a dollar of debt," that was perfectly capable of financing its own medical school. The Flexner proposal even abandoned the firm policy of aiding only those schools willing to commit to full-time clinical medicine. The board, by considering approval of this ill-thought-out project, he concluded, was drifting "far from" its original policies and had "lost sight of [its] guiding stars."[69]

Flexner was brief. He had the votes. He was extremely deferential to Gates, calling his vision "sound and inspiring." But that vision, if confined to endowed schools, could operate only in the East, and that would be neither wise nor fair. To make a nationwide difference, the board had to pursue a policy of cooperating not only with the great endowed institutions but also with progressive state schools that were likely to receive generous and ongoing support. To help only the twenty "first-class" schools was "impracticable and impolitic."[70] There was little discussion. All of those present except Gates voted for the proposal.

Gates was dismayed and angry with Flexner. "How could you!" he wrote Flexner after the meeting; "you have never squarely met one of my arguments!" At least thirty-two states, especially in the South, he charged, could "present . . . a better case than Iowa's." But the fight was over. It was a spectacular victory. He had won the case for a national policy of building strength wherever possible while simultaneously creating strong regional centers of clinical and scientific medicine. The Iowans recognized their debt. The University of Iowa's medical complex, writes the school's historian, "is most properly seen as a monument to Abraham Flexner."[71]

With his Iowa victory in 1922, Flexner had brought about major changes in eight medical schools located in the most populous regions of the United States. All were integral parts of universities, all had won control over clinical teaching at major hospitals, and all were committed to encouraging clinical science. With the exception of Iowa and Cincinnati, where some clinical practice for pay was allowed but discouraged, all had agreed to the full-time principle in clinical medicine. These were to be, in Flexner's view, the model schools that would influence others, that would create a science of clinical medicine, and that would limit the commercial spirit in American medical teaching.

Still other schools, he knew, showed great promise as national leaders in medical education. Not only Harvard, where Edsall was transforming the formerly regional school, but Cornell, Stanford, Pennsylvania, Michigan, and the Western Reserve School of Medicine in Cleveland were destined to be in the forefront of future medical education. The leaders of all these schools were in close touch with Flexner, and most would eventually receive some aid. At Western Reserve, President Charles Thwing typically looked to Flexner for advice on the number of students, the construction of clinical facilities, and the location of buildings in reorganizing his medical school. A compromise was reached on full-time teaching in Cleveland by appointing full-time beginning teachers and retaining the older faculty as part-time instructors.[72] In New York, Flexner was approached in 1920 to assist in bringing the New York Hospital into a closer relationship with Cornell University Medical College. At the University of Pennsylvania, university and medical leaders asked him to advise on their medical school, recognizing, "Pennsylvania must reorganize."[73] No school seeking to improve itself could now afford to ignore Flexner's dominant role in mustering support for change.

In the remaining schools of medicine (seventy-two had closed or merged since 1910), he continued his visits, conferred with leaders, and searched for ways to stimulate efforts at improvement. In all, a dozen more schools were given some help. Many but not all of these schools were in the South, where Flexner's deepest concerns lay. In the West, the University of Oregon was given $113,000 for a medical building and an additional amount for equipment and maintenance, while the University of Colorado, after a Flexner visit, was granted $700,000 for a restructured physical plant and equipment.[74] In the case of every grant, the local school agreed to raise an amount at least equal to that contributed by the Rockefeller philanthropies. None of these second-tier schools, as Flexner thought of them, was asked to adopt the full-time principle, and none received the kind of support given to Johns Hopkins, Vanderbilt, or Rochester.

A total of twenty-five schools were thus given some form of aid, nearly 40 percent of the sixty-six four-year medical schools still standing in the late 1920s. Still other schools were visited and given advice without immediate financial help. In the state legislatures, meanwhile, public appropriations for medical education began to climb. In his years at the General Education Board, Flexner had managed, as he had hoped, to build a loosely coordinated national system of medical schools in place of the "disjointed collection" of schools and hospitals of 1910.[75]

By the early 1920s his authority in matters medical was unquestioned. Every inquiry about medical education was directed to him. No board officer or member would respond to a request for aid or advice without consulting him. When Ray Lyman Wilbur, president of Stanford University (a physician and future secretary of the interior), sought to go around Flexner and appeal directly to Buttrick, the chairman told him: "It would not be wise for us to take this matter up in Dr. Flexner's absence . . . the Board would probably not be willing to take action without a specific report from him."[76]

With his growing influence, he became increasingly jealous of his prerogatives and place in the Rockefeller organization. The young Alan Gregg, then an assistant in the International Health Board of the Rockefeller Foundation, found him "terrifically jealous" of his job and of any apparent incursion on his domain. With Gates's departure Flexner's was the dominant personality among the Rockefeller officers. Few dared to cross him. While Flexner could display enormous tact and patience when necessary, Fosdick recalled that these traits were matched "by a formidable intransigence" and "his unfeigned joy in controversy [which] left behind some wounded spirits."[77] Privately, he took great pride in his achievement in medical education.

The fighting over full-time teaching took its toll. He sometimes wondered whether the struggle was worth the cost. Gradually, sometimes inconsistently, he retreated from his insistence on a strict definition of full-time—the board itself changed its policy formally in 1925—but he remained adamant in his belief that practice for pay, wherever permitted, was demeaning to academic medicine. If law schools were able to get the full attention of lawyers like Dean Roscoe Pound and Professor Felix Frankfurter, he asked, why was it so difficult for medical schools to secure the service of similarly gifted men? As a rule, he wrote President Eliot, clinicians did not have "the same scientific interest," nor did they appear to be made of "quite as stern stuff" as those who had created academic chemistry and academic pathology. In a similar vein, he wrote from Ann Arbor that the clinicians were a "mercenary lot," while the laboratory men were the real heroes of modern medicine.[78]

Beneath the surface, as Flexner was surely aware, currents were shifting in the world of Rockefeller philanthropy. While his authority in managing the vast medical education enterprise and in policy matters affecting secondary and higher education was still supreme, new concerns and new personalities were pushing policy in new directions. The Rockefeller charitable enterprises, once confined to the General Education Board, now included the Rockefeller Foundation, concerned with social and public health problems, founded in 1913; the Laura Spelman Rockefeller Memorial, devoted to the welfare of women and children, launched in 1918; the International Health Board (initially the International Health Division, created in 1909, and now an arm of the Rockefeller Foundation), which had waged an effective campaign against hookworm disease in the southern states; and Simon Flexner's Institute for Medical Research, established in 1902. Many of the objectives of the newer organizations overlapped those of the General Education Board; confusion and clashing personalities sparked turf wars over areas of responsibility; and leaders vied for promotion within the Rockefeller organizations. Staffs increased greatly in size, and Flexner complained privately of the growing "bureaucracy" that hindered swift decision making.

The old guard that Flexner had known so long was fading from the scene. Buttrick, his closest ally, was ailing and would leave the board in 1923; Gates was withdrawing more and more from board affairs; Eliot had ended his long service as a leading board member. By the early 1920s, the entire board was experiencing a major turnover. Rockefeller Jr., who had played so important a role in Flexner's career, was spending less time in hands-on involvement with the family's charities. Flexner's old friend and mentor, Pritchett, too, spent less and less time in Carnegie Foundation affairs. Among the men marked for larger roles in the Rockefeller organization were Wickliffe Rose, a classically trained, courtly southerner who had led the fight against hookworm disease; Richard M. Pearce, a Pennsylvania-trained physician who headed the division of medical education of the International Health Board (and who clashed often with Flexner); Trevor Arnett, an English-born authority on university finance who became a General Education Board officer in 1920; Edwin Embree, a southern-born champion of black education and equal rights who was the Rockefeller Foundation's first secretary and later its vice-president; and, most important of all, Fosdick, a long-time activist in progressive causes, who had replaced Frederick Gates as the Rockefeller family's closest adviser on philanthropy.

The impact of change first struck Flexner in 1923, when Buttrick retired from his leadership of the General Education Board. More than any other person, Buttrick had encouraged, defended, and appreciated Flexner's initiatives for more than a decade. Many expected that Flexner, his oldest and ablest partner, would succeed him, but the board turned instead to Wickliffe Rose, who, according to Fosdick, was "far more of an administrator than Flexner, far less impulsive, and perhaps with better poise and balance."[79] Flexner hid his disappointment stoically, claiming that he had no desire for an administrative appointment. But it was a sharp wound to his *amour propre.* Rose's policies would diverge sharply from his predecessor's, and Flexner found himself at times without the unquestioning support that had marked his first ten years at the board.

In his remaining years at the General Education Board, Flexner alternately struck out in new directions, tried to manage the vast medical education empire he had created, and became increasingly concerned about what his colleagues at 61 Broadway were doing.

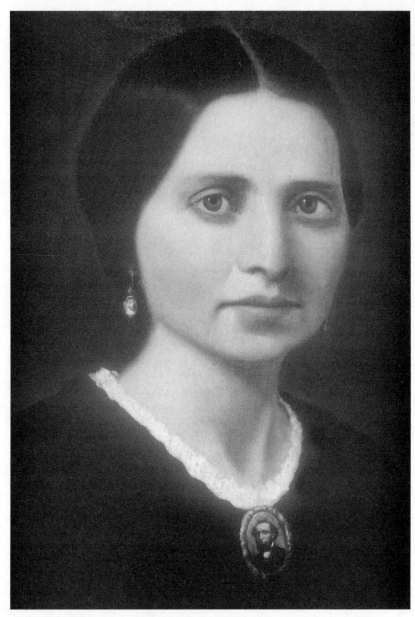

Esther Abraham Flexner. Courtesy M. Saleem Seyal, M.D.

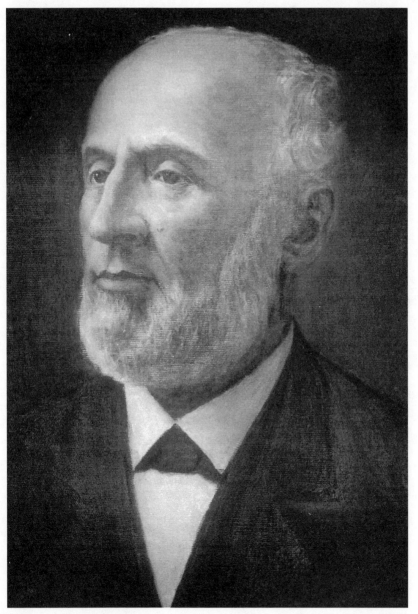

Moritz Flexner. Courtesy M. Saleem Seyal, M.D.

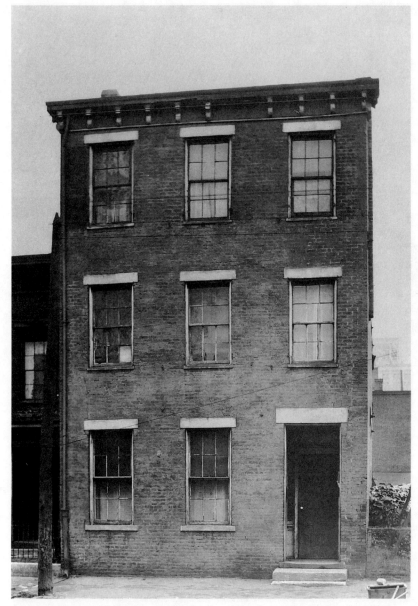

House at 669 Sixth Street where Abraham lived as a young boy. Used by permission of Seeley G. Mudd Manuscript Library, Princeton University.

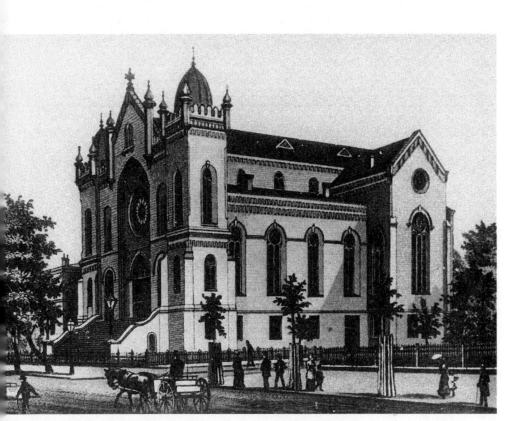

Temple Adath Israel. Courtesy Leo Loeb, Temple Adath Israel.

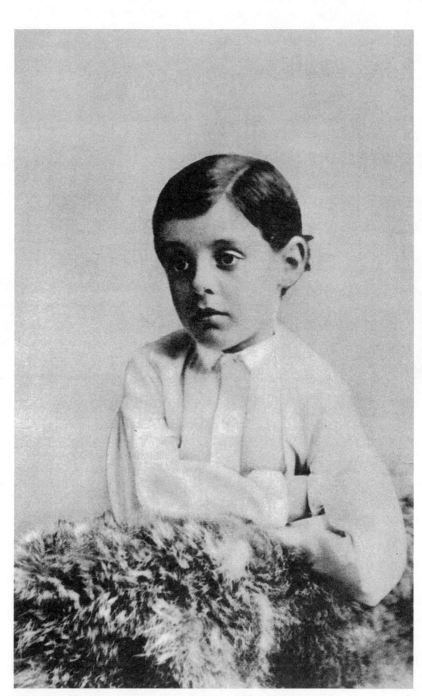

Abraham Flexner at age 7. Courtesy Harry Rosenberg.

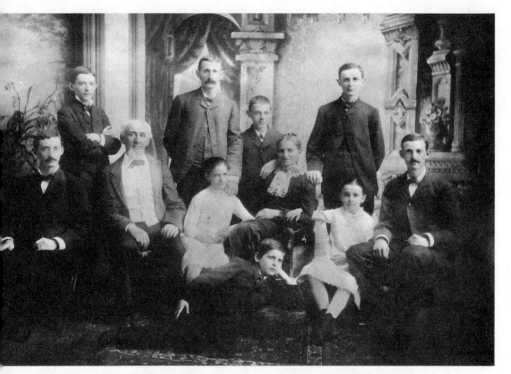

The Flexner Family in the early 1880s. Abraham is second from right *in the last row. Courtesy Harry Rosenberg.*

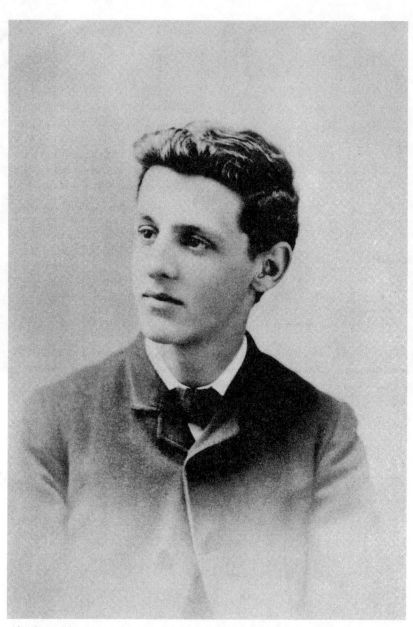

Abraham Flexner at age 17. Courtesy Eleanor Flexner Lewinson.

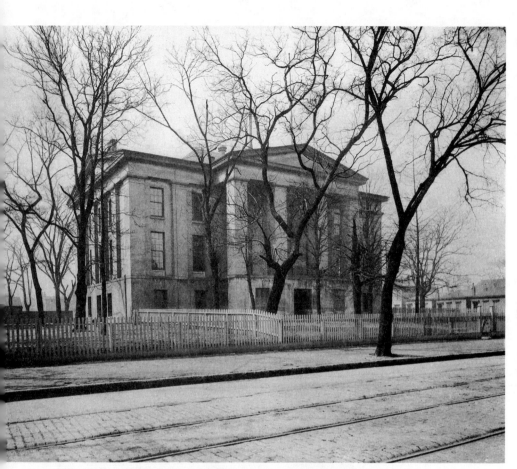

Louisville Male High School, c. 1880. Used by permission of Special Collections, Ekstrom Library, University of Louisville.

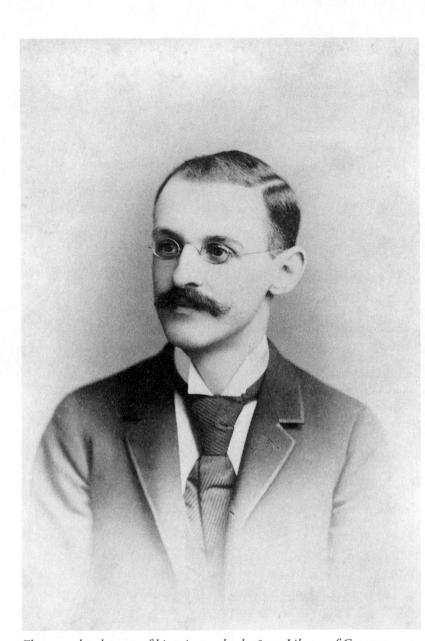

Flexner as headmaster of his private school, 1890s. Library of Congress.

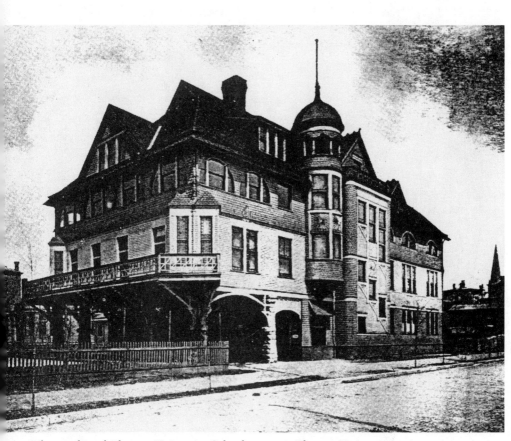

The combined Flexner-University School, c. 1906. Flexner-University School Catalog.

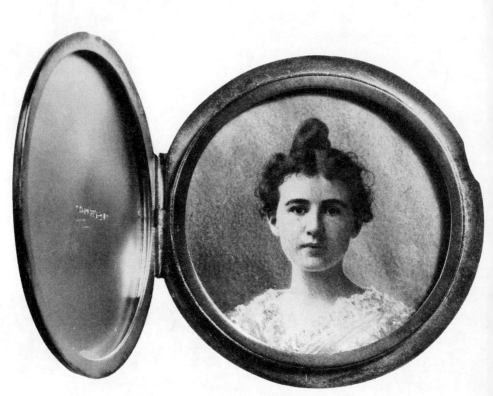

Anne Crawford Flexner. Used by permission of Arthur and Elizabeth Schlesinger Library, Radcliffe Institute.

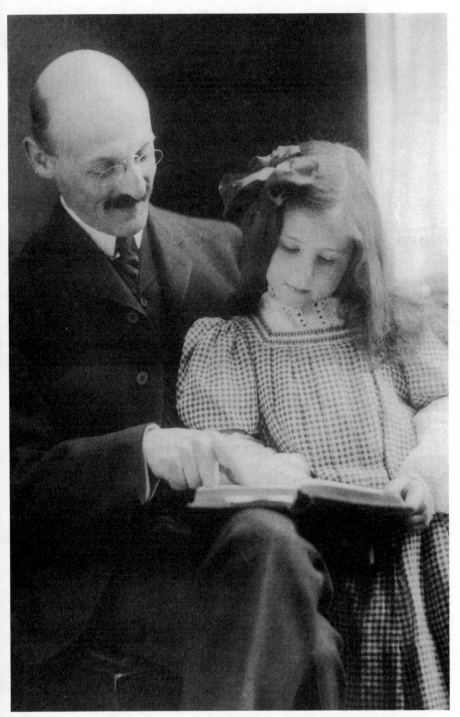

Flexner with daughter Jean, c. 1905. Courtesy Harry Rosenberg.

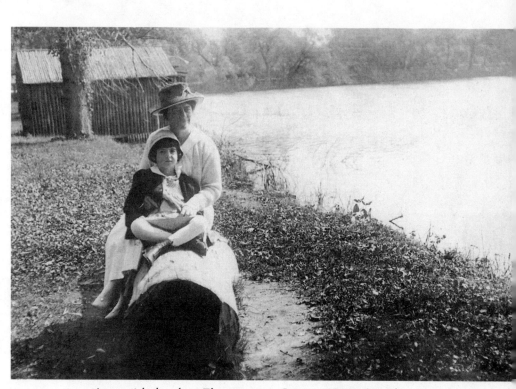

Anne with daughter Eleanor, 1916. Courtesy Harry Rosenberg.

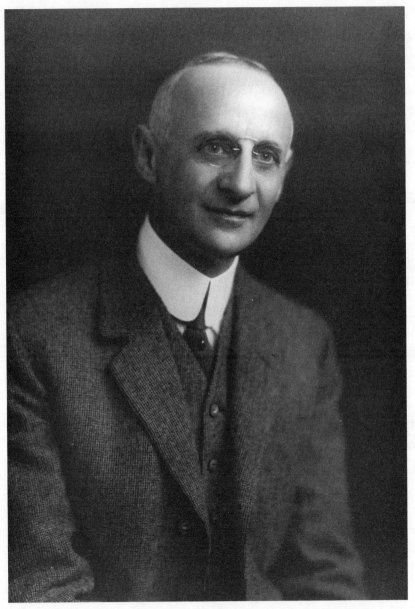

Simon Flexner. Used by permission of Alan Mason Chesney Medical Archives of the Johns Hopkins Medical Institutions.

WEANING TIME

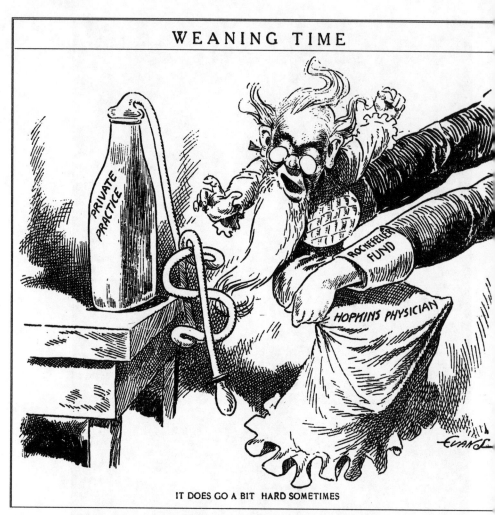

IT DOES GO A BIT HARD SOMETIMES

Cartoon depicting full-time teaching controversy at Johns Hopkins.
Baltimore American, *October 30, 1913.*

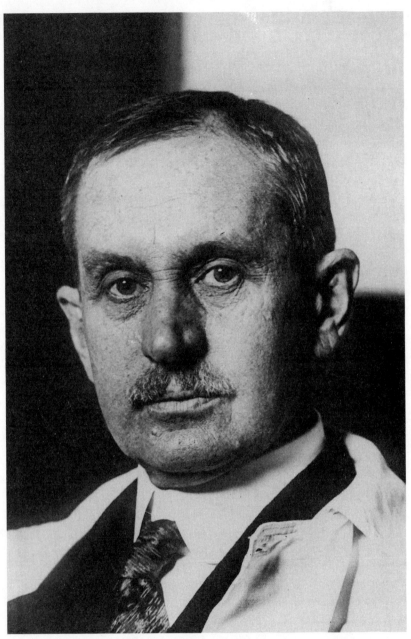

Franklin Mall. Used by permission of Alan Mason Chesney Medical Archives of the Johns Hopkins Medical Institutions.

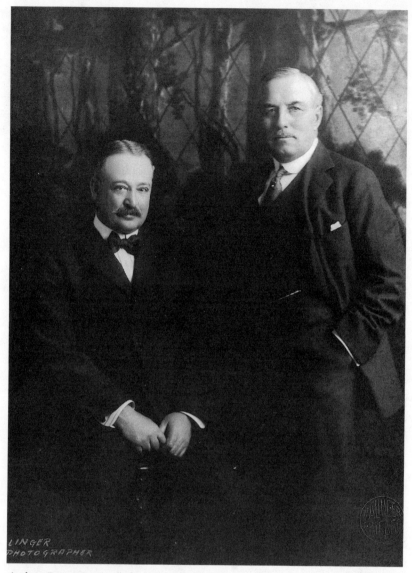

Arthur Dean Bevan (left) *and Frank Billings, titans of Chicago medicine. Used by permission of Rush Medical Center Archive.*

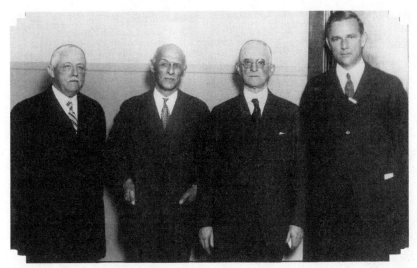

*Creators of the University of Rochester School of Medicine:
President Rush Rhees, Abraham Flexner, George Eastman, Dean George
Whipple. Used by permission of Department of Rare Books and Special
Collections, University of Rochester.*

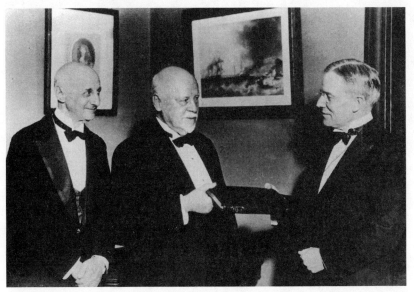

*Simon Flexner, William Henry Welch, John D. Rockefeller Jr. Courtesy
Rockefeller Archive Center.*

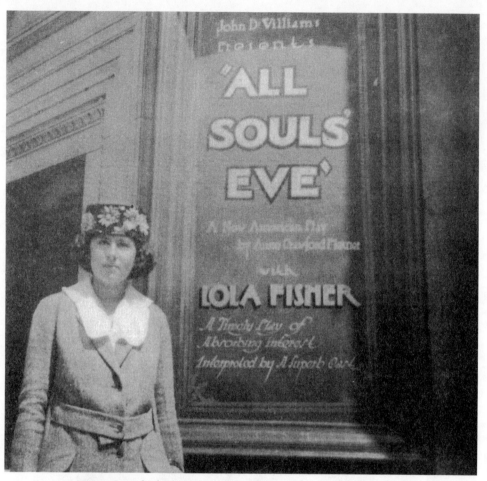

Anne Crawford Flexner at the opening of her play All Souls' Eve. *Courtesy Harry Rosenberg.*

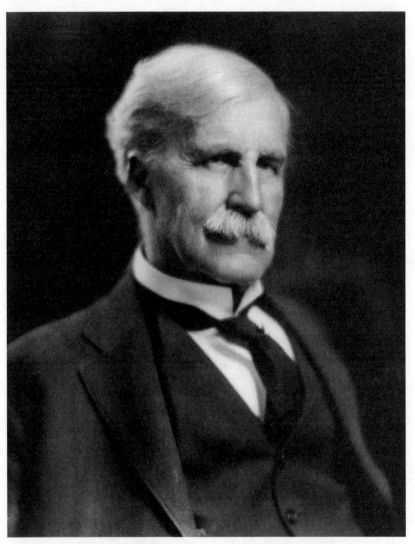

Frederick Gates, influential adviser to the Rockefellers and first chairman of the General Education Board. Courtesy Rockefeller Archive Center.

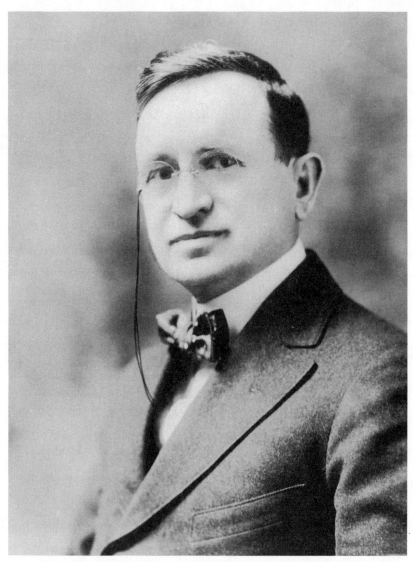

Wickliffe Rose, colleague and rival of Flexner's. Courtesy Rockefeller Archive Center.

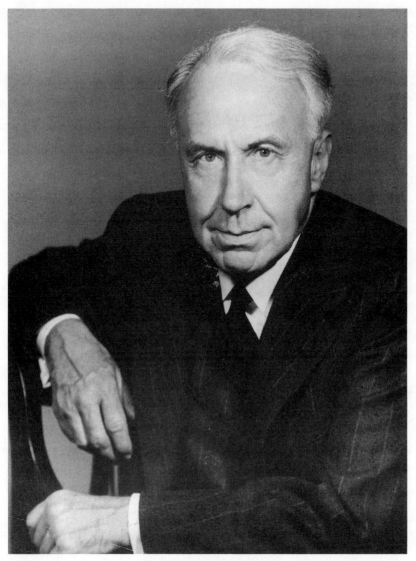

Raymond Fosdick, successor to Frederick Gates as principal Rockefeller adviser, and friend of Flexner's. Courtesy Rockefeller Archive Center.

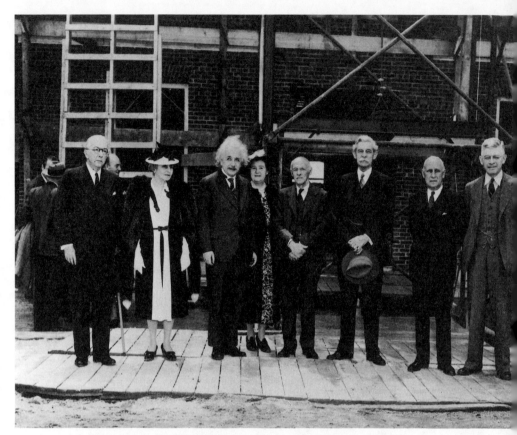

Dedication of Fuld Hall, Institute for Advanced Study, 1939.
Left to right: A. B. Houghton; C. Lavinia Bamberger, Albert Einstein,
Anne Flexner, Abraham Flexner, I. R. Hardin, Herbert Maass, H. W.
Dodds. Library of Congress.

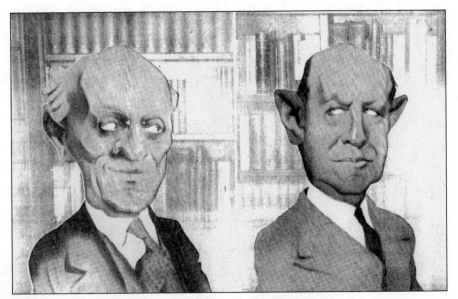

Caricatures of two famous sons of Louisville: Abraham Flexner (left) *and Frank Aydelotte* (right). Louisville Courier-Journal, *February 18, 1940. Courtesy M. Saleem Seyal, M.D.*

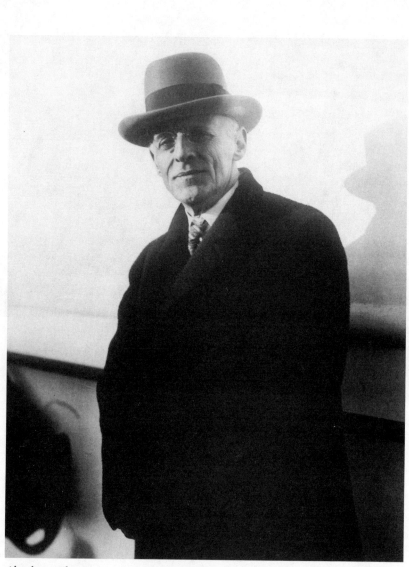

Abraham Flexner, c. 1928. Courtesy Becker Medical Library, Washington University School of Medicine.

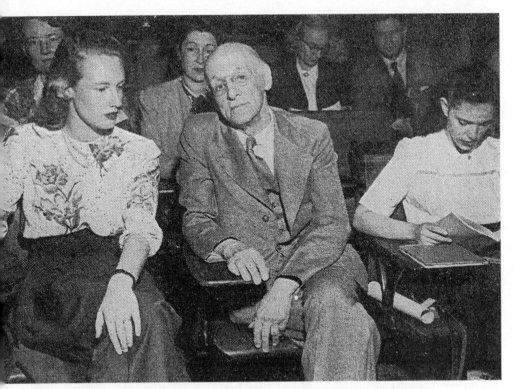

"*Student at 85: Dr. Abraham Flexner, author of the 1910 report which revolutionized American medical education, was 85 last week. The man who raised and spent $600,000,000 through the Rockefeller General Education Board and headed the Institute for Advanced Studies at Princeton sparks his 'retirement' with courses at Columbia, currently in European history and Soviet public administration.*" New York Times, November 26, 1951. Library of Congress.

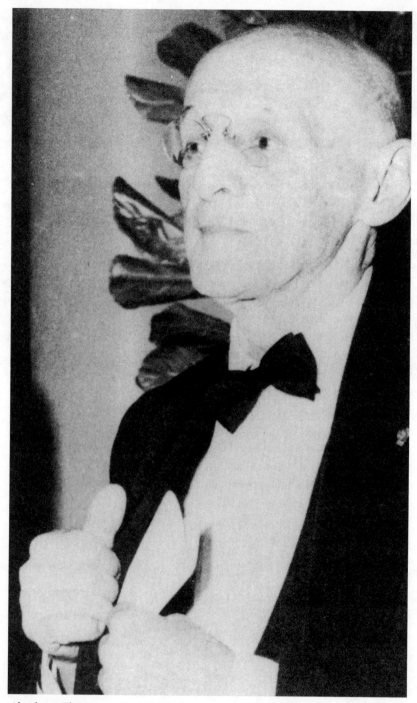

Abraham Flexner receives the Lahey Award in his ninetieth year. Courtesy Abraham Flexner Collection, University of Louisville.

9

A Fall from Olympus

Flexner's grueling work in reforming medical education brought new strains at home. The constant pressures made him more preoccupied, more irritable, and uncharacteristically short with his children. His daughters felt keenly the tension and conflict of these years. Not only was their father constantly busy and away from home for long periods, but their mother frequently made solo trips to Europe for six weeks or two months at a time. When they were together, Anne and Abraham quarreled over their competing commitments, money, and plans for the children.

For the children, the atmosphere at home, Eleanor remembered, was often "disturbing and upsetting." The parents seemed unaware of the effect that their bickering had on their daughters. Her mother seemed always to be in competition with her father, Eleanor said, and this was hard on both daughters. Both recalled that their father was still closer and more attuned to their needs than their mother. A cousin who saw the family in these years thought Anne did not have "the same feeling for family" as Abraham did.[1]

Anne continued to write and produce plays. She spent much time doing the work of the Dramatists Guild, and she started a new social center for actors and stage workers in the New York theater district. She seemed to her family less cheerful and less content with her life than she had been before. Throughout the twenties, she suffered from intermittent bouts of ill health and depression. Sometimes she found relief by taking long trips by herself. Her much-awaited play *All Souls' Eve,* her first in several years, opened in Washington in 1919, but the critics for the most part were not impressed and its run on Broadway was short.

She did not lack for money, however. The royalties from *Mrs. Wiggs* continued to flow in throughout the decade, and thanks to sound investments she was now a moderately wealthy woman. Her husband, however, thought her improvident in her free and casual expenditures and de-

spaired of her ever balancing her bank accounts. She bought two Maxwell
touring sedans—the only cars the Flexners ever owned—but neither she
nor her husband learned to drive. She also bought a remote summer camp
on Lake Ahmic in Canada, 175 miles north of Toronto, after the family
had rented it during the summer of 1920.[2] This proved to be a very wise
investment.

The camp, where Flexner spent virtually every summer for the rest of
his life, was an important part of their existence. The camp was quiet and
rustic—in the family's early years there, water had to be carried from the
lake or a nearby spring and privies were dug several hundred feet from the
house—and family tensions seemed to slacken there. Flexner was able to
relax, fish, swim, read, saw wood, and revel in the solitude. He and Anne,
as well as the children, each had separate cabins.

Frequently, interesting guests came for long stays—historian Allan
Nevins, violinist Efrem Zimbalist, Swarthmore College president Frank
Aydelotte, conductor William Strickland, deputy secretary to the British
cabinet Thomas Jones, and Oxford don E.L. Woodward. The neighbors
were all close friends—the Vanderbilt chancellor James Kirkland, espe-
cially, and a group from the Johns Hopkins School of Medicine: surgeon
Thomas Cullen, medical illustrator Max Brödel, and gynecologist How-
ard Kelly. Kelly often preached the Sunday sermon at a nearby church;
Flexner reported that he was long winded and stuck too closely to his text.
The friends came frequently together for an evening of games or live
music or an afternoon picnic or a fishing party.[3] The camp was a part of
Flexner's life unlike any other, and he cherished it for the rest of his days.
He continued to go there until his ninetieth year.

His two daughters were growing up. In the fall of 1917, Jean was sent
off to Bryn Mawr College, where his sister Mary had enrolled thirty years
before. An excellent student, she majored in economics. Her teachers considered her highly intelligent, dutiful, and ambitious. In her father's mind
there was never any question that both she and Eleanor would lead independent lives. "I want you to lead your own life," he wrote; "I watch you
. . . with confidence . . . with hopes that I hardly dare to let myself formulate." You must know French and German, he told her; you should try
not to overemphasize the study of the past; you must read John Maynard
Keynes's "corking" new book on *The Economic Consequences of the Peace;*
you should seek out the very best places for postgraduate study.[4]

On graduation from Bryn Mawr, she was encouraged by her father to
go to England for further study. At Cambridge University, her father told

her, she would come to know many world-famous scholars. Her interest in labor history and economics, begun at Bryn Mawr, was whetted by a holiday visit to the London School of Economics, where Harold Laski, a leading socialist intellectual, persuaded her to transfer her studies. Her father approved. "The more contact you have with the live wires," her father assured her, "extreme though they may be, the better in the long run."[5]

At the London School, she read Karl Marx, visited trade union officials and leading socialists, and heard lectures by such well-known figures as Sidney Webb, R.H. Tawney, and Graham Wallas. She became active in politics. In the parliamentary election of 1922, she campaigned for Tawney in a run-down slum district in north London. When her father came to visit, they had long discussions about her studies, and he told her that their shared interests meant that they would be even closer friends as adults. He found time to go over her thesis, entitled "Workers' Control in Industry." She reported that he was an incomparable teacher who showed her how to write more "clearly and forcefully, as no teacher of composition had ever done."[6] Later in the decade she would earn a doctorate in labor economics at the Brookings School in Washington, an institution for advanced study founded by her father's old friend Robert Brookings.

Eleanor, nine years younger than Jean, was still an adolescent in the early 1920s. Her father was never as close to her as to Jean. Too young to be a companion to her sister, left for long periods with housekeepers and governesses, Eleanor was less outgoing than Jean, more temperamental, and less interested in her parents' doings and friends. She suffered from rheumatic fever as a child and resented her parents' and teachers' concern that she not "overdo." The two sisters got along badly. Yet she recalled that when her mother was neglectful of her and she had to go to school in "middy blouses," it was Jean who took her shopping and bought her clothes. She came to believe that she was neglected as a child and that this accounted for her later resentments and bouts of depression. In New York, she went to the Lincoln School, where she enjoyed the atmosphere of unusual freedom. Her parents assured her that she would go to college "and be president of the United States in due course!" Unlike Jean, she was deemed unruly and "rambunctious" by her teachers. She thought they treated her more harshly than others out of fear they would be accused of favoring the school founder's daughter.

When she graduated in 1926, she went, at her father's suggestion, to

Swarthmore College. Flexner had earlier given General Education Board support to President Aydelotte's innovative honors program. "I went to Swarthmore," she later wrote, "because obviously it was the best and . . . how could they turn me down?" During her college years and after, influenced by her mother's career, she became involved in the theater, finding part-time jobs in stage work and other tasks. For all her resentment at the lack of attention while growing up, she was fond of her father and realized that he had "an enormous influence" on her. He, in turn, never doubted that Eleanor would find her way and win distinction in her life. Of her and Jean he wrote proudly in 1924, "Yes, they are *truly* vital persons and will, I believe, lead useful lives. They just vibrate with *interests*."[7]

The busy Flexner saw less of his brothers and sisters as he grew older. Only Simon, now at the peak of his power and influence at the Rockefeller Institute, remained close to him. Both now lived in New York, worked for Rockefeller philanthropies, and shared countless interests in developments in American medicine. Each consulted the other about important decisions in their lives, read each other's manuscripts, and corresponded or talked by telephone several times each week. Fortunately for the biographer, most contact was by mail, which was delivered twice daily within the city. A note from one would sometimes be answered on the same day.

Abraham was immensely proud of his brother, who enjoyed even more than he the confidence of the Rockefellers, Frederick T. Gates, and influential leaders in medicine and education. Compared with Abraham, Simon was far less combative, more self-controlled and unobtrusive. He was essentially shy and modest, with no hint of arrogance or complacency. He made no enemies. His achievement in creating a world-renowned center of medical research, his uncanny ability to recruit researchers of promise, and his insistence on harmony among his coworkers had won him unrivaled respect and admiration in the worlds of medicine and philanthropy.[8]

A leader who kept in close touch with his coworkers, he tried to free them from busywork that interfered with research, while keeping up himself an impressive record of investigation. It was he who developed an antiserum for cerebral spinal meningitis in 1907. Later he demonstrated that polio was an infectious disease caused by a distinctive virus. Small wonder that Gates, John D. Rockefeller Jr., Raymond Fosdick, and other Rockefeller officers thought him the most valuable and indispensable of all Rockefeller employees. "If the Trustees of the Rockefeller Foundation had any sense," Gates told Fosdick, "they would give their entire capital fund to the Rockefeller Institute to be spent at the discretion of Simon Flexner."[9]

A third brother, Bernard, was almost as well known in New York as Simon and Abraham. He had come to New York in 1919 after spending seven years in Chicago as general counsel to the utilities magnate Samuel Insull. He had taken a deep interest in the problems of neglected children and was a national authority on juvenile courts. He was counsel to countless liberal movements, including campaigns for workers' compensation and employers' liability for accidents. During the First World War, he was sent by the Red Cross to Romania, where he saw firsthand the wretched conditions faced by many European Jews.

What he found there, he later wrote, shook him "as nothing else in [his] life had done." He realized that he could not be indifferent to the problems of the European Jews.[10] After learning of the British government's Balfour Declaration, which promised Jews a homeland in Palestine, he became a Zionist. At the urging of Louis D. Brandeis (an old acquaintance from Louisville) and Felix Frankfurter, another friend, Bernard returned to Paris in 1919 as counsel to the Zionist delegation at the peace conference.

In Paris, the question of Palestine's future began to consume him. Ahead, he believed, lay "the most trying period" in history for the European Jews. It fell to him to draft the final proposals on the status of Palestine, arguing for a British mandate rather than a Jewish state; the time was not yet ripe, he believed, for an independent state. Upon his return and throughout the 1920s he threw himself into the Zionist cause. In 1925, in what was his most important contribution to the movement, he organized the Palestine Economic Corporation with the help of banker Felix M. Warburg, prominent lawyer Louis Marshall, and future governor of New York Herbert H. Lehmann. The aim of the corporation, he announced, was to promote land development, town planning, new industries, and power development in Palestine.[11]

Of all the Flexners, Bernard was the only one to identify so deeply with his Jewish heritage and to become a leader in Jewish causes. Abraham thought his brother's crusade quixotic, writing a friend, "For the life of me I cannot really believe that the creation of a Jewish state will achieve the good that is expected by the Zionists or that it will do the damage feared by those of a different mind."[12] Although he often saw Bernard socially, Abraham was never as close to him as to Simon.

Abraham reached his sixtieth birthday in 1926. Still remarkably energetic, he was in generally good health except for winter colds and bouts of flu. An article in the *Louisville Courier-Journal* described him as a "small-sized man with a great wide dome of a forehead, a vigorous manner, an active intellect, and every bit of the Flexner capacity for long and patient analysis." Unlike many of his contemporaries, according to the reporter, he was not eager to talk to the press and wanted to stay in the background.[13]

Others found him friendly but distant. The only woman officer at 61 Broadway in these years, Florence Hind, thought him the friendliest of all the men around her. Often he came into her office, she said, and frequently he joined her on the subway ride going home. Once, when they were standing in the aisle, he told her a joke and then put his head on her shoulder, shaking with laughter. "He was always ready to laugh," she remembered. She remarked, too, on his persuasive skills, especially in small groups, though he did not often take part in informal discussions or meetings. He was, she said, a good friend and always "a great joy" to encounter.[14] His personality, it seemed, had not greatly changed. He was both outgoing and private, determined and self-assured, provocative and good-humored. He often seemed to prefer the company of women and bright young people to that of men his own age. Perhaps he was better able to relax and be himself with them than he was with his peers.

His work habits and interests changed little. He kept long hours, worked largely alone, and guarded his time. He continued to prefer conducting personal inspections to reading written reports. He kept up a keen interest in national and world affairs and read widely in history, politics, biography, and the ancient classics. He made scores of friends as he moved across the country, but, except for Wallace Buttrick, he made few close friends among his colleagues. A man of great pride and sensitivity, he continued to shun publicity and public praise. Where others saw him as aggressive or uncompromising, he pictured himself, as the historian Daniel Fox has perceptively written, as "a humble servant of power."[15]

He never acknowledged, even in his autobiography, the great influence he exerted across the spectrum of American learning. Even the initiatives in medical teaching came not from him, he insisted, but from the schools themselves. He was only a "facilitator," an "agent of change." A dutiful humility prevented him from acknowledging a powerful sense of achievement. He claimed instead that he had pursued only "an opportunistic course": "I got what I wanted, because I reduced what I wanted to what I believed I could get."[16] In this he resembled Simon and other members of the family who had early learned to shun the ancient sins of pride and self-promotion.

With Buttrick's retirement, Flexner became more of a lone operator than ever before. He occupied a special place in the Rockefeller philanthropies; he was a legendary figure greatly admired and respected but left largely alone and feared by many of his younger colleagues. He still had— or claimed—a "roving commission" that mocked the boundaries being established among the growing number of Rockefeller enterprises. He acted as if nothing had changed since his early days at 61 Broadway.

Increasingly, he came into conflict with his new chief, Wickliffe Rose, and with the head of the medical education division of the International Health Board, Richard Pearce. A former assistant to Simon Flexner, Pearce was responsible for grants in medical education outside the United States. Rose, as a condition for accepting the presidency of the General Education Board, had insisted on the creation of still another board, the International Education Board, with wide-ranging powers, which he also headed. Flexner, who had roamed widely over medical and educational policies both at home and abroad since his days at the Carnegie Foundation, now found himself hemmed in at times by the confusing and overlapping jurisdictions around him.

The self-effacing but persistent Rose, like Flexner, had won the favor of the younger Rockefeller. He had his own goals for the General Education Board and the new International Education Board, and they differed from Flexner's. With an initial grant of twenty-eight million dollars from the Rockefellers, the new education board was given the power to support projects of all kinds in countries around the world, including the United States. Rose's chief priority, he made clear, was the cultivation of science, especially basic research in the physical sciences. "Make the peaks higher" became his slogan as major grants were given to the California Institute of Technology, the giant telescope at Mount Palomar in California, and the Marine Biological Laboratory and Oceanographic Institution at Woods Hole, Massachusetts. He was responsible, too, for research grants to such promising scientists as Niels Bohr, J. Robert Oppenheimer, and Enrico Fermi. The new board, while useful, Flexner wrote derisively, was "not an education board" but "mainly a scientific research board."[17]

The work of the General Education Board, on the other hand, especially the endowment of promising colleges and universities, was coming to an end, Rose believed. The original principal as well as interest from the early grants had begun to shrivel. Although he made no mention of medical schools, the grants for their support, too, were dwindling as the board, in accord with the original understanding, spent principal as well as interest. Flexner saw the handwriting on the wall and began to spread his interests to other educational initiatives.

Despite the fact that Europe was clearly within Pearce's jurisdiction, Flexner kept up a strong interest in European universities and medical schools. The unaggressive but sensitive Pearce made known his resentment at Flexner's intervention in his bailiwick. "The essential fact," said Alan Gregg, who was then working for Pearce, "was that Abe didn't have a great deal of interest or respect for Pearce's mind or Pearce's ability" and did very little to conceal his attitude.[18] Unlike Flexner, Pearce had little love of Germany and developed a passionate dislike for the German professors he encountered.

Soon after the war Flexner had begun to return to those places, especially Germany, where he had spent so much of his early career. Berlin, he wrote in 1922, "is a sad, sad place . . . It is like a stricken city." The plight of the sciences in Germany he described as "deplorable." "If the work of destruction is not halted," he warned, "the finest intellectual organ ever created will be lost to civilization." At the Kaiser Wilhelm Institute in Berlin he found conditions "distressing beyond words." The best scientists in Germany were living "from hand to mouth." The renowned clinician Friedrich von Müller of Munich could not afford to ride in a streetcar, and his official trips by train had all to be taken in third class.[19]

Unbidden, Flexner prepared a plan to help medical science in the German universities, advising Pearce and George Vincent, president of the Rockefeller Foundation, of the urgency of the situation. He sent long and detailed reports back to the New York offices. While acknowledging to Pearce that he had no authority to speak for the foundation, he nevertheless discussed with German officials the best ways to help. He told Pearce that at least seventy-five thousand dollars was needed immediately to support such key scientists as physical chemist Fritz Haber, anatomist Heinrich Poll, physiologist Emil Aberhalden, and physicist Max Born. On his own initiative, he sought out the American ambassador, Alanson Houghton, later a close friend and chairman of the board of Flexner's Institute for Advanced Study, and won his support for his proposal. As the pressure built for Rockefeller aid, Pearce found himself following rather than leading the rescue effort in Germany. The news contained in Flexner's reports was so "horrendous," Gregg reported, that Pearce was forced to go and see for himself.[20]

As Flexner hurried back and forth across the Atlantic, he kept up a strong interest in European politics and what was happening at home. Often he showed keen insight into events. His views were generally those of a liberal internationalist who believed that Wilson had made crucial mistakes in the postwar era. The president's call for a Democratic Congress in a time when unity was needed he thought "extraordinarily foolish," an act that made certain "the worst possible interpretation" of a negative outcome. Wilson's subsequent failure to name any leading Republicans to the peace delegation he described as "the most amazing example of egotism in all history." With the election of Warren Harding in 1920, Flexner lost all hope for serious U.S. involvement in the postwar world. When awakened by Anne with news of Harding's triumph, he said, "I wanted to go back to sleep again, which is just what the country will do during his administration . . . He is utterly commonplace."[21]

In the postwar world he saw only cataclysmic change. In China, revolutionary Russia, the Balkans, central Europe, and the Middle East, the world was being remade. The Versailles Treaty, he wrote in 1922, "will rank in history as the most idiotic performance ever perpetuated by men." The children of the warring nations could have done "infinitely better." The treaty would lead surely to future conflict, he wrote, because the terms were so severe that they would produce "social and political revolution." Let future historians debate the "moral guilt" of the war, he advised; for now, everyone should remember the words of Grant when he met Lee: "Let us have peace."[22]

Events in Russia seemed beyond explanation or prophecy. The success of the Bolsheviks, he predicted, would not only destroy Russia but be used in Germany to discredit social democracy, thus giving a boost to nationalist and reactionary forces in the former Reich. With the rise of "the wild doings of Mussolini" in Italy in 1922, he likened the Duce's fascism to soviet communism, telling his daughter that "the acme of intolerance" could always be found in "the *extreme* groups." Safety from oppression was found only in the middle, he wrote, "where people vote, talk, are inefficient, to be sure, as popular governments are—but they are *secure*—they go on regardless of individuals."[23]

At home he worried about the postwar fear of radicals. He criticized bitterly the action of the New York legislature in expelling five socialist members. "A more silly and outrageous folly I never heard of! As though it were a crime to *believe* in Socialism!"[24]

Sometime in 1921 or 1922, after several Atlantic crossings, he quietly decided on his next project: he would write a book about the changes in medical education in Europe and America since his reports of a decade before.[25] It was to be a comparative and historical study of how doctors were educated on both sides of the Atlantic. Unlike his earlier studies, it would be not an official report for his employer, but a personal account for which he would seek a commercial publisher. It is a measure of his independence that he sought no approval from any of the foundation officers at 61 Broadway, although he almost certainly told them of his plans. His goal, he said, was to create a definitive analysis that would guide the postwar reconstruction of medical education.

His method was the tried-and-true one of exhaustive travel, personal interviews, and direct observation. While he spent most of his time in Great Britain, France, and Germany, he also visited medical schools in a number of the smaller European countries. Everywhere he had close contact with medical and educational leaders, most of whom knew of his earlier work. At Cambridge, a dozen senior clinicians met with him to review the changes since his testimony before the Haldane Commission. In London, physiologist Ernst Starling told a dinner group that nothing had changed since Flexner's earlier reports. He spent several long sessions with Sir George Newman, the chief medical officer of both the National Board of Education and the Ministry of Health. No one in postwar Britain championed more ardently than Newman the university standard of medical education, which Flexner favored, and Britain's need to emulate recent changes in the United States.[26]

In France and Germany, he was likewise well known in medical circles. Hamburg anatomist Heinrich Poll went so far as to circulate the sections of Flexner's 1912 study relating to Germany in advance of his visit.[27]

He worked intermittently at the book, returning frequently to the United States to deal with other tasks. In all, he spent eight months in study and travel before beginning to write in the summer of 1924. Even before he wrote the first sentence, he was invited by the American Medical Association's Council on Medical Education to report on his findings. At a March 1924 session in Chicago, he attempted a preliminary portrait of what had happened in medical education since his earlier work for the Carnegie Foundation.

There had been no real change, he told the council members, in the European schools. He found some signs that Germany's and Austria's medical schools were beginning to recover from the war. The prewar weaknesses of German medical training—too much emphasis on theory, too much lecturing, classes of staggering size, little bedside experience—persisted and were in fact more serious. There seemed to be no plan to implement the thoroughgoing reforms needed to make German education "more practical." Medical teaching in France, on the other hand, was still almost entirely practical and lacked strong programs in preclinical science. Conditions in French medical schools were "quite stationary," except for Strasbourg, taken from the Germans, which was France's first modern medical school plant. In Great Britain, some changes had been made. The British government was now supporting medical research, and Rockefeller Foundation grants had made possible the appointment of the first full-time teachers of medicine and surgery. But British medical training, in his view, was still on the whole far too practical.

Only in America had there been a real change in medical training. Progress in the United States, he told the council, was "enormously greater" than anywhere else. It affected "every item that goes to make up a medical school." But there were still "great gaps" on the clinical side of the American school, as well as in the preparation of medical students in the "utterly chaotic" high schools and colleges. Teaching in the clinics of America, with few exceptions, was still the work of busy practitioners. In the entire country, he charged, no common meaning could be found as to what constituted a high school education. Beyond that, he added, "What two years of college mean, I defy anybody to say." Both the high school and college were "trying to be all things to everybody."

Democracy, he insisted once more, need not be "synonymous with intellectual mediocrity and inferiority." As for medical schools, the "truly excellent" were still very much in the minority. Even the best showed no imagination. The uniformity of their curricula was "nothing short of an absurdity." Why should the four-year course not be broken up and the notion abandoned that there is only one way to train a physician? Change was coming, but it would take "twenty or thirty or forty years" before it was realized.[28]

His book, *Medical Education: A Comparative Study*, published by Macmillan in 1925, was a serious work of pedagogy expounding on these themes. The major Western systems of preparing doctors he described as divided into three basic types: (1) the practical or clinical type native to France and England, which had grown out of the hospital; (2) the university type developed in Germany, Scandinavia, Holland, and German-speaking Switzerland, which owed much to the fusion of the scientific research of the university with clinical teaching; and (3) the discredited commercial type, cut off from both hospitals and universities, which had started because America needed more doctors than the facilities of that era could train.

Each nation's medical training had its peculiarities. In France, the student was sent into the wards immediately on beginning medical study, and clinical subjects dominated the curriculum. In Britain, likewise, the stress was on the practical and the useful, with students spending two full years or more on clinical teaching. But in Germany much more emphasis was placed on the medical sciences and on the university's responsibility for scientific training. Only the last made sense, Flexner believed, in a time of scientific medicine. By contrast, the faculty of a French medical school, he wrote of the clinical approach to medicine, was made up of a group of practicing physicians and surgeons, who were engaged in training apprentices. French medical training was in no sense university study.[29]

Throughout the book, he repeated his theme of a quarter-century before: the importance of inductive teaching. "Active participation—doing things—is . . . the fundamental note of medical teaching." Students must relate what they see and do to general scientific laws or principles. The teacher thus has two tasks—to teach students to perceive facts and to teach them, further, to generalize about them. "If the student is told too much at the start, he learns generalizations passively or prematurely . . . whereas if he does not get beyond the scope of his own senses, his education . . . will be deficient in depth and comprehensiveness." In the strictest sense, Flexner maintained, all learning was self-learning. Teachers might stimulate or inspire, but "students *learn* more than they are *taught*." The medical school could not begin to produce fully trained doctors; it could only introduce them to the methods of scientific medicine and thus make them "active learners."[30]

Lectures and demonstrations alone never trained the senses or created the ability to generalize. "If the student is to learn how to examine a patient, how to draw an induction . . . how to observe the course of disease . . . he must himself participate continuously in the process, not often enough to acquire skill (that comes only with years), but often enough to learn how." The laboratory and the clinic in this respect were no different. Medicine and surgery were taught just as anatomy and physiology and pathology were taught, that is, by using the eyes, ears, and fingers at the bedside to procure data just as the same senses were used in the laboratory to sort out data and proceed to induction.[31]

Real education, Flexner believed, took place in small groups: it was tailored to individuals, well supported, and expensive. From the organization of his school in Louisville to the launching of the Institute for Advanced Study in 1930, Flexner insisted that learning proceeded best where classes were small, students were carefully selected, and teachers were committed to their students. Only the state or private wealth could supply the abundant resources necessary for the kind of instruction that Flexner admired. Such instruction, he believed, should not be reserved for the wealthy or privileged. In his heart of hearts, he hoped to see the virtues of the class-bound European schools forced into an American equalitarian mold.

The book was an intellectual and pedagogical triumph. No comparable book, as reviewers pointed out, was available in any language. It strengthened Flexner's reputation as the dominant figure in medical education not only in the United States but to a considerable extent in Europe as well. Scores of letters, most of them favorable, from European medical educators flooded into the offices at 61 Broadway.

Soon the book was translated into French and German, receiving favorable reviews in both countries. In Paris an unusually long and critical account, spread over two issues, was featured in *La presse medicale*. From Germany, William Henry Welch reported that the renowned anatomist Wilhelm His had told him of the "immense influence" the book was having on medical education in that country. "To think of an American exerting this kind of influence in Germany," he wrote Flexner, "is to me quite thrilling, and I want Simon and everybody to know—you would never tell them." The British medical journal *Lancet* editorialized that "every thinking man" had to be grateful to Flexner for his insights into medical education in Britain. At home, a *New York Times* writer described him as the one person who "more than any other" was the real crusader in the movement to reform medical teaching.[32]

Friends and colleagues, many of whom had read drafts of the book, added to the praise. Fosdick said that copies of the work ought to be put at "the disposal of professional men the world over." From Baltimore, Dean Lewis Weed wrote that reading the book had converted him to "a more liberal interpretation" of the "lock-step curriculum." Most gratifying of all to Flexner was praise from his old friend and sometime critic, Henry Pritchett, who wrote him that it was "a stunning piece of work" that would "clarify thinking about medical education the world over." "I am proud to have a friend and colleague," he told Flexner, who is capable of such a "masterly" accomplishment. It was a shame, said Pritchett, that Flexner was wasting his time on office details when he could turn out "this sort of thing."[33]

The book brought into focus a number of Flexner's concerns about the direction in which American medical schools were moving. The medical curriculum, he was convinced, was becoming far too rigid and standardized, giving students too little freedom to follow their own interests. As early as 1913 he had warned that the typical medical school closed "down upon the enterprising student . . . with an exhausting and depressing uniformity." In 1921, he had told Harvey Cushing that the imposition of rigid standards by accrediting groups was making the medical curriculum "a monstrosity."[34] Now he wrote that students moved "through medical school in tight lock step, and ha[d] little time to stop, read, work or think." They were "grouped in fixed classes . . . they followed in fixed order, day by day, the same subjects, for the same length of time, in the same year and at the same hour." Future doctors should be educated "by steeping themselves thoroughly in a few subjects, not by nibbling at many."

Of the growing standardization of the American curriculum he could think of nothing "more alien" to the spirit of scientific medicine or to university life. Medical school leaders, intimidated by state licensing boards and the American Medical Association, were not making needed changes. He urged deans and other policymakers to relax requirements, allow more electives, and show more imagination. To David Edsall at Harvard he wrote: "I need not tell you that I favor latitude" in setting requirements. He pressured the faculties at Columbia and Cornell to break up the fixed four-year plan and "encourage students to develop themselves." In a memorandum prepared for a group of medical educators in 1925, he suggested not only giving students more "free time" but allowing students, as in Europe, to drop out for a year to pursue "special studies" or to spend the time at another medical school.[35]

Flexner was concerned, too, about the impact of rigid standards on the remaining schools for African Americans. Throughout the twenties, he carried on a battle with the Council on Medical Education over the education of people of color. The problem was acute. Only two medical schools for blacks, Meharry Medical College and Howard University Medical School, remained to serve a population of twelve million African Americans in the segregated society of that day.

The two schools graduated a total of only one hundred students annually. Even these few could not find internships in the small number of hospitals open to them. Only a handful of black students, fewer than ten a year, graduated from the nation's other medical colleges. The vast majority of schools accepted no blacks. Not a single state in the 1920s gave support to their medical education. In a period of crisis, Flexner believed, it fell upon the foundations and on himself to try to keep alive the remaining schools for blacks. Black physicians themselves understood the role that Flexner played. "We are making our final appeal to you as the most potent representative of the medical profession in America," wrote a spokesman for the National Medical Association, an organization of black physicians, "and also as the Financial Agent whose word is final in such matters."[36]

Of the two black schools, Meharry had the more serious problems. It had been dropped to Class B status in 1914 by the Council on Medical Education. This action threatened the very survival of the school. In states whose licensing boards made Class A ranking a requirement for licensure, the school's graduates could not practice.

In letter after letter to the council, to American Medical Association officials, and to allies like Pritchett and Julius Rosenwald, Flexner argued the injustice of the association's position. "I cannot but think," he wrote Pritchett, "that Meharry is as good an *A* school for the Negro race as half a dozen institutions or more rated *A* for whites." The top-ranked schools in the association's classification, he maintained, were simply the best schools in their regions. The list of Class A schools, he reminded N.P. Colwell, the council's secretary, ranged from Harvard and Johns Hopkins to such weak schools as the University of Buffalo and Emory University. Why not do with the black schools, he asked, what the council was "plainly doing" with white medical schools—varying its standards according to local and regional considerations?[37]

While the General Education Board regarded Howard as the federal government's responsibility, Flexner nevertheless was responsible for several grants to Howard for buildings and endowment. In the case of Meharry, Flexner worked to restore its "A" ranking and to keep the school from closing. A new president, John J. Mullowney, was installed with the General Education Board's blessing in 1921. Mullowney, who had been a missionary in China, saw his work at Meharry as similar to his work in China. He was "greatly impressed," he said, by what Flexner had written about the importance of increasing the number of black physicians.[38]

The problems Mullowney faced were enormous: buildings long past repair, staircases and banisters broken, a library of only 2,500 books, meager laboratory equipment, ill-trained teachers, and a hospital where "asepsis was entirely absent" and where surgery was carried out in "cramped, infectious surroundings."[39] A program of fund-raising and a $150,000 grant by the General Education Board enabled him to renovate several buildings, improve the hospital, and revive morale. Entrance standards were more strictly enforced, and several faculty members were replaced.

Before Mullowney's first year was out, the council's secretary wrote that more improvements had been made during that year than in all the years since the first inspection visit of 1906. Mullowney's relationship with Flexner was important in his efforts at fund-raising. Flexner helped arrange substantial gifts to Meharry from Julius Rosenwald, George Eastman, and Edward Harkness. Steady support continued to come, too, from the General Education Board, so much so that Fosdick called the school "the Board's medical god-child." In time, the total gifts reached more than eight million dollars.[40] It was no surprise when in 1923, nine years after assigning the school Class B status, the council restored Meharry to Class A status.

In one more way Flexner sought to bring new strength to teaching and learning in the black schools. Both Meharry and Howard had difficulty retaining white teachers with superior qualifications, and the schools' graduates had no opportunity for advanced training. Where were teachers to come from? In 1919 Flexner approached Rosenwald, now a close friend, with a proposal that a graduate of Meharry be supported for a year of postgraduate study at a leading medical school and then be sent to the Rockefeller Institute for research experience. In the ensuing discussions, as Rosenwald's interest grew, Flexner suggested that the program be extended to as many as six "workers" in the fundamental medical sciences. During the summer he recruited Welch, Edsall, and Michigan dean Victor Vaughan to serve as a selection committee. He would himself serve as secretary to the committee.[41]

Later in the year he sounded out the members about adding a black physician to the group, suggesting, "It is very important to cooperate with the Negro rather than to do things for him." The response, however, was not enthusiastic. Edsall warned that "an unsatisfactory type" of man might "do harm" by taking the committee's deliberations back to the black community.[42]

The first "Rosenwald Fellows," as they were known, began work the following year. Flexner, however, pushed for the immediate appointment of the top graduate at Meharry, William S. Quinland, to a fellowship in bacteriology and pathology at Harvard. He arranged for Rosenwald to meet him. Quinland, a well-spoken native of Jamaica, was coincidentally working in the Chicago stockyards to earn money for his studies. The Chicago tycoon was much taken with him and agreed to sponsor him at Harvard. In the city's race riot later that summer Quinland lost his job at the stockyards, and Rosenwald hired him at Sears and Roebuck.[43] After three years at Harvard (his fellowship was renewed) he returned to Meharry to head the department of pathology.

The fellowship program did not last long; both Flexner and Rosenwald grew disappointed at the unwillingness of other fellows, unlike Quinland, to return to teaching or public health work in the South. After interviewing the candidates in 1921, Flexner wrote Buttrick that none of them planned to return to the South to teach or do public health work.[44] Most sought more promising careers as practitioners in the northern states. Neither Meharry nor Howard, furthermore, was able to absorb all the new trainees who finished their studies each year.

In the two years of the program's life, not more than a half-dozen fellows completed their training, and only two or three returned to teach or practice in the South. Of all the fellows selected, only one was a woman, Carrie J. Sutton, a Howard graduate who declined her appointment in favor of an internship at the Freedman's Hospital in Washington. In approving her appointment, Edsall expressed doubt that there was "any special place . . . for colored women in medicine, who ha[d] advanced training."[45]

Occasionally, Flexner bent the rules. In the case of the promising researcher Ernest E. Just, a professor at Howard, he urged that an exception be made to support Just's zoology research. Since the Rosenwald program was intended for students, not teachers, he persuaded Rosenwald to set up a special fellowship for Just to be administered by the National Research Council. Flexner himself would serve as liaison. It was the beginning of a long relationship in which the sensitive Just sought Flexner's help and counsel while privately resenting the power and paternalism that Flexner represented. In time he would accuse his benefactor of having blocked his career at crucial turning points and of being "the dictator in all matters concerning Negro education."[46]

If improving the postgraduate training of black teachers in the medical sciences proved difficult, preparing them in clinical subjects seemed nearly impossible. Here the deeply implanted consciousness of race made it all but unfathomable for a teacher in a northern university to give postgraduate training to blacks in hospitals that served white patients. The registrar of the Western Reserve School of Medicine, in a message typical of those Flexner received from others, told Flexner of the great difficulty of finding "clinical material for negroes or men of the dark-skinned races." In seeking advanced training for an obstetrician at Meharry, Mullowney complained that the search was "vastly more difficult" when "white female patients [were] used in the training of Negro physicians." In this case, it was Flexner who found a solution by arranging a General Education Board fellowship for the obstetrician to study in Vienna. Similar fellowships followed. In time, twenty-eight Meharry graduates were given advanced training in Europe and later the United States under Rockefeller auspices. A similar program for Howard graduates began in 1929.[47]

Flexner knew that such programs were not enough. He was concerned that the educational needs of African Americans, now that Buttrick was gone, were receiving less attention at 61 Broadway. He launched an effort to persuade the sympathetic Rosenwald to create a fund for the education of blacks. "You have acquired a prestige in the field of Negro education," he told the philanthropist, "which ought not to be wasted and which perhaps no one else will ever again acquire." No more important task confronted the nation, he said, and the time was now ripe to take forceful steps. The greatest need was for more and improved schools, in both urban and rural areas, and for greater opportunities in higher education. Starts had been made, but "much more" could be done.

The problem of black education, he said, had become much more than "simply a southern problem." For in the great cities of the North an African American was "a Northerner as well as a Southerner" and suffered equally from discrimination. It was obvious, he wrote Rosenwald optimistically, that blacks would ultimately have as wide a range of educational opportunities as whites, but timely help was necessary. Perhaps he saw himself as the leader of a new enterprise now that his role at the General Education Board was becoming less certain. In a long letter to Rosenwald he set forth the objectives and structure of an organization for black education.[48] The proposal was vague, ambitious, and probably unrealistic, given the range of Rosenwald's existing commitments to the education of African Americans. Flexner pushed hard nevertheless. Further discussions with Rosenwald were held, and the idea continued to be mentioned from time to time, but no evidence exists that the Flexner initiative ever came close to realization.

Flexner's program to enable black medical schools to train teachers better was matched by a larger effort to create medical scientists for the many new positions that were opening in the rest of America's medical schools. At a meeting of foundation officers in 1921 it was agreed that Flexner should prepare a plan to meet the serious shortage of qualified teachers. With "characteristic verve" and following "somewhat unorthodox and irregular procedures," in the words of Fosdick, Flexner conceived a scheme to send promising medical scientists abroad for prolonged periods of study. He arranged with the National Research Council for the General Education Board and the Rockefeller Foundation to give fifty thousand dollars each to a program of fellowships for promising scholars interested in teaching and doing research in medicine.[49]

In all, forty-eight scholars were subsequently chosen, including Harvard neurologist Stanley Cobb, Vanderbilt internist Hugh Morgan, and Herbert Gasser, Simon Flexner's successor as head of the Rockefeller Institute. It was a prestigious program and the beginning of organized postgraduate study for medicine's future researchers and teachers.

With the rapid improvement of medical training in the 1920s another issue began to preoccupy Flexner. How well was the nation being served by the smaller number of physicians being educated in the fewer and more expensive schools of medicine? Many critics blamed his 1910 report for the disappearance of practitioners from many small, rural towns and the rising disparity in medical attention among regions and groups in the country. Doctors were flocking to the urban centers, where wealth, public transportation, telephone service, hospitals, and specialists made practice more convenient and profitable. Physicians were, after all, "sensible people": they "do business where business is good and avoid places where it is bad," said a 1920 study.[50]

In 1921 Flexner asked two members of the General Education Board staff to undertake a careful survey of the distribution of physicians across the United States. Under his supervision they collected data for the next two years. Unlike in the 1910 study, considerable attention was paid to student access to medical school and the ratio of medical graduates to regional populations. Their report showed a serious gap in access to medical care between America's cities and the nation's small towns and rural areas. Those living in cities had almost a two-to-one advantage over those who lived in small towns. Medical schools needed to take into account their impact on the supply and distribution of the nation's doctors, the authors warned. Despite the disparity between town and city, the nation was nevertheless still oversupplied with physicians, the report concluded.[51]

By the mid-1920s, as medical education declined in importance amidst the expanding and overlapping initiatives at 61 Broadway, Flexner spent less time on such questions. Most of his medical school reorganization work now lay behind him; the book on comparative medical education was in print; the program of medical fellowships was running smoothly; and most of the monies set aside for medical education had been spent. Flexner was given a new title in 1925—director of studies and medical education—which reflected his new and uncertain responsibilities. He chose to interpret the change optimistically as meaning that he had a wider mandate "to investigate new lines of activity, such as forestry and jurisprudence." He would now be able to "stay home mornings with a clear conscience," he told Anne, and concentrate on "really creative, intellectual" tasks. "I am seeing only people concerned with the larger projects," he said, and "my mail dwindles accordingly."[52]

Among the "larger projects" he now undertook was a renewed attention to the direction and purpose of the American college and university. Since his days in Louisville he had been convinced that the system of higher education in the United States was deeply flawed and contradictory. Nothing that had happened had changed his mind. Colleges no longer served a clear purpose, he believed, and the university was increasingly an ambiguous mixture of advanced study and career training. In his work on medical education he had attacked the poor preparation of doctors, their lack of a broad basis of liberal learning, and the inordinate length of their training. He continued to blame the colleges, too, for the tight control they exercised over the secondary curriculum.

Pritchett was jubilant when he learned that Flexner was returning to his own favorite themes. "I am tremendously interested," he wrote his old colleague, "that you have come back to the thing over which I have been hammering, namely the need for a re-examination of the [whole] education system." Colleges and universities in America were not likely to become "true intellectual centers," he said, without "a reconstruction of the secondary school which they ha[d] done so much to corrupt."[53]

In a provocative address at Vanderbilt in 1925, Flexner laid out his case against the American secondary school. Ask a Frenchman what the end and aim of the lyceé were, he challenged, and "you will get a definite and uniform response." The same was true of the German gymnasium. In both cases the object was "the selection and training of brains." But ask an American high school or college official the purpose of instruction, he said, and "you will get nowhere!" Unlike American high school education, secondary education on the European continent was serious; "it *counts*," he said. One could not enter a university, a profession, the army, or state service without it. In America, by contrast, schools and colleges were wide open to students indifferently trained, and no value was attached to intellectual distinction. A professional school could not begin to insist on high entrance requirements without risking its very existence. Although an able student could get a much better education in an American college than ever before, average students neither had their intelligence challenged nor gained mastery of any important field of knowledge.

Was citizenship or character education now the chief end of college education, as was frequently claimed? Then how could it be explained how this or that course produced a finer citizen or a better character? Was selecting and training intelligence in some way undemocratic? It depended, he said, on how democracy was understood. In his conception, democracy was not a matter of numbers or of "lung power." A democratic society, more than any other, he insisted, needed the best possible intellectual leadership. "To the extent that the colleges level down they injure and frustrate democracy." What democracy in education really meant, he maintained, was the removal of "all artificial barriers and advantages—wealth as well as poverty, race, color, every possible biological accident and social prejudice."[54] Democracy meant access to good education, not its watering down to accommodate everyone.

Flexner's strictures were met, as always, with a mixed response. Frank Aydelotte, president of Swarthmore and now his close ally, told him that he thoroughly agreed with him but that the revamping Flexner suggested was "not a very popular thing to do."[55] In the last several decades, public attitudes toward education had begun to harden. Many now asked what specific changes in American schools, even if desirable, were possible at this late date. The American high school and college, for better or for worse, had opened up to an ever-wider constituency, and intellectual training was only one of a range of ends and purposes.

Although he disliked the term, a "leadership elite" would preserve America from intellectual mediocrity, Flexner believed. Other aims of education such as character education or occupational training or community service, he argued, were important but should be handled by other agencies. The role of the college and university was to nurture the minds of the nation. They ought not themselves go into the marketplace, said Flexner, "and do a thriving business with the mob." Democracy, it was true, demanded opportunity for all, but why should the community's need for teachers, businessmen, nurses, and others be added willy-nilly to the burdens of the university, the basic purposes of which were research and advanced study? The university, he charged, had become a service enterprise offering a variety of programs to meet specific societal needs and had largely abandoned its historic mission to train students in how to learn and think. It was "an educational department store containing a kindergarten at one end, and Nobel Prize winners . . . at the other, with all possible variety and forms of schooling and training in between, and a mail order annex besides."[56]

What then should an American university look like? As early as 1922 he had impressed Fosdick, Rose, and Rockefeller during a staff retreat with an idea about universities that was "so unusual," in Fosdick's words, that he was asked to put it in the form of a memorandum.[57] In the entire United States, he then wrote in the memorandum, there was no "real university" but only overgrown colleges that were in reality nothing more than secondary schools. These colleges or universities made much of social activities and competitive sports and were "in constant danger of being swamped by boyish activities." Such famous old colleges as Harvard, Yale, and Columbia had all developed graduate departments, to be sure, and now called themselves "universities," but not one of them existed "even mainly, not to say altogether," to do serious work at a high scholarly or scientific level. Colleges and universities were always at "cross purposes."

Nowhere did America bring together a like-minded faculty of productive scientists and scholars with a student body of mature and independent young people. Only Johns Hopkins and the University of Chicago had even made serious attempts to create a real university; both had succumbed to the need to prepare undergraduate students. "*If the Johns Hopkins University or the University of Chicago had been established in 1920,*" he emphasized, "*instead of 1875 or 1890, neither institution would have an undergraduate department.*"

What could be done at this late date? His "unusual" idea was to enable either Johns Hopkins or the University or Chicago, or perhaps both, to rid themselves of undergraduate study and establish an "American university" of scholars free of "social, athletic or other worldly distractions" and able to concentrate on "their own productive work." Once in existence, such a university would be so attractive to serious scholars and students that others would follow, and the university with its graduate schools would separate itself from the undergraduate college.[58]

It was a breathtaking proposal. Both Johns Hopkins and the University of Chicago had sizeable undergraduate divisions, which were far less expensive to operate than their graduate programs. To reverse direction now would take courage, leadership, and a great deal of money. For the next several years Flexner's idea was seriously discussed among the policy-makers at 61 Broadway. The normally cautious Vincent called the proposal "admirable" and suggested that the undergraduate program at Chicago, in particular, might be gradually discontinued.[59] The General Education Board went so far as to authorize two million dollars to help the University of Chicago drop its first two years of undergraduate work, until the untimely death of Chicago president Ernest D. Burton stalled the negotiations.

Flexner was more interested in the possible reform of Johns Hopkins. He spent considerable time in Baltimore with university president Frank J. Goodnow and members of the faculty and board of trustees. Goodnow was able to persuade the trustees in early 1926 to adopt a plan to eliminate the first two years of undergraduate study and to merge the last two years with the graduate school. Flexner made public the Hopkins plan and clearly expected to be asked to raise the ten million dollars needed to make the change. The money would not come from the General Education Board, Rose made clear, in declaring that no further grants would be made to institutions as a whole. Flexner, however, was persistent and badgered his colleagues to support the plan.[60] He was confident that, if necessary, he could raise the money from other sources. At this juncture, however, President Goodnow became suddenly ill and retired from the Johns Hopkins presidency. His successor, unfortunately for Flexner, was firmly opposed to the Goodnow-Flexner Plan, as were a number of the faculty, and the idea was quietly dropped. A few years later, still convinced of the need for a purely graduate institution in America, Flexner was able to persuade a new set of donors to found the Institute for Advanced Study at Princeton.

The other large area of responsibility that Rose's reorganization left open was the humanities. Rose's own interests lay heavily in the sciences; under his leadership a great burst of new grants went to specific scientific undertakings. He had little interest in the social sciences but was more tolerant of General Education Board support for humanistic study. He was content to give the responsibility for humanistic projects to Flexner, who moved quickly to stake out the new territory. In a lengthy memorandum from 1924, Flexner outlined what he saw as the prevailing indifference of foundations and universities to the humanities. What was needed to redress the balance, he argued, was large sums for support of humanistic teaching and research in universities. He advocated, too, the support of field investigations and university presses, the encouragement of scholarly societies in the humanities, and fellowships and grants for students and younger scholars. To Simon he complained that the work of the General Education Board had become "too lop-sided—all medicine and science." The humanities were being "left out in the cold."[61] And so for the next four years, until he left the board in 1928, he was heavily involved in the first significant humanities programs undertaken by the Rockefeller enterprises.

His first initiative came through a chance contact with Aydelotte. He had known Aydelotte since both were teachers in Louisville. Aydelotte had consulted him at the Male High School about learning Greek to prepare for an application for a Rhodes Scholarship. Aydelotte had won the scholarship, had finished his education, had been named secretary of the Rhodes Trust, and had come to Swarthmore in 1921 determined to begin an Oxford-type honors program. When Flexner invited him in early 1924 to head a General Education Board committee to investigate the teaching of college English, Aydelotte demurred, telling him of his preoccupation with his planned honors program. Flexner then asked him if he had enough money to give the program a fair trial. When Aydelotte responded that he did not, Flexner said, "Why don't you ask us for money?"[62]

Flexner quickly arranged a five-year subsidy ranging from twenty thousand to sixty thousand dollars a year, and the Swarthmore honors program, the first of its type in America, was well begun. More grants followed. In his first few years at Swarthmore, writes Aydelotte's biographer, nothing was more important to him than his encounters with Flexner, whom he found a "like-minded, stimulating co-worker and an extremely congenial friend."[63] A decade later, Flexner brought him onto the board of the Institute for Advanced Study, where he was Flexner's closest ally and eventual successor.

In late 1926 he called together in Washington an unprecedented conclave of scholars to consider the needs of the humanities. A distinguished Princeton classicist, Edward C. Capps, was invited to take the chair. The tone of the meeting, as reported in the minutes, was one of discouragement. Leaders of universities were not supportive of the humanities, and the scholars themselves were not aggressive in promoting their interests. Some of those present told Flexner that it was "the first time in their lives that anybody had turned a sympathetic ear" to their concerns.

When pressed, they listed their needs: more money for appointments, travel, publication, secretarial help, and fellowships for graduate students. Flexner remarked repeatedly on "the unaggressiveness of the group." When the meeting adjourned, he began to lay out a program of institutional and faculty grants, as well as support for libraries and university presses.[64]

How could aid best be given to the humanities? Flexner was convinced that, compared with the sciences, a shortage of teachers in the humanities fields was the rule. To train more teachers in such traditional subjects as ancient and modern languages, art history, archeology, and medieval history he encouraged a proposal from Princeton University to build these departments and add new facilities. More than three hundred thousand dollars was approved by the board for endowment, facilities, and publications at Princeton, which soon announced that it had a "humanistic laboratory" in art and archeology.[65]

A still larger amount was given to Harvard to endow the university's Fogg Museum of Art and to support faculty research in ancient and modern languages. The University of Chicago was notified that it would receive a quarter-million dollars for "developing the humanities." He also prepared the way for similar appropriations to Yale, Columbia, and the University of Michigan. Special grants of $150,000 and $125,000, respectively, were given to the American Classical League and the American Council of Learned Societies. In the latter case he said that he wanted to see if cooperation were possible in the field of humanistic study as it had been in the sciences.[66]

At Johns Hopkins, where the venerable William Henry Welch was about to retire, Flexner hit upon an idea to combine a more humanistic environment for physicians with a new recognition of Welch as one of the most cultured and literary American physicians. He approached Welch in the early months of 1925 about the creation of a new medical library and a chair in the history of medicine, which Welch would inaugurate. "You should spend your loafing years lolling about in a chair of the history of medicine," he wrote him. Welch was "enormously gratified," he told Dean Lewis Weed, to find that the idea had come from Flexner and agreed to talk it over with him at his New York office. After several discussions with Flexner and others, he was persuaded. The history of medicine, Flexner and Welch agreed, was a field in which science and the humanities could be brought together.[67]

In other ways, too, Flexner sought to bring historical and humanistic depth to American medical training. He convinced the board to support the translation and publication into English of a number of "medical classics," especially Theodor Billroth's influential *The Medical Sciences in the German University* and Claude Bernard's groundbreaking *Introduction to the Study of Experimental Medicine*. There was no real conflict, said Flexner, between the rigorous methods of science and the broad cultural values of the humanities. It was just as important, in his judgment, for physicians to be humanely educated as that they employ their "severest intellectual effort" in their scientific study.[68]

By far the greatest impact Flexner had upon the humanities was in the field of archaeology. In the winter of 1925–26, he departed for the Middle East on what he described as his "first winter holiday." In Cairo he became well acquainted with University of Chicago Egyptologist James H. Breasted and several of his associates. Nightly they dined together at the Semiramis Hotel, where, according to Flexner's later account, "the room rang with laughter" as they told stories about their past doings. With the irrepressible Breasted as his guide, he journeyed up the Nile and spent many days in the Valley of the Kings. "Day after day, as sunset approached," Flexner recalled, "we would mount our donkeys, ride out to Karnak, climb one of the easily accessible walls, and watch the sun drop down with sudden brilliance behind the distant hills."[69]

Flexner became enchanted with the charming Breasted and his ideas for further archaeological work throughout the Middle East. Flexner committed himself to raising four hundred thousand dollars for a new library and other facilities for the University of Chicago's facility in the Egyptian desert. On his return home he persuaded Rosenwald and the General Education Board to share the costs of the new construction. But this was only the beginning. Breasted proceeded to exert the same mesmerizing influence on the other officers at 61 Broadway. "When he talked about Ikhnaton," remarked Fosdick, "even the shrewd and wily Buttrick was moved by his eloquence." The General Education Board's total grants to Breasted's Oriental Institute in Chicago passed $3.5 million; when added to other Rockefeller board gifts, the total support reached, in time, an astounding $11 million. The institute, with this kind of support, became the leading center of archaeological research in the world.[70]

Flexner made one more important stop on his winter tour. After leaving Egypt he spent several weeks in Greece touring the sights of ancient Greek civilization. His knowledge of Greek and interest in the classics spurred an "immense interest" in what he was seeing. He became closely acquainted with the director of the American School of Classical Studies at Athens, Bert Hodge Hill, who told him that the Greek government had recently opened the possibility of excavating the great marketplace of ancient Athens, the Agora, a project that would be too expensive for the government to undertake. The Agora had been for nearly a thousand years the vital center of Athenian political and commercial life, the place where Socrates had walked and talked. When told that the cost of the daunting enterprise would be between $2 million and $2.5 million, Flexner said he would see what he could do. On his return to New York, he arranged a luncheon with John D. Rockefeller Jr. to make an appeal for the project. He told Rockefeller, as he remembered it, "that immortality was within reach of the person who financed this enterprise." Nowhere on earth, he said, was there such an opportunity for American scholars.[71]

Rockefeller, after some consideration, agreed to donate in annual installments the amounts needed to begin the excavation. Through the International Education Board, grants totaling five hundred thousand dollars were funneled to the School of Classical Studies for its archaeological work. Rockefeller's support continued throughout the life of the project. "I shall always owe you a debt of gratitude," he told Flexner in 1932, for bringing "this opportunity for cooperation in Athens to my attention." Although Flexner's direct role was much smaller, the International Education Board also gave one million dollars for the support of archaeological work at the American Academy in Rome. By the time he left the General Education Board in 1928, according to two recent scholars, he had "left an immense legacy [in the humanities] behind him."[72]

In his last years at the General Education Board, Flexner took on, in addition to humanistic projects, a variety of special assignments. Some were incredibly ambitious. In 1926, he was asked by the Laura Spelman Rockefeller Memorial Fund to investigate practical methods of promoting peace in Europe. Concern over rising tensions in Europe—especially after the publication of an article by Winston Churchill called "Shall We Commit Suicide?"—was being discussed at 61 Broadway. Rockefeller officers, especially Fosdick, were distressed at what they saw as the futility of efforts in the field of education when at any time "a war could destroy more than decades of effort [could] possibly make good." Flexner's response to the assignment was not optimistic. "Let us not deceive ourselves," he wrote, "a long struggle lies before us. We shall work no miracles." With Fosdick, Rose, Rockefeller Jr., and the latter's son, Nelson

Rockefeller, Flexner journeyed to Geneva to discuss an anonymous gift that might promote the cause of peace. When the others left for home, Flexner and Rose were left to continue talks with the permanent members of the League of Nations Council. Out of these talks came the decision to build and equip a great library where international conflicts and issues could be studied by both league officers and visiting scholars.[73]

The following year he was working on a quite different project. He was asked by his old friend Robert Brookings for advice on how to merge several of his initiatives into a new research organization in the social sciences. In a ten-page report, he urged Brookings to have his new institution focus on research and a "long vision" rather than practical goals. The institution should be unified in theory and in organization, with a single board of trustees, a single facility, and a single head. Thus organized, he told Brookings, the Brookings Institution could affect social studies "very much as the Rockefeller Institute ha[d] affected the medical sciences."[74]

Flexner seemed at times to have little inkling of how much the ground had shifted beneath him at 61 Broadway. As the years passed, he, like many leaders before him, was left behind. He continued much as he had earlier, using his own initiative, working pretty much on his own, ignoring jurisdictional boundaries, and brooking little opposition. To the outsider his power seemed greater than ever, and few dared cross him in public dispute. His public reputation had steadily grown, and his name was known far beyond educational, foundation, and medical circles. He must have seemed untouchable among the galaxy of foundation executives that flourished in the late 1920s. He was aware, of course, of the mushrooming number of programs at 61 Broadway and of the confusing boundaries between them, and he sometimes complained that an anonymous new bureaucracy was being created.

"The work of the Boards has grown rapidly and been highly 'organized,'" he wrote in 1925, with the result that "no one knows anybody." Everyone was so busy on specific projects that there were practically no casual contacts. He suggested a program of "Monday lunches" for board officers to encourage more interchange but found that there was little interest in such gatherings. The new breed of "executives" and "administrators" ("I am really not exaggerating the extent to which we are getting to be viewed and to view ourselves that way") never did things themselves; "they just get other people to do them," he said. The typical new assistant was attached to a particular division and "there he [would] stick." No time was given to thought, planning, or personal initiative. Not a free moment

could be found for "intellectual or social play" for the newly hired "coun-
terjumper" who "has to punch a time clock." The creative period at the
General Education Board, he feared, was over, but he said that he was not
depressed; "my own term—the number of years still left," he explained,
"is too brief for me to bother."[75]

It was briefer than he expected. With the multiplication of boards and
projects, even Rockefeller Jr. was not able to read all the reports of the various organizations or to keep in touch with their activities. He decided in
1925 to bring in an outside consultant, attorney and friend Frank S. Staley, to review all the Rockefeller philanthropic enterprises and to propose
an organizational chart for all of the officers. Only Flexner apparently dis-
sented from Staley's broad description of the activities of the Rockefeller
boards. The section on the Lincoln School he found "inadequate and
rather misleading"; the summary of medical education was "entirely mistaken"; and the section on legislation was "all wrong."[76] Nevertheless, Fosdick, the man closest to Rockefeller and his special assistant, was now
given the assignment of trying to reduce the overlap and conflict among
the five separate Rockefeller boards.

The greatest expansion had taken place in the International Health
Board and in the Laura Spelman Rockefeller Memorial, where the young
and headstrong Beardsley Ruml was pushing an ambitious program of social research. As one colleague put it, Ruml gave away twenty-five million
dollars to university centers studying social problems "before he could be
stopped."[77] Rose, meanwhile, had moved rapidly to fund scientific research with the twenty-eight million dollars given him for the International Education Board. Conflicts abounded. Medical education was the
concern of both the General Education Board and the International
Health Board, especially its Medical Education division. Several of the
boards were interested in public health, in scientific research, and in nurs-
ing education. Social problems were studied willy-nilly by the Spelman
Memorial and by the Rockefeller Foundation.

Flexner was particularly disturbed by the fragmentation of the General
Education Board, by its shift away from broad educational issues, and by
the fact that Rose was giving support to scientific research directly, rather
than as a part of graduate and professional education.[78] It was no longer
clear in some cases who was in charge or making decisions.

The heaviest pressure for administrative reform came from the Rockefeller Foundation, where Vincent chafed at his lack of power. He was especially concerned over the actions of the International Health Board,

which was nominally under his jurisdiction. Fosdick was appointed chairman of a committee to make recommendations for change. Although convinced that major "surgical" measures were needed, he was able to effect only a minor change that left Vincent more clearly in charge. But Rockefeller and Fosdick, now persuaded that more change was necessary, moved to study the other Rockefeller boards and to grapple with the vexing questions of overlap and competition.[79] How might the several boards be reorganized and consolidated around clear social and educational objectives? Fosdick asked the senior board officers. How could order be brought out of the existing chaos?

Flexner took the assignment seriously. He responded with a thirty-page memorandum in January 1927. In it he attacked vigorously the Rose reorganization of the General Education Board, arguing that science was not "a proper division" of the General Education Board because science could not be developed in a college or university as a "thing by itself," separate from the rest of the university. Further, in the case of medicine, giving grants to individual faculty members, he believed, undermined the ideal of a medical school that was completely integrated into a university. His own division of "Studies and Medical Education" likewise made no organizational sense, he argued, since it was created in the first place only because of his "accidental presence" on the staff. Even so, he had not been allowed to work in such areas as legal education, secondary schooling, or teacher training—areas for which he was well prepared. Indeed, since being made head of the division, he complained, he had not conducted a single study.

Nor was there anywhere in the present structure a place for urban educational problems, such as the plight of black education in the northern cities. The International Education Board, which Rose had created and led, belonged, in his judgment, more naturally in the Rockefeller Foundation with such agencies as the International Health Board. The General Education Board and the International Education Board were in fact "two separate streams that [did] not mix." Also disturbing was the incursion of Ruml and the Spelman Memorial into the work of university departments of social science, thus relegating to themselves "a slice [of] the American college and university field." The poor coordination within the General Education Board among the sciences, humanities, and medicine was "thus further aggravated." The only real solution, he believed, was to bring the Spelman Memorial into the higher education division of the General Education Board.

In Flexner's view, all Rockefeller philanthropies working in the United States should be consolidated in the General Education Board, while the Rockefeller Foundation carried on educational and health work in the rest of the world. Flexner finished with a characteristically blunt assessment of his colleagues. All the reorganization in the world, he warned, would make little difference without first-class people. Ideas, not money, were at the heart of philanthropy. Mediocre persons who read and think very little, he wrote, "cannot scent just where progress is likely to take place." While a billion dollars might be "tied up" in New York's foundations, "no billion dollar group of thinkers and administrators" could be found. The Rockefeller group, while better than others, lacked capable workers and young people of promise. He ended with a plea to his colleagues to be less "amiable" and "docile" and to be more outspoken, direct, and critical in their deliberations. Important ideas, he insisted, required spirited and honest debate. "I deplore," he said, "the usual timidity of the Board."[80]

It is small wonder that Flexner's generally sensible proposals for reform were lost in the *ad hominem* attacks on his colleagues. "In Abraham Flexner," said Alan Gregg, "we had free insurance against complacency." Flexner may well have been right in his evaluation of the intellectual caliber of his associates, but his views were bound to leak out (if they were not known already) and to diminish the effectiveness of his ideas. As in previous disagreements, he mistook tact for weakness and insisted that candor, even bluntness, was necessary for effective discussion. Confident in his own intellectual ability, he was not able to understand why others did not welcome the intellectual combat that he so relished. Gregg made essentially the same arguments as Flexner concerning staff weaknesses in his memorandum to Fosdick but recommended gently that they be overcome by "greater concern in the choice and training of officers and their assistants."[81] But Flexner was moved by a sense of moral urgency and a longstanding belief that the issues before the Rockefeller boards were too important to spare feelings. It is easy to see how he carried with him an aura of superior idealism that offended and often alienated those he worked with.

By the time he wrote his memorandum, he was facing mounting criticism for his management of the far-flung enterprises in medical education. With the monies for reform running out and the spirited backing for his bold initiatives dissipating, he found himself more and more on the defensive. His heart went out of the fight for full-time commitment to medical teaching as school after school struggled to get out from under the restrictions. He was bitterly disappointed at the retreats, compromises, and outright abandonment of the full-time principle.

More schools were moving toward some variation of the Harvard geographical plan. Frequently he would lash out at those who defected from the ideal of a purely academic model of medical teaching. But the tide was moving steadily against him. In 1923 Dean Winternitz at Yale told him of growing faculty discontent over the handling of the fees paid by patients; the following year the General Education Board trustees authorized a revision of its contract with the University of Chicago, which had found it impossible to implement a strict full-time plan; at Vanderbilt the new dean, Canby Robinson, insisted that "clinical men be allowed to collect fees"; in 1925 Flexner and the General Education Board were forced to back down from a threat to sue Columbia after the medical faculty voted to abandon the full-time agreement; and even the University of Rochester, Flexner's own creation, was preparing to abandon strict full-time teaching.[82]

At Harvard, Flexner's nemesis Edsall continued to struggle against Flexner's policies and was winning more friends and allies, even at 61 Broadway. Richard Pearce, an opponent of Flexner, was Edsall's former colleague and close friend, while Alan Gregg had been Edsall's student at Harvard. In the course of the 1920s Edsall was elected a trustee of both the International Health Board and the Rockefeller Foundation, greatly increasing his influence over Rockefeller policies. Funds began to trickle in to the Harvard Medical School. Flexner nevertheless continued to view Edsall's proposals skeptically and to stir the Harvard dean to genuine anger. "Mr. Flexner would block giving any considerable sum to this institution," he told Pearce concerning a new proposal, "as he has repeatedly blocked me in my requests."[83]

In the same year, two of Edsall's colleagues at Harvard publicly attacked Flexner's management of the monies for medical education. The gentle and highly respected professor of medicine Francis Peabody, long hostile to the full-time clinical teaching principle, wrote that Flexner's successes had weakened "the soul of the clinic." Teaching in the clinic was now "overorganized," bound by strict rules on the handling of patients, and was often sterile. He pleaded for a more patient-oriented, less academic place to teach medical students and for "more of the spirit that gives life."[84]

In an even sharper attack, bacteriologist and popular writer Hans Zinsser lamented the growing power of foundations, particularly the General Education Board, over educational decisions within the university. Too many conditions were attached to each medical school grant, Zinsser complained. There was real danger, he warned, that control over medical education was passing from the universities into the hands of "a permanent or, at any rate, self-perpetuating body of gentlemen." Chief among this "body of gentlemen," charged Zinsser, in a barb obviously aimed at Flexner, was "a capable scholar who has made himself one of the foremost lay students of medical education." What to do? Simply remove the conditions imposed on each grant, said Zinsser, as the International Health Board had done.[85]

Although Flexner's board had made this possible in 1925, he continued to press for longer trials of full-time teaching strictly defined. His reaction to the Zinsser article was typical: "I do not consider Zinsser's article is any more deserving of serious attention than Bryan's views on evolution."[86] While steadily retreating from his battle to crush the commercial spirit in academic medicine, he continued to fire rearguard salvos at those who sought to weaken the full-time policy.

More serious than these outside attacks was the growing number of Rockefeller officers who were willing, albeit usually privately, to criticize Flexner. Gates, although no longer an active board member, kept up his repeated blasts at Flexner's stand on aid to public universities. In a blistering paper read at a board meeting in 1925 he not only criticized the violation of longstanding policies by "recent officers, inexperienced in the art of educational giving" but voiced regret over the decision to put "more than one salaried officer" on the board. Flexner, everyone knew, had been the first such officer, after Buttrick, to sit with the board. In a private letter, Gregg, who greatly admired Flexner, challenged him for belittling the opponents of strict full-time teaching, which, he argued, only spurred them to defend their views "more fanatically and successfully." The strong-willed secretary of the Yale Corporation and General Education Board member Anson Phelps Stokes told Flexner that they had "been somewhat too rigid" on full-time teaching and that many thought the board was interfering with the freedom of universities to determine their own policies. The Rockefeller Foundation president, George Vincent, was likewise concerned about public reaction to full-time teaching, but Flexner said he was "not so sensitive about the thing" as Vincent was. During the negotiations with Columbia, his old comrade-in-arms Pritchett urged him repeatedly to compromise.[87]

Flexner was keenly aware of the discontent among his supporters but was determined to stand firm long enough to give his policies a fair trial.

If he had to compromise, he made it clear, it would be only on terms as close as possible to his own. He intended to remain steadfast, even defiant, in the face of the gathering storm.

Why was Flexner so rigid? His earlier triumphs had been based on the "elegant simplicity" of his reasoning and the remarkable clarity of his writing. Compromise and accommodation had never been his strong suits. His moral certainty, furthermore, permitted little "tolerance for uncertainty." Much of his life had been spent in working with children, who offered little resistance to his ideas. In his background, too, as Steven Wheatley has written, were the many uncertainties he had himself overcome: his father's failure, the poverty of childhood, the anti-Semitism of a changing society. "His need to be self-assured must have been too great for him ever to have considered the alternative."[88]

As the plans for reorganization of the Rockefeller boards moved inexorably forward, Flexner grew less confident that his programs and ideas would survive. For nearly two years, Fosdick wrestled with competing ideas for reform put forward by Rose, Vincent, and Flexner. Vincent wanted a single comprehensive foundation that would absorb all the boards into distinct divisions of graduate education and research, professional programs, applied science, and education at all other levels.[89] Rose's concern, on the other hand, was to make scientific research or "the advancement of human knowledge" the principal goal of a reorganized Rockefeller Foundation.

Fosdick wavered in his thinking until the fall of 1927, when he came up with his own plan: the Rockefeller Foundation was to be the major instrument of Rockefeller philanthropy, concentrating on research ("the organization of knowledge") with subdivisions of physical science, social science, humanities, and the arts. The General Education Board, much reduced in scope, would be responsible for only elementary and secondary education, black education, and teacher training. Programs in applied knowledge, such as medicine, law, and agriculture, would fall under the auspices of the Rockefeller Foundation.

Thus the two principal sources of Flexner's power in the late 1920s, the humanities and medical education, were to be taken from him.[90] The International Health Board, which had caused so much confusion, was put on the road to extinction, while the International Education Board was transferred to the Rockefeller Foundation. As for the Spelman Memorial, most of its endowment was moved over to the Rockefeller Foundation as it was gradually phased out.

What was left for Flexner? It became clear that he would be left with management of only the small remaining funds from the 1919–20 gifts to medical education. The General Education Board, furthermore, as reconstituted in Fosdick's scheme, violated Flexner's core conviction about education: that teaching, research, and professional training were inextricably intertwined. Even worse, the head of the new General Education Board, to replace the retiring Rose, was to be Trevor Arnett, a younger man who had crossed swords with Flexner both in his earlier stint as a General Education Board officer and later as a vice-president of the University of Chicago. Arnett told Fosdick that he simply would not take the job unless Flexner was removed from the staff. "Something will have to be found for Abe," Fosdick wrote Rockefeller, "or he will have to be retired."[91]

As events at 61 Broadway were taking this threatening turn, the troubled Flexner provoked a family crisis over the proposed marriage of his daughter Jean. Relations with Anne were already frayed because of her abrupt trips abroad, now more frequent, and her handling of money. He was distressed that they were living beyond their income and that she was away so much. He was worried about the future. He had trouble sleeping and grew more irritable. "In the most trying months of my life," he wrote her, "I have had to fight it out alone." He said that he did not want another argument that would tear him "to pieces once more." He found himself, he said, "against a stone wall on almost every side and somewhere the wall must give way, or I will." Then came the spring 1927 revelation that Jean, to whom he was very close, was deeply in love with a fellow student at the Brookings school. Her father, who wanted no interference with his daughter's promising career and who "wouldn't have been satisfied with anyone" Jean chose, according to her sister, hurriedly arranged a European tour in a classic effort to stave off an unwanted alliance.[92]

It didn't work. "The long absence," she reminisced, "decided me the other way." On her return, she quickly moved to marry her friend as her father tried desperately to prevent it. Flexner even went to visit her intended's parents but failed to persuade them to intervene. He refused to attend their September wedding. Anne, who was out of the country, moved on her return to heal the breach. By the following summer Jean and her husband, a young historian named Paul Lewinson, were welcomed to the Flexner camp at Lake Ahmic. Soon the father-in-law, now convinced that Jean would continue her career, began to take an interest in Paul's work. He read carefully and made suggestions on Paul's dissertation, later published as a groundbreaking study of black suffrage in the South.[93] Although the relationship was strained at the outset by Flexner's boorish behavior, it was to become more civil in succeeding years. His strongly emotional reaction was a symptom of the personal crisis that he was experiencing.

During the winter months of 1927–28 Flexner's morale reached a new low as it became clear that the plans for reorganization were hardening into reality. The decision to terminate the General Education Board's programs in medical education and the humanities, which now seemed firm, removed the last vestiges of Flexner's power and influence. His humiliation was deepened by the realization that future work in medical education would fall to his old foe at the Rockefeller Foundation, Pearce, for whose talents Flexner had only contempt.

He was not surprised when Rockefeller Jr. invited him to lunch on March 29, 1928, to inform him of the proposed changes. Gently, he told Flexner that he was "the real difficulty," that while all recognized his value, they did not wish to put Flexner "as a subordinate to Mr. Arnett, a younger man [and] . . . that they wished to unify the work in medical education." Rockefeller proposed that Flexner resign as of July 1 and become a member of his personal staff at the same salary. Flexner's immediate response was that he did not think that he "could be happy or useful in that way." He proceeded to challenge the reorganization: the consolidation of the work in medical education, the lack of suitability of Pearce to carry on his work ("he did not have the personality"), and the "schematic organization" that ignored the key role of people and ideas. Rockefeller promised "to hold the matter in abeyance," as Flexner "had given him a great deal to think about."[94]

But the die was cast. While Flexner was not surprised by Rockefeller's softly worded ultimatum, he was stunned at what he regarded as the insensitivity to the contributions he had made over the last fifteen years. "It is no simple business," he wrote to Anne, who was in Paris, "to sit by and see your life's work strangled or mutilated." Simon and Bernard came to console him after the meeting with Rockefeller, and he met with Fosdick the following morning. All agreed with his own judgment: as he told Rockefeller, "The honorable course for me to pursue [is] to withdraw and to leave the new organization every opportunity to make good." He would be given his full salary until he reached 65, Rockefeller told him, and a generous pension thereafter.[95]

The way in which he had been treated continued to rankle him. "My mind has not ceased to marvel," he wrote, "at either the folly or the brutality of what has been done." To Anne he lamented: "I am clear that I am not wanted—indeed only docile and mediocre talents are required." He was downhearted and bitter. How could he have failed to see what was happening? He felt that his associates at 61 Broadway had betrayed him. "Let us wait and see what five years hence will be said about the wisdom of those who have participated in the debacle." As late as December he was writing that the "Hopkins-Flexner regime" in medical education would "be summarily replaced by a Pearce-Edsall-Harvard regime," which meant selecting individual researchers rather than institutions as the best way to promote progress. And who was to make the selections? "Persons who every day get further from the realities."[96]

Publicly, he maintained an imperturbable calm. He was determined to recover from the blow that had been dealt him. He told friends that the separation had been amicable and assured his former colleagues that he would not cause trouble: as he told Fosdick, "I wish to be as helpful as I can and I shall do everything in my power to make the way smooth in the future." In a printed letter sent out "To My Friends," he wrote: "Mr. Rockefeller offered me a post of equal dignity and importance but . . . I felt my presence under the new conditions might prove an embarrassment to those who had the responsibility of conducting the new organization."[97]

It was the closest he came to revealing his true feelings about his departure. Consistency in his beliefs and dignity in the face of adversity were his foremost concerns. It was against his nature to engage in public recrimination, although the press badgered him for any hint of what had happened. Even without his cooperation, the New York papers covered his leaving beneath such headlines as "Board Denies Rift with Dr. Flexner" and "Mystery of His Resignation Unexplained." The *New York Times* called him "an educational knight-errant" who was "a wholesome challenging force in the world." In a public statement, the General Education Board stressed that his retirement was "wholly voluntary" and that he was leaving "after many years of remarkably successful service" with "the unqualified good wishes" of Board members and staff.[98]

It was providential that his resignation was announced while he was in England giving the prestigious Rhodes Trust Lectures at Oxford University. Not only was he far away from American reporters, he threw himself into the Oxford experience with an enthusiasm that surprised even his family and friends. He was making a remarkable recovery. His topic was an old favorite—the comparison of universities in Britain, Germany, and the United States. The lecture hall was filled to overflowing as he gave one of the most candid and controversial series of lectures in the normally placid history of this event. He was lionized by the dons at Oxford, was feted at college dinners, and became lasting friends with a number of his hosts. Out of the lectures came the most talked-about book on higher education of the interwar years and, indirectly, the launching of the Institute for Advanced Study at Princeton. Nothing could have done more to salve his wounded feelings in that fateful spring of 1928 than the experience at Oxford.

10

Phoenix Rising

The abrupt departure of Abraham Flexner from the General Education Board brought to an end his remarkable years of social engineering in the field of education. No foundation official of his time (or since) left so large a mark on so many levels of American learning. From inauspicious beginnings, he had moved steadily across the worlds of higher education, management, and philanthropy to become "one of the most influential managers in the history of American philanthropy."[1]

Into a decade and a half he had crowded a series of pioneering surveys of state educational systems, the creation of a model progressive school, a major reorganization of the nation's medical schools, a campaign to promote clinical research in medicine, a landmark study of medical training in Europe and America, important steps to further the education of African Americans, fundamental challenges to the direction and purposes of the American college and university, and a broad program for foundation support of the humanities. "No finer piece of constructive work," in John D. Rockefeller Jr.'s characterization of his service, "has been done in any of our philanthropic boards."[2]

Many of his associates saw him as one of the "giants" of American philanthropy. The large sums of money he had managed so shrewdly for the Rockefeller enterprises were multiplied many times over through a mastery of the arts of challenge gifts and matching grants. He had become an organizer, a fund-raiser, and a cheerleader without peer in the cause of American education. With his departure from the General Education Board, an era ended.

His unusual grasp of the possibilities of philanthropic management, in the words of the historian Steven Wheatley, "expanded the range of philanthropic power and created a new standard of national policy making." He was instrumental in transforming foundations from loosely structured, informal organizations working on largely local problems to 213 national institutions attempting to bring major changes to the field of education and to society as a whole. He helped create the model for a new type of national leader who owed his allegiance to neither government, nor business, nor the academic world. His entrepreneurial and boldly innovative style alienated many but got results. When he left the General Education Board, the *New York Times* opined that he had become the nation's "educational knight-errant," ready to speak out "plainly about education in high places." He had had the temerity to ask whether Americans really value education. His "bright record of achievement," said the *Times,* ought to have an epilogue, for he had been "a wholesome challenging force in the world."[3]

Others wondered, too, whether there would be an encore to his crowded years at 61 Broadway. He was, after all, only 62 years old. Simon wrote him from England, "The general, large interest in your retirement and future career . . . [is] acute." Briefly it was rumored that he was under consideration for the presidency of the Johns Hopkins University, but his colleagues at 61 Broadway learned that the Hopkins committee had passed him by.[4]

His warmest admirers believed him well rid of the entanglements of the new Rockefeller structure. The outspoken Alfred Cohn, chief of the Rockefeller Institute hospital and a stout backer of Flexner's ideas, told him that he had "a sense of great relief" that Flexner would take no part in the reorganized Rockefeller philanthropies. At Oxford his success would put him in a far better position "to point out what direction education in America should take." "To me," Cohn encouraged him, "you seem . . . to represent Phoenix rising from these very dead ashes."[5] Letters of support poured in from George Eastman, Julius Rosenwald, Robert Brookings, and dozens of other old friends who assured him that his creative years were not over and that new opportunities were at hand. Already the word was spreading of a plan to turn the Rhodes lectures into a powerful new book on American and European universities, and of a further honor given him at Oxford to deliver the Taylorian lecture that fall.

During and after his time at Oxford, he alternated between bursts of optimism and periods of depression over his recent treatment. His normally placid temperament gave way to emotional ups and downs. "I feel better in some ways," he wrote Anne in early 1929, "my hand is steadier . . . but sleep is still fitful and difficult." A few weeks later he told her, "I have never been so weary in my life and tho' I flare up when in action, I sink into an armchair here by the fire when I get back and sit listless for an hour or more." But to his brother Bernard, who was very close to him

in the months of crisis, he denied that the events at 61 Broadway preoccupied him: they had "so far receded that I do not think of [them] any-
more." He was turning his mind to other projects, he said. "If I can find
means of carrying them out, perhaps the debacle will prove a blessing in
disguise—well disguised, however."[6]

Very important in his emotional recovery was support from Anne. She
spent as much time as she could with him at Oxford and during his travels for the forthcoming book on universities. "I am writing . . . with a full
heart," he wrote her in May 1929, telling her that he was bringing gifts
that would "humbly" express his appreciation for her and his plan to "lean
on" her in the years ahead. The abrupt change in his fortunes seemed to
bring a sharp upturn in his marriage. A year later he was writing: "I who
have written books and never failed for words, am struck dumb when I
try to tell you what you and your two girls mean to me. I feel that I should
like to live forever, keeping things among and between us, as they are."[7]

The term at Oxford had come at the suggestion of his good friend
Frank Aydelotte, the American secretary of the Rhodes Trust. He named
Flexner and the physicist Robert Millikan as possible American candidates
to the governing committee at Oxford. Flexner, he told the committee,
was responsible for "all the best in American medical education at the present time" and was "in some ways the most trenchant thinker on educational questions in the United States today." The first Rhodes lectures had
just been given by Sir Robert Borden, the wartime prime minister of
Canada, but had attracted only a small audience. The committee was understandably anxious to draw attention to the lectures and was considering
nominations of Albert Einstein, South African leader Jan Smuts, French
statesman Georges Clemenceau, Italian historian Benedetto Croce, and
others.[8]

The lectureship was first offered to Einstein, who declined for reasons
of health. The offer then went to Flexner. After Flexner's acceptance, Einstein changed his mind but was asked to defer his appointment to a later
year. It was thus no insignificant honor that had come to Flexner; he was
joined in the years immediately following by such international figures as
not only Einstein and Smuts but astronomer Edwin Hubble and French
historian Elie Halévy.[9]

One of the reasons for Oxford's surprising choice of Flexner may have
been a stipulation that the lecturer must remain in residence a full term
and be freely available for provocative discussions with undergraduates
and dons. Flexner's well-known fondness for intellectual exchange, as well

as his reputation as an innovative teacher, doubtless figured in the selection. He would be "enormously useful," Aydelotte told the Oxford Committee, "in the kind of conversations being planned with dons and professors." Further, he was well known to many at Oxford from his previous visits and had maintained close friendships with a number of its faculty. The appointment was well received, and he and Anne were welcomed as "never in [their] lives" by the Oxford community.[10]

Life at Oxford was an enjoyable round of receptions, dinners, and get-togethers with students and faculty. He was thoroughly charmed by the secluded colleges and their green-covered lawns, the quaint academic customs, and the unhurried pace of town life. The chairman of the Rhodes Trust, Sir Otto Beit, gave a reception and dinner in Flexner's honor in his London home. Guests included Lord Haldane (before whose committee Flexner had testified twenty years before), Mrs. Stanley Baldwin (the prime minister was detained), classicist Gilbert Murray, historian E.L. Woodward, Deputy Cabinet Secretary Thomas Jones (now a good friend), and the Duchess of Athol. "Such surroundings do seem specially designed by Providence," wrote Anne, "after all that Abe has recently been through."[11]

On another occasion they were guests of Lady Astor at Cliveden, where he and Winston Churchill, goaded by their hostess, got into "a grand scrap." Churchill asked him what he thought "ailed England." Flexner replied, "It's governed by amateurs," which drew howls of laughter. From Lady Osler came an invitation to take tea with old friends. Scarcely a day went by that they were not invited to a luncheon or dinner. They were able to rent a small cottage belonging to a professor of Latin; according to Anne, they had "come to anchorage in a beautiful haven." The rent was six guineas a week, "linen and plate supplied."[12]

Flexner had been warned not to expect a large audience at the lectures. "Oxford is 'fed up' with lectures," a fellow at All Souls College (where Flexner was made an associate member) told him; "you will have a good audience of persons curious about you at the first lecture; by the last the audience will dwindle to nothing." But as he told members of his family, almost the reverse happened. "I had a good audience at No. 1," he reported, "a much better and more distinguished one at No. II and the hall was packed, 'standees' lining the walls at No. III."[13]

For those who had not heard Flexner before, his lectures were something of a revelation: they were remarkably candid, often amusing, and thoroughly provocative. Based on his wide experience and careful preparation, the lectures dealt with a subject not often dealt with in universities—universities themselves, and specifically the characteristics of the English, German, and American varieties. The enthusiastic reception restored his shattered self-confidence. "I wonder if you realized how big an audience you had, for Oxford," wrote the paleographer E.A. Lowe; "we have been edified and honored by your performance." The warden of New College, H.A.L. Fisher, a former minister of education, told him he was immensely pleased with Flexner's "brilliant and impressive course of lectures." Both the Rhodes Trust chairman, Philip Kerr (later, as Lord Lothian, ambassador to the United States), and Frank Aydelotte, who had arranged to be present, told him, according to Flexner, "that nothing like it had ever happened before."[14]

The lectures must have seemed familiar to Aydelotte and others who knew Flexner's views. They were not made public because of his request to the Rhodes trustees that he be allowed to convert them into a book. The lectures were given in May, "always a bad time for getting audiences," according to notes kept by the secretary of the trust.[15] He prepared carefully, mixed humor with analysis, and spoke in a clear and distinct voice. At the outset he talked about the "idea of a modern university," then moved in the second lecture to a description of the American university, and closed with an analysis of the British and German universities.

His most devastating critique was of the American system. America, he charged, had weakened its earlier commitment to advanced study and research by mixing university purposes not only with undergraduate teaching but with vocational and service programs. The British and German universities, by contrast, had maintained the centrality of serious study. The Germans, in particular, had kept their universities separate from vocational and general liberal studies; they were unique places of original research and advanced preparation for teaching and leadership. Clearly Flexner preferred the German model, although he found much to criticize in it as well.[16]

The lectures sparked a surprising amount of interest in the United States. The press published many reports on them, along with critical comments from university presidents, who understandably resented the public attacks on their institutions, especially before a foreign audience. Flexner's resignation from the General Education Board was not announced until May 24, after the last lecture had been given, and speculation arose immediately that he had been fired for his controversial views. Several newspapers reported that Flexner had criticized the United States and Britain for spending millions on war instead of on education and that he had attacked the "freak degrees" given by American universities to future "advertisers [and] plausible bond salesmen."[17] Were these attacks the reason for Flexner's sudden departure from the General Education Board, the press asked?

Both Wickliffe Rose, representing the board, and Bernard Flexner, representing his brother, disavowed any connection and stressed that the resignation had come well before his trip to Oxford. Flexner did not help the situation when he told a reporter from the *New York Post* that he had "quit to criticize" the modern systems of education.[18]

What would he do after the lectures were finished? One paper speculated that he intended to remain in England "indefinitely." In fact, Flexner was himself unsure and dreaded returning to the United States. He had something of a reprieve in being asked to return to Oxford in the fall to give the Taylorian lecture, and he could spend further time abroad working on the revised Rhodes lectures—but what then? "New York is the place for you," he told Anne, but "it is dubious for me. I dread it— largely because it looks empty as far as I am concerned . . . It may not even be the best place for me to write my book." To Bernard he confided, "I cannot live in a vacuum. I must have occupation and I must have contacts." Even Simon had failed to help him in his hour of need, he said, although he understood his brother's "delicate position" as a Rockefeller officer and trustee. Only a couple of letters had come from him. "Why his pathological timidity and self-regard," he wrote angrily of Simon, "should be permitted to so undermine our relations at such a period of my life passes my comprehension." At bottom he was unsure how former colleagues and friends would receive him after the humiliating termination of his job. "I do wish I had some sign," he told Anne, "as to what the town is likely to offer me. I cannot be idle in it."[19]

After the term was finished he spent the summer with Anne and the children at their camp on Lake Ahmic, where he rested and then began preparing the Taylorian lecture. He spent little time in New York and saw few of his old friends and colleagues. He was, however, in close touch with Eastman about an idea that had struck him while at Oxford. His friendship with Eastman had grown steadily through the twenties, and the philanthropist had come to rely on him for advice about projects that interested him. In the middle of the decade, Eastman had asked Flexner to explore the possibility of building a free dental clinic in London modeled after the pioneering clinic he had opened in Rochester.[20] He had also conferred with Flexner about gifts to Meharry Medical College and the Brookings Institution.

Now Flexner sought to encourage Eastman to provide endowment for a visiting American professor at Oxford who would each year expound on "American ideals, American conditions, [and] American experience" to undergraduates and the wider community. The professorship would be something of a "fair exchange" for the scholarships provided to Americans by the Rhodes Trust. It would be administered by Frank Aydelotte's Association of American Rhodes Scholars.[21]

Eastman liked the idea. Flexner drew up the necessary papers, and the chair was established in 1929. As part of the arrangement, Eastman agreed to provide a comfortable home for the Eastman professor. The visiting American, he told Aydelotte, must have "a place to live in which he will not have to wear a shawl over his back while he is eating his breakfast, or wait ten or fifteen minutes to get some hot water at the tap." The first Eastman professor was the Harvard English professor John Livingston Lowes, followed by such well-known scholars as Wesley Mitchell, Felix Frankfurter, Arthur Compton, and Simon Flexner.[22]

In October Flexner returned to Oxford briefly to deliver the Taylorian lecture. His subject was "The Burden of Humanism," which he defined as living in an industrial and science-dominated world that had largely "destroyed the puny notions within which religion, philosophy, and history once led a relatively easy intellectual existence." Science had proven to be a two-edged sword that "gave wings to the human spirit" but also brought out "the worst that is within" people. The inexorable march of science was indifferent, "whether the outcome is a new philosophy of creation or hideous instruments of destruction for the next war." The science of bacteriology, which wiped out typhoid in peaceful communities, also "made possible war on a previously undreamed of scale."

Likewise, industry, while it had made life better, was "more or less ruthless." The same entrepreneurial spirit that made food and clothing plentiful and accessible made "peons of African natives and thoughtlessly destroy[ed] Oxford's superbly beautiful countryside." Science and the machine were "efficient, not sensitive."

It was the job of humanism to provide a means of weighing alternative choices, to hold to a system of values "outside science as such, outside industry as such, and yet ultimately operative within both." Above all, humanism must raise questions of value and worthwhileness. It must look at not only the distant past but the present. No longer could the humanities scholar be content to withdraw from the world. What was needed was a "more fearless conception" of humanistic studies, one that included an examination of contemporary political, industrial, and scientific dilemmas. Literature, language, and history were not ends in themselves but ways of understanding the human passions that lay below contemporary events. "That is the burden," he concluded, "that rests upon the shoulders of humanism in a world that will become a chaos if men do not strive to understand both themselves and one another."[23]

Even as he finished his stay at Oxford, he was immersed in plans for the book on universities. For the rest of 1928 and much of the following year he retraced his earlier steps across Europe. He visited a dozen or more universities, renewed friendships, and talked endlessly about the changes under way at many institutions. He returned to his tried-and-true method of investigation. As he explained it to Anne, he talked to as many as twenty people each day, all of them speaking "from the angle of [their] own subject and experience," while he was "comparing, thinking up new relationships, thinking out suggestions, problems, possibilities." When he went to bed each day, this process continued, keeping him awake, he told her.[24]

From Oxford he journeyed to France, where he spent considerable time in Paris, and then on to Hamburg, where he compared notes with his friend Heinrich Poll, who had recently been in America. He then went to Berlin, where a surprise awaited him, then visited other German universities, and finally came back to Oxford, where he began to outline the book.[25]

The surprise in Berlin came while he was in conference at the office of the minister of culture. The visit was interrupted by the dean of the medical school, who had just learned that Flexner was in Berlin. He had rushed to tell him that several weeks earlier the Berlin faculty had voted to give him an honorary degree in medicine, the first ever awarded to a layperson. According to the dean, no discussion of medical education "now takes place that does not start from the exposition of your views"; "no one else has ever treated the subject with such thoroughness, objectivity and comprehensiveness." The faculty had decided on the action without knowing that Flexner was in Europe and would be coming to Berlin.[26]

The news was reported in the United States, and many of his old colleagues at 61 Broadway, including Rockefeller Jr., wrote to congratulate him. The warm recognition helped to overcome the dread he felt about returning to New York. Simon wrote him that "the grand news" had pleased all his friends and former colleagues and should be "most gratifying" to him. Simon called the honor "quite as wonderful as it is deserved."[27]

During his stay abroad he found time for reading, relaxing, and attending plays and concerts. He wrote Bernard that he had finished John Drinkwater's biography of Charles James Fox, the liberal British leader, and had been rereading Jane Austen and Boswell's *Johnson*. He was also reading "a couple of hours of French" each day. While in Berlin he was enthralled by a concert given by the twelve-year-old Yehudi Menuhin, who had "a lovely round face with a beautiful smile and a white jacket, short black trousers and socks, his lower legs half exposed." His violin "sang out above the orchestra with the voice of angels." He arrived home "stirred to the bottom of [his] heart"; "only a few times in a lifetime can one be so moved," he said. "I was glad," he told Anne in an uncharacteristic outburst, "that he was an American, glad that he was a Jew."[28]

He also maintained his interest in European politics. The unrest in Germany and the weakness of allied policy weighed heavily upon him. He commented uneasily on the growing number of anti-Semitic incidents occurring in Germany. He kept up a steady barrage of criticism of British and French politicians. To his friend Tom Jones, who as deputy cabinet secretary was close to the men in power in Britain, he wrote frankly of his low opinion of British and French leadership. Of the British foreign secretary, Sir John Simon, he said, "He knows nothing of Germans or Germany and has very limited imagination and sympathy." He accused the allies of being "largely responsible for both Hitler and Papen." The French in particular, by their harsh policies and distrust, "had pursued precisely the wrong policy" for "vengeance and hatred are not only wrong: they don't pay." While traveling in Germany, he was strongly impressed by the mayor of Cologne, Konrad Adenauer, whom he described as "one of the masters of the new Germany—if America and the Allies will permit a new Germany to be made."[29]

He tried once more to interest the younger Rockefeller in the plight of the German universities as an investment in "international good-will and cooperation." He suggested that a fund of at least fifteen million dollars be raised in the United States. He again enlisted the support of former ambassador Alanson Houghton, now returned to his post as president of the Corning Glass Works, who praised the proposal, saying, "No equal expenditure of money can render a greater service to humanity." But Rockefeller, after a long lunch in late 1929, told Flexner that despite finding the idea very "appealing," he was loath to intervene personally so soon after the restructuring of his philanthropic endeavors.[30]

Flexner also supported strongly a proposal that Rockefeller make a gift to the Louvre, which was in serious disrepair in the years after the war. "As I walked through the long galleries a few months ago and peered into the little rooms in which the curators were at work," he wrote Rockefeller, "I was struck by the modesty and simplicity with which these great scholars, wearing threadbare clothes, worked in dark corners, illuminated by small lamps."[31]

While in Europe as well as during his trips home, he continued to seek support for several of his favorite projects. He turned successfully to Rosenwald to assist in William Henry Welch's efforts to start an Institute of the History of Medicine at the Johns Hopkins University, and he also persuaded him to help German physiological chemist Emil Aberhalden continue his research program at the University of Halle. The Rockefeller Foundation, he told Rosenwald, was not "prepared to step in" on such projects, so it was "a case of now or never." He also lobbied Rosenwald and the General Education Board for further assistance to the Swarthmore College honors program. "Oxford and Swarthmore," he wrote President Aydelotte, "are indeed the two places which I should like during the next few years to help, for they both have tremendous possibilities of enlarged usefulness."[32] The Swarthmore campaign for a larger endowment, despite the growing economic crisis, reached its goal.

As the months passed, he began to regain something of his old energy and confidence. He discovered that he was not without influence despite his severance from the General Education Board. Even his relations with his old colleagues at 61 Broadway began slowly to improve. He was consulted by Trevor Arnett, Edwin Embree, Raymond Fosdick, and others about continuing the support to the medical schools he had promoted while on the board. To the schools that had begun to back away from previous commitments to full-time clinical medicine he sent sharp rebukes. The officers at 61 Broadway, he advised Richard Pearce and Arnett, had a "moral obligation" to carry out his unfulfilled commitments, especially to Vanderbilt and Meharry Medical College. The General Education Board should treat Meharry "generously," he told them, and "make appropriations adequate to establish a good Medical School on a sound basis." Both Meharry and Howard needed better facilities for intern training and needed to establish postgraduate programs. Once the Vanderbilt program was completed, he urged support for Tulane University's school of medicine, in order to create still another strong school in the South.

At Johns Hopkins, more help should be given to the new history of medicine department, he told his former colleagues. In the case of Harvard, he saw no reason for either the General Education Board or the Rockefeller Foundation to honor Dean David Edsall's request to match gifts to the Massachusetts General Hospital. Harvard was still an institution, he believed, that sought constantly to use its special position to evade commitments and obligations expected of others. For the most part, the Rockefeller leadership followed the advice and suggestions of their long-time colleague. He was even asked in 1932 to write the history of the General Education Board, but he declined.[33]

He kept up a steady barrage of correspondence with medical leaders despite his "retirement" from public life. Although he now had little power to influence the decisions of philanthropic organizations, deans and presidents continued to seek his advice and approval. When William Henry Welch reached eighty and prepared to retire from the new chair in the history of medicine, Dean Lewis Weed asked for his evaluation of Henry Sigerist of Leipzig as his successor. Flexner responded enthusiastically about the potential appointment. Flexner also began a survey, apparently at his own initiative, of medical graduates of leading universities who had attained the rank of professor at other institutions.[34]

Even those who were weakening their full-time clinical programs found it necessary to consult with Flexner. Many came to dread the scolding missives that came from his pen as he quarreled with changes he disapproved. To Franklin McLean, dean of medicine at the University of Chicago, who was considering changes in the original full-time plan, he wrote that the school and its hospital were at risk of abandoning the purpose for which they were founded "in order that [they] might become profit-making institutions." An influential professor at the University of Pennsylvania, Alfred N. Richards, who was advising the new president, was told, "Unless the University ceases in-breeding on the clinical side, it will continue to shrink in relative importance, as I believe it has been shrinking for the last thirty years."[35]

Even his old allies, Milton Winternitz at Yale and Rush Rhees of Rochester, faced his dissatisfaction. Winternitz was blamed for "the absolute sterility" of his pediatrics department. "When will you people learn," he scolded, "that you can't make a scientist out of a non-scientist by giving him a title?" Concerning Rochester, which was altering its commitment to full-time teaching, Flexner wrote President Rhees, "I hear rumors, which, I hope, are unfounded towards some inclination to weaken your full-time clinical organization." If the clinicians were not "busy enough," he continued sarcastically, it had to be "for the lack of ideas." Nothing that had happened since the school's beginning, he told Rhees, "would justify such a disappointment to those who played a part in securing its establishment." And when G. Canby Robinson, whose appointment as dean at Vanderbilt was largely Flexner's work, left for another position, Flexner chastised him for leaving a school into which he had "put so much energy and intelligence" and joining those "who after founding it helped pull it to pieces."[36]

In 1929, when asked about a new survey of medical education being carried out by a prestigious group of medical professionals headed by Yale hospital administrator Willard Rappleye and including such notables as Dean Edsall and President A. Lawrence Lowell of Harvard, President Ray Lyman Wilbur of Stanford, bacteriologist Hans Zinsser, and representatives of the American Medical Association, the American Council on Education, and the National Board of Medical Examiners, Flexner dismissed the committee's work curtly. "It isn't worth reviewing in your Annual Report," he told the secretary of the Carnegie Foundation, "for it is without significance—an obvious, common-place mostly second hand compilation of opinions and quasi-statistics, not beginning [anywhere] and lead[ing] nowhere. No one will read it—it is too dull and jerky."[37] His judgment was too harsh. He underestimated the study's worth as a detailed portrait of the state of medical education in the late 1920s. He failed to note, too, how closely Rappleye's recommendations followed his own. But his prediction of its impact proved essentially correct. The final report had little impact on the teaching of medicine, and its broad recommendations were quickly forgotten.

He became more outspoken, too, in his views on ethnic and racial conflict. It was a time of Jim Crow and racial lynchings in the South and campaigns against immigration and ethnic minorities in the North. In a commencement speech to Jewish social workers in September 1928, he asserted, "Far from regarding the mixed composition of races in this country as unfortunate, I regard it as fortunate, and as an advantage of which not enough use has been made." There was, he said, "no subject on the face of the earth about which more nonsense [had] been uttered than the subject of racial characteristics." He doubted whether there had "ever been anywhere a Nordic race." It was just as absurd to apply terms like Christian, Jewish, Protestant, or Catholic to this nation. He urged the graduates to remember that they were "Americans as well as Jews" who had a duty to mitigate the ethnic and racial differences around them. A writer in the *New York Times,* reporting on the speech, praised him for speaking out against the idea of "pure-blooded race" and for knocking out "the Nordic straw-man."[38]

His new activist role also led Flexner to join the board of Howard University in 1930. His backers, notably Julius Rosenwald, were convinced that someone of Flexner's experience was needed to deal with the school's financial needs and tangled relations between the board and the administration. Almost immediately he was named to work with committees on financial support and on the university's organization and operation. Two years later he was elected chairman of the board in the middle of the most tumultuous events in Howard's history. To a friend he wrote that conditions at Howard were "in considerable confusion" and that the board needed to be thoroughly reorganized, with younger men familiar with "modern educational problems and experiences" brought into service. "At my time of life," he wrote, "I do not see that I can do anything beyond this."[39] Affairs at Howard would nevertheless take much of his time over the next three years.

By the summer of 1929, he felt confident enough of his reception to return to New York, where Simon gave him the use of two rooms at the Rockefeller Institute. Here he began writing the much-awaited book on universities. It had been the talk among educators ever since the controversy over his lectures at Oxford. Further, he had written dozens of provocative letters to university leaders questioning this or that practice and giving them an opportunity to rebut his impressions. As chapters and galley proofs were completed, he sent copies to educators in Europe and America for their comments and corrections. As he worked quietly in the institute, he came to know a number of its scientists—chemist Phoebus Levene, virologist Tom Rivers, and experimental surgeon Alexis Carrel. Through Carrel he became acquainted with Charles A. Lindbergh, who began working with Carrel in 1930 on his glass pump to keep alive organs outside the body. Lindbergh later came to rely on Flexner as his principal adviser in the charitable disposition of his New Jersey estate after the famous kidnapping.[40]

As he began to set pen to paper, he was eager to keep his friends apprised of his progress. To his friend Tom Jones in Britain he wrote that he was "bending all energies" to revamp the lectures he had given at Oxford. "I am having a lot of fun especially with my own country, which is much madder than I expected," he wrote. Later he added, "If I can wake up a few [Americans] and then give a slight punch in the ribs to a few Englishmen and Germans, my three years will not have gone for naught." He wrote to Rosenwald that he expected to be "skinned alive" by American university presidents. European university officials who had seen the proofs, on the other hand, urged him "to speak out with the utmost candor." To a friend at Harvard he confided that his only purpose was to raise questions. "In the next few years," he prophesied, "the great university presidencies will all be filled with young men who may know a subject, chemistry or law or God-knows-what, but who do not know education either in this country or in Europe." In his book, he said, he wanted to "forewarn" people about what could happen. Henry Pritchett, on learning of Flexner's intended approach, cautioned him against firing "at point blank range" and told him to "come down to earth in [his] suggestions about university reform."[41]

The advice was not taken. Flexner wanted to be provocative. When friends expressed concern about the pungency of his language or the stress he laid on harrowing examples of educational practice, he replied that he had to jar readers and stimulate debate to make any impact. Later, in his autobiography, he insisted that he had "told the truth" and given "full credit for all that was good" in American universities. Critics did not like his book for one reason, he said: "I riddled with facts, sarcasm, and documents the outright and shameless humbuggery that was proving profitable at teachers' colleges; in home study courses at Columbia, Chicago, and even my own beloved Johns Hopkins; in correspondence courses competing with work on the campus; and in the absurd topics for which the Ph.D. degree was given."[42]

As the publication date neared, he outlined his views in a comprehensive address to the American Philosophical Society. In the traditional sense of a university—a place of advanced learning and teaching—there was, he said, "not a single university in the United States." While there were scores of scholars who rightly belonged in a university, they nowhere determined the character of the institution. "An American university," he charged, "is a miscellaneous aggregation, devoted to secondary education, college education, technical education, vocational education, professional education, and disinterested scientific and scholarly teaching and research." The term "university" was so broad-based as to lose all meaning. He thus anticipated Clark Kerr's famous definition of the "multiversity" thirty-three years later but in a context totally different from Kerr's requiem for the traditional university.[43]

In 1930 Flexner could still argue that to be true "seats of learning" universities must have certain characteristics: they "must be small, not large

. . . flexible and easygoing rather than efficiently mechanized . . . comfortable places for the queer and the unusual . . . [and] must avoid, as they would avoid the plague, every influence that tends to subject them to standards that may be relevant in business." Flexner thus set his face against the democratization of the university idea, but, as he was to learn, it was too late. An avalanche of social and political change had opened the universities to programs and students undreamed of in Flexner's youth. His ideas about learning and higher education had changed but little since his days in Louisville, but the world around him had come to accept a very different view of the university. He was too enamored of the Johns Hopkins University of 1884, said Clark Kerr, and too little of the Harvard of 1930.[44]

The book nevertheless provoked the most intense debate on the purposes of a university since the late nineteenth century. His measured but blunt outburst spurred the beleaguered defenders of the traditional university to a final stand and stirred the champions of the modern in higher education to a vigorous defense. To Clark Kerr the book was "a classic in the literature of higher education" by preserving in its purest most completely reasoned form the idea of a modern university.[45] It was a remarkably candid, at times brutal, reasoned attack on what Flexner saw as the misdirection of American universities.

The charges he made have continued to echo through the years, especially in the corridors of liberal arts conclaves. He blasted the proliferation of occupational schools and schools of education that stressed technique and theory rather than learning. He railed against the growth of big-time athletics, student governments, and other activities that made a mockery of serious learning. He assailed the growth of a mammoth bureaucracy to administer the whole. He took strong exception to the emphasis on "service" that took scholars away from the pursuit of learning. Service, he said, was a very important goal of modern life, but it should be the byproduct, not the purpose, of a university. Universities needed to be more than mainstays or props of the status quo, he insisted; they needed to criticize and analyze underlying trends.

The proper role of education in a democratic society, he believed, was to enable individuals "to exercise [their] powers in helping to determine the precise form" of the next "social revolution." At the heart of every university, he maintained, was the advanced study of the liberal arts and sciences, the graduate school, certain professional schools based on science and scholarship, and selected research institutes that created new knowledge.

Basic to this view was his longstanding conviction, acquired at Johns Hopkins and in Germany, that intellectual inquiry, not job training, was the purpose of the university. Only a university so dedicated, he asserted, could lift society out of mediocrity toward excellence. Particularly savage were his critiques of the large number of dissertations pouring out of the universities. He ridiculed such topics as "A Time and Motion Study of Four Methods of Dishwashing," "Style Cycles in Women's Undergarments," and "Variations in Demand for Clothing and Different Income Levels."[46]

He never doubted that other institutions were needed to provide training for engineers, technicians, social workers, nurses, journalists, musicians, businesspeople, and people in the dozens of other occupations vital to a modern society. But instead of creating and improving schools offering training in such occupations, as in Europe, the United States was moving every preparation for a career demanding more than a high school education under the wing of the university. Both scholarship and training for a career thereby suffered from the amalgamation. "Is there no incongruity or incompatibility," he asked, "between the pursuit of culture and ad hoc training for a simple job?"[47] Quality in a university was not measured by size, either the number of programs or the number of students. Learning remained for Flexner, as it had for forty years, an activity best carried out in small groups under a caring teacher.

His championship of the centrality of the faculty in a university and his denigration of the new class of administrators endeared him to generations of scholars and scientists. American university professors, he wrote, were "wretchedly underpaid" while huge sums were being spent on supervisory officers, on athletic facilities, and on student amenities. "Athletic coaches are more highly paid than professors," he chided, while the professoriate was becoming "a proletariat, lacking the amenities and dignities they [were] entitled to enjoy." While "glorious buildings" and "concrete stadia accommodating fifty or one hundred thousand enraptured students at a football contest" had sprung up on every campus, the university was pleading its inability to pay decent salaries.[48] No modern friend of the academy can fail to find satisfaction at some of his thrusts.

For Flexner, natural scientists, humanists, and social scientists were the only real university faculty. While natural scientists, on the whole, were doing well and had a bright future, humanists needed much more support. Social scientists, too, needed to be encouraged to a degree that they had never been in the English or German university. The empirical and experimental methods used so successfully in the natural sciences were not yet applied sufficiently in the social fields of study. The humanities, on the other hand—languages, literature, philosophy, history—were indispensable to understanding the values by which human beings lived. All of these fields, he wrote, needed to be more rigorous, more "scientific." They needed to become beehives of "creative activity, productive and critical inquiry."[49]

Flexner hoped that his devastating critique would awaken the American public to the evils of mass education in the university, much as his survey of medical education in 1910 had awakened people. But 1930 was not 1910, and the movement to open up America's universities had far too much momentum to be stopped. America's colleges and universities were more open and varied than those of Europe. They offered instruction in far more subjects. Ahead lay the spectacular revolution in access and the proliferation of programs that grew out of the Second World War. By the time of his death, in 1959, the American system of higher education would be as different from what it had been in 1930 as it was from that of the undeveloped countries of Asia and Africa. The years after Pearl Harbor transformed the landscape of American higher education—not only in size (a dozen students in college for every one in 1940) but in spirit, programs, governance, and social role.

Flexner was raising his banner in a losing cause that would later seem out of character for the crusading progressive of earlier years. Flexner's progressivism, like his admiration for the German university, was rooted in a turn-of-the-century Jeffersonian vision of individual intellectual attainment. Like German educators, he placed a high premium on meritocracy, order, efficiency, and the role of elites in society. No country, Flexner believed, was in more need of specialized intelligence than the sprawling, chaotic, and decentralized America of the early twentieth century.

The future of the nation depended, he insisted once more, on the realization "that democracy is not synonymous with intellectual mediocrity and inferiority."[50] It depended on an open society where able individuals were free to develop their talents. But how to ensure the predominance of the expert and the well prepared without arousing the latent egalitarianism of America's democratic ideals? In the case of the university, how could its mushrooming purposes and programs, all responding to egalitarian or commercial pressures, be pushed back into the bottle of the Johns Hopkins model of 1880? The crusade, he must have recognized in his heart, was quixotic. He wanted nevertheless to demonstrate how wooly the concept of a university had become and how much he believed had been lost in the transformation. In particular, he wanted to expose newer educational practices that smacked of fraud, quackery, or misrepresentation.

Flexner's book, entitled *Universities: American, English, German,* published by Oxford University Press in New York, was widely and respectfully reviewed. It aroused a great deal of interest and stronger feelings than perhaps any other book on higher education in the twentieth century. Not untypical was one reviewer's conclusion that it was "the most stimulating and thoughtful book in the field of university education . . . since Cardinal Newman's." No major newspaper or journal of opinion failed to give it a prominent place in its columns. Often it was the subject of front-page news stories as prominent educators defended themselves against the author's charges. In the *New York Times,* the book's publication was announced in a five-column story under such headings as "Flexner Denounces 'Sale' of Education," "He Criticizes Columbia," "Many Courses He Classes as 'Rubbish.'" Two weeks later the *Times* praised the book in a front-page story that invited educators to strike back at his arguments.[51]

They needed no such invitation. A group of Columbia administrators in journalism, business, and university extension indignantly called Flexner's ideas "medieval," rebuking him for not knowing that they were "living in the twentieth and not in the fifteenth century." Across the country, Flexner's critics and defenders found outlets in the metropolitan press and in academic journals. "I have been bombarded by telegrams [and] long distance calls," wrote a Louisville columnist, "for an opinion on the indictment Abraham Flexner has drawn of several American universities."[52]

Flexner seemed to delight in providing critics with particularly damning instances of questionable practices in the nation's leading universities. The response of the Columbia administrators was aimed at his indictment of that school's "trivial" and "inconsequential" offerings in teacher education, which occupied over two hundred pages in its catalog. He had scorned, too, the university's "profit-making" in correspondence and home study courses. He skewered his old critic, Nicholas Murray Butler—"the vainest human being in existence," he called him privately—for his grandiloquent description of Morningside Heights as "one of the four most sacred and most inspiring spots in the world"; the remaining three were the Mount of Olives, the Acropolis, and the Capitoline Hill at Rome.[53]

He ridiculed the way the University of Chicago had "wretchedly compromised" its training of physicians. The university had managed to maintain two separate medical schools, one on the campus and the other at Rush Medical College. This made high standards impossible. Elsewhere on its campus, the university accepted high school credits in stenography and bookkeeping for admission. Why not "manicuring, hair-bobbing, or toe-dancing?" he taunted. He had written President Robert Maynard Hutchins, who generally shared his views, for an explanation of these practices but got no response. "These damn fellows make me sick," he told a friend.[54]

Harvard and Yale were not spared. The school at Cambridge, he warned, had created a graduate school of business that was committed not to serious scholarship but "to furnish[ing] advertisers, salesmen, or handy men for banks, department stores, or transportation companies." Students of business should indeed study such subjects as the psychology of sales, he said. But they ought not be taught how to fool the public; they should understand the harmful consequences "when a jingle like 'not a cough in a carload' persuades a nation to buy a new brand of cigarettes." Such utilitarian skills as salesmanship or advertising, which were aimed only at sales and without "noble purpose," did not belong in a university. Indeed, he thought they poisoned the very air of a place of learning. Yale was likewise ridiculed for its emphasis on buildings rather than scholarship and for its proposed interdisciplinary program in human relations. "I honestly think," Flexner told Anson Stokes, "if Yale had less money and fewer new buildings, the chances are that it might be a greater university."[55]

Critics scarcely knew how to deal with a blunderbuss attack from so renowned and powerful a figure. The book combined shrewd and careful analysis with a no-holds-barred denunciation of what were presented as typical practices in the American university. Most reviewers praised its candor, its keen historical sense, and its transatlantic comparisons while dissociating themselves to greater or lesser degree from the overall thrust of the argument.

Faculty reviewers and professional book critics liked the book more than members of education colleges or university administrators had. As one reviewer explained it, "Mr. Flexner's book has been so widely read, chiefly because he has stated a point of view pleasant to a large group of professors who have more interest in scholarship and research than in the need for inspired teaching." The literary critic Robert Shafer found it "unanswerable, fundamental, and final" in its analysis. Albert Bushnell Hart, a distinguished historian at Harvard, gave limited praise to the book, applauding its exposure of the "preposterous" lengths to which the elective system had been taken. It was "an uncomfortable" book, he said, that reflected poorly on a number of leading universities. A leading scholar of French history, Albert Guerard, found the work "a searching discussion" that transcended "the bounds of mere pedagogy." In a private letter, the renowned historian Charles A. Beard thanked Flexner for "telling the truth about our 'higher hokum' in education." Every honest man, he told Flexner, "knows you are right, but you have the courage to say it and say it with words as hard as cannon balls."[56]

College administrators were far more critical. The former president of Lafayette College, John Henry McCracken, called it "utter nonsense" that Flexner found such favored schools as Swarthmore free of the vocational taint of other colleges. He cited examples of vocational-type offerings from the Swarthmore catalog. According to L.D. Coffman of the University of Minnesota, the ideal university "does not exist, never has existed, and never will exist." In the future, as in the past, wrote Coffman, new studies will come into the university "because new needs have arisen" and "the university will teach what the people want." He was right, of course. Amidst the storm of attacks and counterattacks, a writer in the *Saturday Review of Literature* advised: "Don't content yourself with the newspaper stories of this book and its wild-eyed reception by defensive pedagogues. Buy it and read it yourself. It is penetrating, provocative and deliciously humorous."[57]

Of all the reviewers, Flexner responded to only one. In the *International Journal of Ethics,* John Dewey wrote a respectful account commending Flexner for saying "things that needed to be said" about "the absurdities, superficialities, and extravagances" in American universities, but he took him to task for assuming that "the cultural and the vocational" in education must always be in conflict. He found himself agreeing with Flexner, he said, in regard to specific criticisms but unhappy with the book's general argument. The American people, he wrote, "are blindly trying to do something new in the history of educational effort." They were being "forced by facts" to develop a universal education in which "the vocational quality [was] pervasive." Flexner's criticisms, while warranted, failed to take account of the currents in American life that made this trend inevitable.[58]

Flexner's respect for Dewey reached back to their first contacts in the 1890s, despite a dislike for Dewey's "obscurity" and lack of a "sense for style." He now wrote Dewey for further clarification of the ways in which Dewey saw the cultural and vocational in American education overlapping. "Is it possible," he asked Dewey, "that there is enough cultural interest in being housemaid or street-cleaner or barber or stenographer to satisfy a human being, or must not education undertake to supplement vocational activities by the development of tastes in music, literature, art, etc.?" Dewey's reply must have been reassuring, for Flexner thanked him for his "kind and detailed" letter, announcing that he agreed that there was a region in which vocational and cultural activities were "closely intertwined." After reading Dewey's letter, he said that he did not believe that his "general attitude" about the future of education in America was very different from Dewey's.[59] While this was perhaps true in the narrow sense that both expected a different kind of university in the future, the two men clearly differed about whether such a change was needed or desirable.

Flexner's book gave a tremendous boost to his reputation and public celebrity. In scores of faculty offices, literary discussions, educational meetings, articles and journals, and letters to newspaper editors his name was invoked more than that of any other educator. In Europe, where his book was translated into French and German, a lively debate sprang up over the differences he saw between the New World and the Old. He had been only two years "in exile"; he was now back in the limelight facing audiences larger than ever before. His life was not yet over, after all.

Still hoping for a chance to create a "real university" and to stifle the critics, he yearned for an upbeat climax to his long career. He hinted strongly that this climax might be near. In the closing pages of the book, he advocated "the outright creation of a school or institute of higher learning, a university in the post-graduate sense of the word." Such an institute would be "slight and inexpensive" to administer; scholars themselves would participate in its government; and it would be run by a president "come down from his pedestal." Such a "modern American university"— a true "society of scholars"—would attract "the ablest scholars and scientists" and the "most earnest students." Small in size, it would exert a "propulsive power out of all proportion to its size," just as the Rockefeller Institute had.[60]

As if on cue, while Flexner was finishing the opening section of his book, he was approached by emissaries of Newark department store magnate Louis Bamberger. They sought advice about a large charitable gift. Bamberger and his sister, Caroline Fuld, had sold their company to Macy's in 1929 and were looking for a way to show their gratitude to the Newark community. They had in mind the creation of a Jewish medical school in Newark, one that would combat the discrimination against Jewish students in the New York area. A doctor friend of the Bambergers,

E.M. Bluestone, who was skeptical of the plan, suggested that Flexner be consulted. Thus came the two emissaries, both attorneys—Samuel D. Leidesdorf and Herbert H. Maass—to the Rockefeller Institute to get Flexner's advice.

It was quickly evident that Flexner thought the idea foolish and impracticable. Newark did not have a good teaching hospital; it was too close to New York to offer any real competition; it could not provide a strong university to house such a school; and he was opposed in principle to any discrimination save on the highest professional standards. From his experience, he told the attorneys, men and women of the Jewish faith or origin were not facing discrimination.[61] While manifestly untrue, certainly in the metropolitan area, Flexner saw the issue in national terms, professing to believe that talented Jews could find a place somewhere in American medicine. Furthermore, as he wrote later, "it would not be good for [Jewish] medical students to be associated [solely] with other Jewish medical students just as it would not be good for Christian students to be associated solely with Christian medical students." The same was true of students of color.[62]

As he talked with the two men, the pages and galley proof of his book lay open before him upon his desk. Suddenly, after finishing the medical school discussion, he asked his visitors, "Have you ever dreamed a dream?" He proceeded to describe his idea of a purely graduate university devoted to learning and research. Like Eastman, Brookings, Edward Harkness, and Rockefeller Jr. before them, the two men were caught up in Flexner's vision of a new departure in American education. By all accounts he was alternately charming, persuasive, and humorous, impressing them with his carefully thought-out plans and his high ideals. They left with a copy of his opening chapter in hand, promising to read and discuss it with the Bambergers.

Soon after, Flexner was invited to the Bambergers' suite at the Hotel Madison, and negotiations were set in motion to create an Institute for Advanced Study. In May, he learned that the Bambergers were prepared to give him five million dollars to start the enterprise and "select the best brains and train them in all the solid scientific and scholarly fields of interest." According to Flexner, he explicitly told them, "There shall be no distinctions whatsoever in the student body, in the faculty, and in the board of trustees based upon race, religion, or sex." Coming from "two Jews of liberal spirit and lofty purpose," he said, he hoped that it might "do something to encourage tolerance in this country—and perhaps in other countries."[63]

"It makes a rather thrilling climax to my career," he confided to Rosenwald. A month before the book was published, the news broke. Understandably, it added to the aura of celebrity around him. The new venture,
said the *New York Times*, quoting him, "will be a university without rules
and will centre about a small faculty of distinguished teachers rather than
an expensive building." A new round of stories and interviews appeared in
the popular press and opinion journals. "Here is the prospect of a real University," said a writer in the *New Republic*, "shorn of spectacular sideshows
and compromises with babbitry; a place where genuine scholars will work
in an atmosphere as ideal as intelligent foresight, wise policy and ample
funds can provide." Once more he was news. So much mail and so many
requests for interviews piled up, he told Aydelotte, that he was forced to
cancel a planned dinner with the Swarthmore president.[64]

In November, as the book appeared, the *New Yorker* did a profile of the
man it called "Robin Hood, 1930." The "kindly, smooth-spoken old doctor," the story began, had "fleeced innumerable rich men, and expects to
continue as long as they will let him." But the "depredations" were for the
benefit of humanity and the victims soon became his accomplices. What
was this "hypnotic highwayman" like? The author called Flexner "a lean
gentleman with no hair on his head . . . with features that may be described as spiritual: a very delicate mouth; a fine long aquiline nose that
flowers into spirited nostrils; a large, placid forehead that hints at the
quality of the intellect behind it; and eyes whose constant expression is a
concern for the welfare of what they behold."

What was he interested in? His range of interests was "Elizabethan,"
said the writer—"domestic and international politics, art, literature, and
music." Nor were his interests in the humanities merely "pleasant and
bloodless," for he was "a fierce partisan and a passionate antagonist."
Flexner, the author stated, "takes every opportunity to decry our Janus-
faced morality, our herd-like conformity, our lowest-common-denomina-
tor amusements, our worship of bulk." Such a man had become "an
institution" that could not be "suddenly dissolved." And so he was em-
barking, at age 64, on a new career "to realize one of his noblest dreams: a
school for graduate study, a snug harbor for students, a Green Pastures for
those who would play with wisdom and learning for their own sakes."[65]

11

A Last Hurrah

Flexner's triumphant return to the limelight after his no-holds-barred attack on American universities dismayed those who had come to fear and loathe him. In the twenty years since the release of his medical report, he had steadily won enemies. "I know how university presidents feel about me," he lamented; "they think I am a little Jesus Christ." All his life, he said, he had gotten both more praise and more abuse than he deserved. Since his book on the American college in 1908, he had been unremittingly attacked by such figures as Nicholas Murray Butler, A. Lawrence Lowell, and Arthur Dean Bevan. Now he was about to launch a revolutionary venture in higher education and could expect little encouragement from educators.

He was "haunted," he had to admit, that he had never been "on the inside" of any college or university. He feared that this could be a serious weakness. But he would not dwell on it, he said, for that would leave him "paralyzed in both speech and action." To his friend Frank Aydelotte of Swarthmore he confessed: "I am only a theorist in dealing with higher education while you have been an active and successful agent."[1] As he set out on the new adventure, he was filled with both confidence and trepidation. It was his last chance to make a mark on the world of education.

In a telling piece of self-analysis, he tried to place his educational views on a liberal-conservative scale. Many of his critics, he wrote, thought him deeply conservative, even reactionary, for his wish to go back to the pure research university of Daniel Coit Gilman's day. But others found him radical for his ideas on student learning, secondary education, and medical schools, and his general willingness to upset the status quo. In a letter to Justice Louis D. Brandeis (whom he had known in Louisville) he betrayed his contradictory impulses in starting the new enterprise. He would use as his model the Johns Hopkins University of a half-century earlier, he told Brandeis, but at the same time he would "smash precedents freely, and nobody [would] stop" him. "In many ways," he confided to

Simon, "I would regard myself as a conservative," but that would not account for a penchant for new ideas or for "the element of pugnacity in my make-up, without which I should probably be teaching school in Louisville today."[2] Small wonder that liberals and conservatives alike have claimed him since; while he championed radical causes, he clung to ideas that had served him well in the past.

He was determined to move carefully in planning the new school. He wanted to make no mistakes. "I haven't a conviction that I am not willing to sacrifice," he declared, "because I want to do the thing right."[3] In Louis Bamberger he had a patron who was modest, quiet, almost shy—a man of shrewd business sense who listened quietly before taking a firm position. He had built one of the nation's great department stores and contributed much to Jewish and non-Jewish charities alike. A generous man, he gave out a million dollars in bonuses to his senior employees when he sold his company to Macy's. Now seventy-five years old and in good health, he was semiretired and took long vacations with his sister, Caroline Fuld, who shared the ownership of the family fortune.

Both Bambergers were much taken with Flexner and seemed perfectly willing to follow his judgment in laying the groundwork for the new enterprise. They were content, he told Anne, to let him "proceed in the most deliberative fashion." Indeed, they seemed reassured when he told them he wanted to go "very, very slowly." Bamberger had gone so far as to say: "I do not care whether you do anything at all during my lifetime. I only want it to be right when we do it."[4]

Flexner was asked in May to head the new institute. After mildly protesting that he was too old, he accepted. He was to be paid a salary of twenty thousand dollars, and provision was made for his travel and secretarial expenses. "I realize that I cannot expect to give many years to it," he remarked, "but much will depend upon getting a few of the right men and women in the first place and still more upon associating with it someone who can be trained to carry it along."[5] Already he had in mind Aydelotte, an early appointee to the board of trustees, as his successor.

The Institute for Advanced Study, as it would be called, bore the unmistakable imprint of Flexner's thought. From the beginning he had emphasized to the donors his conviction, dating from a memorandum he wrote in 1922, that a university was above all "a free society of scholars and students devoted to the higher training of men and to the advancement of knowledge." It was first and foremost a haven, a quiet retreat, a fortress of learning. At its heart was the faculty, who needed only "simple surroundings," protection from interference, generous professional remuneration, little supervision, and freedom from any obligation "to entice or compel students to work." "I shall seek a few first-rate men," he said, and "give them ample salaries on condition they hold up their end of the job."[6]

Such a "paradise for scholars" would provide "the new stimulus, the new ideal" so badly needed in American higher education. As for the small number of students he anticipated, there would be none of the "disastrous luxury" lavished upon them by contemporary universities, a pampering that had turned them into "sybarites" instead of the "spartans" they ought to be.[7]

The similarity to the Rockefeller Institute run by Simon was deliberate. Like Simon, he saw himself as "a master talent scout" who would "collect brilliant strays, loners, and eccentrics," scholars who would flourish in the heady atmosphere of the institute. Like his brother, too, he saw his institute as "a series of autonomous departments, with each fiefdom shaped around a resident genius"; Abraham would keep close tabs on the central budget.[8] His academic paradise would have no formal teaching curriculum, no academic credits, no regular students. It would exist only to give a sheltered freedom to a talented elite to learn, to teach, and to exchange ideas. Eventually, even doctoral students would be excluded from the haven, as they were at the Rockefeller Institute, to the dismay of some faculty members. Remote from the practical affairs of the normal university, the institute's scholars, like those of Simon's institute, would be urged to spend their time on only pure research and projects that would advance science and human knowledge. Down the road he saw the institute exerting a powerful effect on the development of American higher education.

In choosing trustees and a location, he was stunned to find that the Bambergers had strong ideas of their own. The articles of incorporation, at their insistence, called for a location "at or in the vicinity of Newark."[9] Indeed, it was the founders' hope that the new venture would be housed on their thirty-acre estate in South Orange, New Jersey. Flexner could think of no advantage to a Newark location and was dismayed by its lack of a great library, a neighboring university, and a quiet atmosphere. Only gradually, with the added weight of trustee and scholarly opinion, was Flexner able to persuade them to consider the advantages of a university location in Princeton, some forty miles south of Newark.

The choice of Princeton was made over the quiet opposition of the donors. They could not deny that the small university town met the criteria of a magnificent library, a community of scholars, and room for expansion. Princeton University was agreeable and offered the use of space in one of its new buildings. But the location of the institute in a conservative Ivy League setting signaled that there would be limits to Flexner's break with tradition. He clearly reveled in the association of the institute with one of the nation's most prestigious universities. His association with the president and deans of Princeton was close and personal. He was apparently unbothered by (and may even have welcomed) the fact that the Jewish-led institute (nine of its fifteen trustees were Jews) would be located in a place known for its low-key anti-Semitism. "Princeton," said Albert Einstein, "is a wonderful little spot, a quaint and ceremonious village of puny demigods on stilts."[10]

In the choice of trustees, too, Bamberger had definite views that clashed sharply with those of Flexner's. The latter wanted trustees of educational experience, including prominent professors, who could provide active guidance in shaping the institute. This was a highly unusual idea in 1930. As he explained it, the board should include "an adequate representation of the faculty" and a group of knowledgeable "outsiders," as well as "a number of businessmen." His end view, he said, was "to curb the powers and influence of the Director and to bring before a jury of laymen the views of academic insiders and academic outsiders."[11] But the department store executive was used to a corporate board of management and wanted business-minded trustees who would guard the donors' interests.

Flexner never got the cadre of "academic outsiders" he wanted. In addition to Flexner, Bamberger informed him, he and his sister would serve on the board along with his nephew and three of his associates. This was half of the board. A number of Flexner's suggestions of distinguished academics, such as classicist Edward Capps at Princeton and literary scholar John Livingston Lowes of Harvard, fell by the wayside. Bamberger concurred on the rest: Frank Aydelotte; Alanson Houghton, the former ambassador; Alexis Carrel and Florence Sabin of the Rockefeller Institute; Lewis Weed, the Johns Hopkins anatomist; Herbert Lehman, lieutenant governor of New York; and his old friend from his student days, Dr. Julius Friedenwald (who was a cousin of the Bambergers).[12]

Flexner was well acquainted with all of them and had worked with them on various endeavors over the years. Although this was not the board he wanted—its makeup would cause him problems later on—he was hopeful that he could work with its members.

Over the early discussions hung an uncertainty about finances. It gradually became clear that the deteriorating financial climate after 1929 was making the Bambergers far more cautious than Flexner had imagined they would be. The stock market had collapsed soon after the Bambergers had sold their department store, and now the expected recovery had failed to materialize. As they saw the value of their investments plunge, they became gloomy and worried about the future. Their advisers urged them to limit their contributions until the picture became more clear.

Less was said about a "small university" and more about an "institute" of limited size. Indeed, the final draft of Flexner's book, completed after the discussions were well under way, now questioned "whether the term 'university' can be saved or is worth saving." The chapter on the American university ended, somewhat ambiguously, with a description of "a school or institute of higher learning, a university in the post-graduate sense of the word."[13] Flexner was clearly adjusting his sights to the diminished circumstances.

A month after the book's publication, the board was called to its first meeting. Flexner announced that the institute, though small and limited in scope, would nevertheless be "a graduate university in the highest possible sense." It would be, in essence, a truncated version of the graduate university he had tried to reshape at Johns Hopkins and the University of Chicago while at the General Education Board. The work would begin in whatever fields "men and women of genius, of unusual talent" might "be found willing to be associated" with the institute. The first task, he told the board, was "to discover the talent" that would make the institute successful; this would take time. He intended to survey outstanding scholars and scientists all over Europe and the United States for counsel and suggestions, for it was "of extraordinary and fundamental importance" that they "make no initial mistakes." He pleaded for patience, saying that their steps were to "be tentative, provisional, experimental" so as not to "bind and embarrass" those who would succeed them.[14]

The board followed his wishes. Two years elapsed before he announced the appointment of the first faculty members. During that time he crisscrossed the country talking to educators and scholars, exchanged lengthy letters with scores of advisers, and made several leisurely trips to Europe.

He talked often with his brothers, especially Simon, Bernard, and Jacob, with long-time friends like Aydelotte, Julius Rosenwald, Robert Brookings, Alfred Cohn, and Tom Jones, and with Raymond Fosdick, George Vincent, and Trevor Arnett at 61 Broadway. Simon, particularly, was a dependable critic. He counseled his brother against further public statements ("You have now passed from critic to actor"), urged him not to consider having the institute award graduate degrees, and recommended that he keep fluid his plans for the organization and government of the institute. He advised: "I do not even think you ought to commit yourself now to the permanent retention of a lay board of trustees, however constituted." If his brother succeeded in attracting the outstanding scholars he sought, Simon counseled, "they ought to have a very important share in working out" the institute's form of government.[15]

Bernard was likewise involved in advising his brother. He served as a conduit, too, for the ideas of his good friend Felix Frankfurter, whose Harvard Law School post put him at the center of a widespread network of politically engaged graduates. At Bernard's urging, the sharp-tongued and forthright Frankfurter met several times with Flexner, often playing the role of devil's advocate. After "a jaw of about seven hours" in March 1931, Frankfurter told Bernard that he thought one of the best services he could render was to enlarge upon Flexner's difficulties and "make him intensely aware of them." He was uncompromising with Flexner, he said, that the institute must have "easy access to a great library" (the location was still not finally decided) and that he must spend more time in visiting such American centers of learning as the California Institute of Technology. "He has to get Europe out of his system," he wrote, and "realize that the Institute has to be hewn out of his brain, and fundamentally out of American resources and with reference to American conditions."

At another session he argued that Flexner's growing preoccupation with creating a school of mathematics as his first subject was misdirected and that "the so-called social sciences alone would furnish a test of courage and capacity." He had tried, he confided to Bernard, to "penetrate his thick skin with a sense of the awfulness of his job. I made him feel . . . that he has about as much intellectual responsibility as confronts anyone in the whole domain of education today." It is small wonder that Flexner found these sessions somewhat irksome and not "nearly as definite" as those he had with others.[16] They presaged much sharper disagreements in the future.

In March, following his second meeting with Frankfurter, Flexner embarked for Europe for a series of conferences on the institute. He had spent much of the previous spring and early summer there discussing the galley proofs of his book and the institute's preliminary plans. Now he set out to interview in depth those whom he believed to be most knowledgeable regarding the organization, subject areas, governance, and possible faculty members for the new institute.

At Oxford he spent time with the historians he knew, E.L. Woodward,

Arnold Toynbee, and H.A.L. Fisher, as well as his old friend, the warden of All Souls College, W.G.S. Adams. The views of Toynbee, in particular, as we shall see, carried much weight with Flexner. In London he was especially interested in the ideas of political scientist and socialist Graham Wallas and economists William Beveridge and Henry Clay, economic adviser to the Bank of England. He strongly admired Beveridge, who, like Tom Jones in Britain and Flexner in America, was one of a small group of public figures who drew equally on academic, governmental, and philanthropic contacts in framing policy changes.

On the Continent, Flexner went to the Sorbonne and the Collège de France. The loose and informal structure of the latter, like that of the Rockefeller Institute and All Souls College at Oxford, reinforced his sense of what the new institute should be. He went on to the German universities, especially Berlin, Hamburg, Heidelberg, and Bonn. He finished with visits to Rome and Geneva, whose interest for Flexner lay in its attraction for students of the international economy.[17]

By the end of the tour, he told Simon, "I believe I see . . . how to make a small, modest, experimental start at a high level."[18] He was now convinced that he would need to begin with one or two subjects, probably mathematics and economics, and continue to move slowly in view of the deteriorating world economy.

He came home flooded with advice, some of it conflicting. He was in his element, questioning the ideas he had heard, inviting criticism of particular ideas, and sorting through scores of letters and notes from his interviews. Of all those whom he had seen in Europe he seemed most taken with Wallas and Toynbee and their reactions to his plans. He had begun his journey with the strong conviction that his small band of scholars should be insulated from the mundane concerns of politics and events outside the institute. They should be freed from everything but pure thought, scholarly research, and intellectual exchanges with their colleagues. But Wallas and Toynbee, like Beveridge, Frankfurter, and later the historian Charles A. Beard, challenged his ideal of the disinterested scholar cut off from all distractions. Especially in the social sciences, in the words of Toynbee, scholars coming to the institute should not "cut their roots" to the society outside. Instead, they ought to emulate the faculty of the early royal academies in moving freely back and forth between cloistered study and service to the state. Wallas likewise argued that the scholar should be not only a part of society but an informed participant in it, helping to shape its reform. An economist or political scientist who

"worked all his life at books and teaching," he told Flexner, would necessarily "slip into unrealities."[19]

But he got opposite advice from others, especially Joseph Schumpeter,
a brilliant professor of economics at Bonn and former minister of finance
in Austria, who joined the economics faculty at Harvard the following
year. Schumpeter warmly endorsed the idea of the isolated scholar. In a six-
teen-page handwritten letter following his visit—Flexner called it "one of
the most remarkable letters in my life"—Schumpeter was effusive in praising Flexner for his "true vision of the University." More remarkably, he
said, Flexner was able and willing "to *act* upon his vision." The "scientific
worker" in economics, as in the natural sciences, Schumpeter told him,
made progress only out of "passionate love for problems for their own
sake" and "never from practical need." As an economic theorist, he believed that a knowledge of mathematics (and even theoretical physics) was
crucial for real progress in economics. The problem for economists was not
too little involvement with the *"hackneyed prejudices"* of politics and business but the need to teach hundreds of career-minded students and carry
on practical work of no interest to economics as a science. The true scholar
in economics, as in other fields, needed to teach, not in the drudgery of
routine classes, but in "pure science for the sake of pure science."[20]

The conflict in views between Schumpeter and the English scholars
bothered Flexner. Should he seek to build a corps of pure scholars in the
social sciences or try to make a useful contribution to resolving the world-
wide economic collapse? His uncertainty was apparent at a 1934 board of
trustees meeting: at one point he said that the institute should appoint
economists who had "been in contact with practical problems of business
and government," but later he urged that as research scholars they should
be kept "aloof from practical life" and not "diverted to the performance
of current tasks."[21] He found it impossible, as it turned out, to find persons with just the right mix of practical experience and the genius to make
original contributions. The creation of the School of Economics and Politics, which he had hoped to inaugurate at the outset, was thus delayed
until 1935, and it would bring him more disagreement and heartache than
any other program.

On his return from Europe, he continued to meet and correspond with
his American advisers. For counsel on humanistic study, he looked to his
ally Aydelotte, an authority on English literature, and especially to Princeton archeologist Charles R. Morey, who became a close friend and con-
fidant. He eventually hoped to be able, he told one of the trustees, to have

a person at the institute like the historian of science George Sarton, who could develop "the humanistic aspects of scientific development" and thus bridge the gulf between science and the humanities.[22] For further advice in economics, he turned to financier Paul Warburg, to leading university scholars, and briefly to Supreme Court Justices Brandeis and Oliver Wendell Holmes. In history he sought counsel from an old friend, Edward M. Earle of Columbia, a specialist in diplomatic history who was now ill with tuberculosis in Colorado, as well as historian Charles Beard, constitutional scholar Max Farrand of the Huntington Library in California, and especially J. Franklin Jameson, a friend from his Hopkins days and a respected leader of the historical profession at the Library of Congress.

No adviser engaged his attention more than Beard. Only three years before, Beard and his wife, Mary, had published *The Rise of American Civilization,* which had broken new ground in setting American history in a broad context of "civilization." Fired from Columbia in 1917 for his critical views on silencing dissent during the First World War, he had been a founder of the New School for Social Research in New York and now worked as an independent scholar in New Milford, Connecticut.

When Beard wrote to congratulate him warmly on his book on universities, Flexner responded by asking for his "interest, aid and counsel" in planning the new institute. He and Anne were promptly invited to dinner by the Beards, and their long first meeting grew into a close friendship between the two couples. "Perhaps my long experience with the inside of the academic game," he told Flexner, "may be of use—negative at least." The institute, if it were to do anything for higher education, Beard said, must "incorporate in its foundation documents" the ideas in Flexner's book.[23]

Two of Flexner's ideas about the institute, in particular, were the subject of long discussions between the two men. Beard found Flexner's vision of a small band of isolated, largely self-governing scholars unrealistic and impracticable. "I dissent from your fundamental proposition," he wrote Flexner, "that if a group of scholars could be comfortably housed, something of significance to thought and mankind will happen. Death, intellectual death, may happen, as it did in many a well-appointed monastery in the middle ages." He questioned Flexner's choice of All Souls College as a model; his own study there convinced him, he said, of "how remote these cloistered scholars were from the substance of things." He encouraged Flexner to have the institute focus on the study of civilizations, their interconnectedness, their ideals, and their tendency to decay. "Politics is rubbish without economics," he declared; "economics is futile without politics; literature that does not reflect movements of the human spirit is dead at birth; the applications of science without ethics are unthinkable."[24]

Flexner welcomed the "pummeling" he received from Beard but insisted that he had no intention of setting up a monastery. Beard's fear of narrow and insignificant scholarship was understandable, he responded—he, too, wanted to avoid sterile scholarship—but what of "specialists" like Darwin, Carrel, Millikan, or Einstein "who specialize in the significant?" What he had in mind, he told Beard, was "vaguely and loosely defined schools into which anything would fit provided" they obtained "a first-rate intelligence."[25]

Beard's other major objection was to Flexner's scheme for informal self-government by the faculty. "Would it not be presumptuous of me," Flexner had asked Beard, "to try in advance to lay down rules or to formulate anything?" What did world-class scholars want anyway "over and above association with one another . . . and absolute freedom to follow [their] own lives to the end?"[26]

But Beard told him that a firmer hand was needed at the helm, for "first-rate scholars can be as narrow-minded as any Babbits." From his own "bitter experience" he could not agree that "the scholars would work out their code." "My answer," he said, "is that they will not." What had happened at Columbia "when the storm broke and the university began firing professors without notice or hearing?" Even the good men, like John Dewey and James Harvey Robinson, Beard charged, "scurried around like bewildered rabbits, talking, protesting privately, and cursing the trustees . . . they were utterly unequal to the occasion."[27] Flexner, he urged, must exert leadership and lay down broad ruling principles, especially on academic freedom.

"I understand why you shrink from leadership," said Beard, "but you are taking leadership when you want to collect scholars and let them alone." "I want you to be a kind of teacher to the academicians," he said.[28] Here was another issue that would cause Flexner endless difficulties in the years to come, and Beard would remind him of these early warnings.

Beard, now Flexner's closest adviser, offered counsel on other matters. He urged Flexner to "chuck mathematics and take economics" as his beginning subject. He understood but rejected Flexner's claim that mathematics was the easiest way to start because it took "only a few men, a blackboard, and some chalk." This was "defeatist" reasoning, in Beard's view, because it shirked the tough issues facing the academy. Mathematics, after all, could be taught as well in Moscow or Berlin or Rome as in Princeton. Economics, on the other hand, was "the hardest subject" because it dealt "with the inexact." It put a person "smack up against the whole business of academic freedom."[29] He tried also to convince Flexner that the high salaries and "decent living conditions" he planned for the institute should be written into the bylaws, for if they were not, they would be defeated by scholars who would "devise assistantships and various ways for splitting funds in the interest of expansion."[30]

Flexner did accept some of Beard's counsel. He modified considerably his views on the scholar's role in society; he fought against trustee resistance for guarantees of faculty control over their own affairs; and he secured board agreement that the institute should begin with economics as well as mathematics if it proved possible. But he did not prevail with the board in a number of instances, and he was not fully persuaded by Beard.

Further, he was essentially alone in planning a vast new venture on a worldwide stage, buffeted by conflicting advice, strong trustee opinions, donor intransigence, and the views of prospective faculty members. It is a marvel not that he failed to accomplish everything that he hoped but that so much of the final outcome reflected his own long-held convictions. Those who saw him in this period were impressed by his steadiness and equanimity amidst the avalanche of clashing views.

One further experience had a marked impact on his thinking. At the urging of Simon and Bernard, as well as Frankfurter, he left in February 1932 for a trip of several weeks to the West Coast to visit the California Institute of Technology in Pasadena. Caltech, as it was popularly called, had sprung into prominence after the First World War as a center of basic science and engineering headed by the renowned physicist Robert A. Millikan. In a very short time it had attracted a number of the nation's top scientists and won financial support from foundations and private donors.

Fortunately for Flexner, Beard was a visiting professor there at the time, and they had further opportunity for long discussions. Also in residence during his visit was Albert Einstein, a towering figure in the world of physics, though Flexner initially had no intention of calling on him. It was Thomas Hunt Morgan, about to win the Nobel Prize for his studies on heredity, who urged him to call on the eminent physicist.

Most of his time was spent with Morgan, with astronomer George Ellery Hale, and with Millikan. All three left a deep impression. Millikan was not only the doyen of American physicists but perhaps the most skillful entrepreneur in American science. His achievements in attracting outstanding scientists and widespread financial support to Caltech were nearly miraculous. Millikan's close friend Hale, a genius at instrumentation in science, was likewise a builder of great observatories and institutions. And the quiet Morgan, a nephew of the Civil War raider John Hunt Morgan, and like Flexner a native of Kentucky, was a pioneer in genetics who had created at Caltech an undepartmentalized group of scholars in biology.

Flexner came away from Pasadena ready to act. Millikan and his group, he said, "are a really very distinguished body, and their graduate work is in the field of science very much the sort of thing that I hope to attempt in other fields." He told the board of trustees that he wanted, like Millikan, to select "a small number of eminent men who [surround] themselves with a few really promising disciples." Such small groups of able scholars, he said, would "in due course assist in the regeneration of the American graduate school."[31]

Of his visit with Einstein he said little to the trustees, but he was clearly surprised by the physicist's enthusiasm and interest in the planned institute. "He caught the point of the new Institute more quickly," he wrote, than "anyone with whom I have talked." Of his own accord, he confided, Einstein had said that when the institute was ready "he would come and stay" there. This revelation would tend to belie Flexner's later insistence that he had "no idea" that Einstein might be interested in joining the new institute. But we can well believe, as he told Jean, that "it was a thrilling end" to his visit.[32] The two men agreed to meet later that summer at Oxford.

Eight months after his trip to California, Flexner announced the creation of the School of Mathematics with the appointments of Einstein and the Princeton mathematician Oswald Veblen. Both were to be paid $15,000 annually, the same salary as Princeton's president. He had met that summer with Einstein at Oxford and later in Berlin. In June Einstein assured him of his intention to come to Princeton. "Ich bin Feuer und Flamme dafür [I am on fire with the idea]," Flexner recalled him saying.[33] Einstein was already convinced that the Nazis would rise to power and that he had no future in Germany.

Veblen, in contrast, had been in close touch with Flexner throughout the long period of planning and preparation. A tall, immensely self-confident, take-charge man, Veblen had definite ideas about the proposed institute. He was one of the nation's most influential mathematicians, a former president of the American Mathematical Society, and had helped make Princeton a world center of mathematical research. He had long hoped to build a "mathematical institute" where scholars would spend less time in teaching and more in pure research.[34] Flexner had furthered that ambition while at the General Education Board when Princeton applied for support in creating professorships in mathematics, mathematical physics, and other sciences.

Veblen may also have been attractive to Flexner because of the mathematician's famous uncle, the heretical economist Thorstein Veblen, who had skewered American higher education several decades before Flexner. Veblen shared with his uncle a number of traits that Flexner admired—a tough, combative mind, a suspicion of academic administrators, and a contempt for business interference in the university—though unlike his combative uncle, the nephew carried on his crusades quietly by stubbornly refusing to "be forced from the field of battle."[35] None of his institute appointments would cause Flexner so much vexation and frustration as that of the strong-willed mathematician.

Veblen was not Flexner's first choice for the appointment of an American mathematician. Before considering Veblen's appointment, Flexner had decided that he must try to balance his selection of Europeans, many of them refugees from Nazism, with the appointment of leading American scholars. In mathematics those he consulted had strongly recommended George D. Birkhoff, a prominent researcher in dynamics and relativity at Harvard. When he met with Birkhoff, he found that the Harvard scholar held ideas about the planned school of mathematics that were similar to his own. The mathematical group should be small, he advised, informal, built around "one or two mathematicians of great and undisputed genius," staffed mainly by "younger men giving promise of unusual talent." No thought should be given to balance "among the various fields of mathematics."[36]

Veblen, in contrast, urged the creation of an entire department of nine persons in various age groups, a size "large enough to perpetuate a tradition." The strength and balance of the whole, in his view, was more important than the presence of outstanding individuals. In February 1932, clearly taken with Birkhoff, Flexner made the first offer of an institute position in any field to him, four months before his agreement with Einstein. Birkhoff quickly accepted but then had a change of mind. Harvard put immense pressure on him to stay at his post. He asked for more time, then accepted once more, but finally declined.[37] It was a bitter experience for Flexner, who had already told the Bambergers of the appointment.

Flexner was now anxious to make at least some appointments. He had promised the trustees he would act soon. While in Germany that summer, visiting Einstein once more, he also went to Göttingen, held by many to be the world center of mathematical study, where he was especially impressed by the eminent geometer Hermann Weyl and where Oswald Veblen was coincidentally a visiting lecturer.

After long discussions with both men, he made a tentative offer to Weyl, who was immensely interested. Weyl, he wrote, "saw [at the institute] possibilities for research" that could not be duplicated anywhere else in the West, but he had deep family ties and was loath to leave his homeland. On the other hand, he told Flexner, "It is, nevertheless, difficult now to feel at home in Germany, for no one knows what is likely to happen politically or financially." Flexner's deep aversion to what was happening in Germany, where he had many friends and where he felt increasing sensitivity as a Jew, led him to try to convince Weyl of the dangers ahead. He left Göttingen determined to make Weyl a strong offer as soon as he could get trustee approval.[38]

Veblen, meanwhile, was tenacious in his quest to join the institute, which surprised Flexner. Flexner had hesitated in pursuing him because of fear that such an appointment would damage the close working relationship with Princeton University, which he thought critical to the institute's success. But Veblen sought to convince him that his joining the institute would strengthen rather than weaken the ties between the institute and the university. The work in mathematics would be made even stronger by the alliance, he argued, and Princeton would benefit as much as the institute. Cooperation would necessarily be close between the two groups of scholars. Indeed, the university was about to offer the use of space in the university's Fine Hall, which housed the department of mathematics, for the new school of mathematics. Before leaving Europe, Flexner wrote Veblen that if the Princeton authorities "interposed no obstacles," he would have his appointment.[39]

Flexner now believed that he had in Einstein, Weyl, and Veblen three outstanding appointments to launch the institute. Einstein and Veblen had both accepted, while Weyl continued to hold off on a final commitment. At the October board meeting in 1932, news of the Einstein and Veblen appointments and creation of the School of Mathematics was released to an avalanche of favorable publicity. A long front-page story in the *New York Times,* with large photographs of Einstein and Flexner, was devoted largely to Flexner's ideas about the school and the institute. Editorials and favorable commentary appeared across the country. Beard congratulated him on achieving his purpose "in grand style." With Einstein, he wrote, "You have not only an unquestioned master but also a rare human spirit. It's splendid." He even conceded that Flexner may have been right "in starting with a man and a subject beyond controversy."[40]

The Bambergers, too, were enthusiastic about these first steps. "I trust you will not overtax your strength in this great work," Louis Bamberger wrote him. Among his correspondents, only Frankfurter was critical, chiding him for thinking he could build "an almost cloistered austerity in scholarship and learning" by "seeking Einsteins" for his "society of scholars." However he tried, Frankfurter warned, he would not be able to "keep Einsteins off the front page."[41] He was right.

Over the next few months there were mounting disagreements with Veblen. Veblen was bent on building the mathematical group as quickly as possible. He had little patience for Flexner's concept of a deliberate incremental growth that encompassed the other programs planned in economics and the humanities.

He clashed sharply with Flexner, too, over his efforts to bring further members of the Princeton department into the School of Mathematics. "Merely moving men from one place on the checkerboard to another," Flexner told him, "does not modify the general situation in respect to scholarship in this country." The director did finally agree, with the approval of Dean Luther Eisenhart of Princeton, himself a mathematician, to the appointment of Princeton's James W. Alexander to the mathematics group. An outstanding topologist, Alexander was Veblen's close friend and collaborator and shared many of Veblen's ideas about the future of mathematics. Both of them were known, too, for their critical views about the support of mathematics in the university, harboring "feelings of great discontent with the University and its administration." Resentment began to grow among Veblen's former colleagues, and an "air of intrigue hung thickly over Fine Hall."[42]

In the meantime, Weyl had cabled his acceptance from Göttingen, bringing a balance once more between foreign and American appointments. But Weyl, whose wife was Jewish, continued, like Birkhoff, to have second thoughts. More than once he wired Flexner of a change of mind. Flexner recounted the twists and turns in the exchange: "He accepted by cable in principle, shortly afterwards he declined. Soon after he reconsidered and accepted. Not long after that he declined and three hours later accepted, saying that this time his decision was 'irrevocable!'" Soon he was begging to be released, and again Flexner agreed. "He is plainly a neurotic person," he said, "not in good health."[43]

At this juncture, Veblen pressed for the appointment of another European. This time it was the widely respected and gregarious, Hungarian-born John von Neumann, already interested in machine computing and game theory, who was then teaching half-time at Princeton. Flexner at first resisted, feeling more and more sensitive about taking away members of the host university's faculty. He was concerned, too, about the need to recruit American scholars. "If we do not develop America," he asked Veblen, "who is going to do it?" Among America's 120 million people there must be some mathematicians "worthy of development."[44]

But with Weyl's seemingly final decision to remain in Europe, Flexner decided to take a chance and offer the position to von Neumann. While Dean Eisenhart agreed to the offer, many others in the administration and faculty did not and thought Flexner had gone too far. So negative was the university's response to this third Princeton appointment, in fact, that the Bambergers themselves were forced to make a commitment to the university president that the institute would hire no further members of its faculty. Even when Erwin Schrödinger, the Berlin physicist who shared the Nobel Prize in 1933 and was close to Einstein, wanted to come to the institute rather than Princeton, Flexner refused: "Under no circumstances will the Institute compete with the University for any one."[45]

But Veblen had largely had his way. He had outmaneuvered Flexner in creating a mathematics faculty that was largely his own design. No one could dispute that it was a strong group certain to bring world attention to the institute. Within a very short time, more than 80 percent of all mathematical fellows of the National Research Council, a First World War offshoot of the National Academy of Sciences, were choosing to study at either the institute or Princeton.[46]

As Flexner prepared to open the school of mathematics in the summer of 1933, Weyl once more changed his mind. With Hitler in power, he and his wife now wanted to get away from Germany "today rather than tomorrow." The Bambergers were opposed to renewing the offer to him, but through Aydelotte (a favorite of the donors) Flexner succeeded in winning them over. The beginning faculty in mathematics was now complete—Einstein, Veblen, Alexander, von Neumann, and Weyl—and the school was formally opened in early October 1933, nearly four years after Flexner's first meeting with the Bambergers. "I have a feeling," he told the board, "as if the mist has risen, that what we saw more or less dimly as a vision is beginning to stand out clearly defined in the sunlight."[47]

Flexner now began to turn his attention to planning the schools in economics and politics and in humanistic studies. But Veblen continued to press him to make further appointments in mathematics, to keep salaries very high and uniform, and to start preparing to move the institute to a separate building away from the Princeton campus.

Flexner seemed patient with the importunate mathematician and constantly assured him of his value to the institute and of his own high regard for him. "No professor in the country," he assured Veblen, "feels more strongly than I do about the importance of higher and more dignified salaries." He took him to the Rockefeller Institute so that Simon might convince him that having a small group of research-minded scientists would be better than having a conventional university department, but the visit had little effect. Contrary to Veblen's wishes, Flexner made it clear that doctoral students were not to be admitted to the program. When Veblen demurred, he told him bluntly, "I don't want to begin giving the Ph.D. degree, for I don't want to involve the staff in theses, examinations, and all the other paraphernalia. There are plenty of places where a man can get a degree. Our work must be beyond that stage."[48]

The idea of a completely postdoctoral institution struck Veblen, as it did many, as untried and questionable. When Flexner found that Veblen was admitting doctoral students and incorporating their studies into those at Princeton, he took the matter to the board, and the practice was stopped.

Gradually, he grew firmer in turning down Veblen's repeated requests for changes in institute priorities and policies. He was especially brusque about Veblen's constant urgings to start work on a separate building. "I should find it difficult to get up any enthusiasm now," he wrote Veblen in late 1934, "on the question of site and buildings." Over and over he cited the maxim of his mentor, Daniel Coit Gilman, that "men and ideas," not imposing buildings, "make universities." Repeatedly, he tried to reassure Veblen of his confidence in him: "I value you perhaps more highly than you have ever been valued in your life," he told him.[49] He never told Veblen of his many differences with the donors over money and programs, while Veblen for his part never became reconciled to Flexner's plans and management style.

It was embarrassing to Flexner that when the school finally opened neither Einstein nor Weyl was there. On hand for the beginning were only the three men—Veblen, Alexander, and von Neumann—who already called Princeton home. Flexner had tried hard to have Einstein present when the term began, but the physicist had pleaded that he had urgent commitments to fulfill in Europe.

By the time Einstein arrived in late October, concerns were growing over his safety. He had been warned while abroad that he should not return to Berlin, where his property and savings had been seized. He and his wife had changed plans and rented a cottage on the Belgian coast, where British agents had been assigned to protect him. It was rumored that the Nazis had put a price on his head and that his life was not safe even outside Germany. His wife, Elsa, wrote the Veblens that they would like to land secretly in America so that "neither press nor photographers" were present.[50]

Flexner hurried to Washington, where he met with the undersecretary of state and other officials who agreed to a private landing at the quarantine station in New York. They advised him that if Einstein arrived quietly, gave no interviews, and tended to his work, he would be "in no more danger" than anywhere else. But "if he keeps himself in the public eye," according to Flexner's account, "there is not a country in the world in which . . . he is safe." Secretary of State Cordell Hull wired Flexner of his approval of the arrangements. The director was greatly concerned about a planned appearance by Einstein at the Albert Hall in London before departing for America and enlisted the help of his brother Bernard and trustee Felix Warburg to have the lecture cancelled, but it was not.[51]

Flexner was now determined to bring Einstein to Princeton without publicity and to keep him out of the public eye after his arrival. "There is only one way to procure quiet and *safety* for Einstein," Flexner wrote to a prominent New York judge, Julian W. Mack, who wanted Einstein for a New York rally, "and that is by saying 'No' without exception to all invitations." "I should not make an exception of Jesus Christ," he said, "not to say, the President of the United States." To Einstein he sent a note to be given him on debarkation: "Your safety in America depends upon silence and refraining from attendance at public functions."[52]

Here was laid the groundwork for a festering quarrel between Flexner and Einstein. Einstein called it the "little war in the beer glass." Flexner genuinely believed that Einstein was in danger, and this concern reinforced his determination to protect him and the institute from publicity. Frankfurter, who had no great liking for Einstein, had warned that Einstein's appointment might mar Flexner's vision of a quiet, scholarly retreat, but Flexner could not have anticipated the huge public interest that came with his subsequent targeting by the victorious Nazis. By the time of his departure from Europe, he had become a living symbol of resistance to the brutality and stupidity of Hitler's regime. He could not, he believed, withhold his voice from the effort to expose Nazi atrocities and to rally resistance to them. "In these times of danger to Jewish and liberal interests," he told Flexner, "one is morally forced to take on many things that in normal times could be avoided."[53]

The two men were on a collision course. It was aggravated by Flexner's fear that Einstein's outspokenly liberal and internationalist views would alienate the conservative Bambergers and other members of the board. As a Jew himself, one who very much shared Einstein's concerns over refugees and Western policies toward Germany, he found himself repeatedly torn over the scientist's public stance on controversial issues. Constantly, he weighed his desire to aid refugee scholars and support liberal policies against his determination to steer the institute away from the shoals of political involvement. He knew, after all, that this was his last chance to shape a place of learning according to his deepest convictions.

The landing went smoothly, if unhappily for those who planned a gala reception at dockside. Mayor John O'Brien, lawyer-activist Samuel Untermeyer, and hundreds of prominent citizens were left standing in the rain, while the Einsteins were whisked away from quarantine to Princeton. As promised, Flexner shielded them from the press, visitors, and a flood of invitations. "It is really not necessary," he informed Elsa Einstein, "for you or your husband to answer every invitation that comes to you."[54] As he had been doing for months, he declined politely but firmly every invitation for Einstein to speak, to meet with visitors, or to be interviewed.

Then, on November 3, two weeks after his arrival, a call came from Marvin McIntyre, press secretary to President Franklin D. Roosevelt. Flexner was asked to convey an invitation to the Einsteins to come that evening to the White House and have lunch with the president the following day. For reasons of his own, Roosevelt, under pressure from Rabbi Stephen S. Wise and other Jewish leaders, needed a public symbol of his sympathy for the cause of German Jews. Flexner refused, telling him, somewhat disingenuously, that by Einstein's own request he was avoiding public engagements.

Later that night McIntyre phoned, getting him out of bed to repeat the invitation. An annoyed Flexner told him "that a person of Einstein's eminence might well be given more than a few hours notice to lunch with even the President." Einstein, moreover, must not be used as a political symbol, he told the secretary. A few days later he received a note from the White House saying that on reflection the president agreed with him.[55]

When the Einsteins learned of the invitation (it was repeated and accepted), they were furious. Flexner, they charged, was interfering in their private lives in this and other matters. Flexner responded with some heat that he had done his best to protect their privacy and security but that "he would refrain in the future from any intervention at all." He also warned that anti-Semitism existed in places outside Germany, even at Princeton, and that American Jews needed to take care not to exacerbate it. "It is because I am a Jew myself and wish to help oppressed Jews in Germany," he told Elsa Einstein, "that my efforts . . . are absolutely quiet and anonymous." At stake, he declared, was "the most effective way of helping the Jewish race in America and in Europe." Again and again, he urged the scientist "to have absolutely nothing to do with the press" and to avoid public appearances, such as a proposed violin performance by Einstein at the Waldorf-Astoria to raise money for Jewish refugees. "I know America far better than you or he," he told Elsa Einstein. Such publicity was certain to continue and would in the long run harm her husband's work and that of the institute.[56]

As relations worsened between the two men, Einstein went so far as to decline an invitation to dinner with Flexner. "After your behavior towards us last week you will hardly be surprised," Einstein noted. Einstein then took his complaints to the board of trustees, outlining his disagreements with Flexner and threatening to leave the institute.[57]

A chastened Flexner quickly retreated, doing his best to restore the tattered relationship. On December 11, he talked with Einstein at length and later reported to the Bambergers that "all the little misunderstandings" between them had "been completely removed." Flexner and his wife were promptly invited to a "Deutsches dinner" at the Einsteins the following night and accepted "eagerly." Now, reported Flexner, "everything is lovely, and the goose hangs high."[58]

The rapprochement was apparently real, for Einstein accepted few engagements thereafter and cancelled a number of honorary and part-time appointments that had greatly troubled Flexner, particularly at the Collège de France and Oxford University, as well as in Spain. The scientist also made it clear that he agreed with Flexner that he should no longer continue to accept short-term appointments at Caltech, where he had frequently gone in years past. Millikan had been particularly aggressive in importuning both Einstein and Flexner that the physicist's continued visits were in the interest of both Einstein and science. "The truth is," reported Flexner, that Einstein is "happy and tranquil here . . . [and] that he begins to realize that I was right when I ventured last summer to suggest that he should concentrate on the Institute."[59]

By May, seven months after Einstein's arrival, all the wounds seemed to have healed. Flexner wrote Simon of an encounter between the two men just before Flexner left for another trip to Europe: Einstein "came over in the rain Thursday night, against my instructions, to bid me goodbye." The scientist had confessed that the past year had been "the happiest of his life." Flexner had come to realize, he wrote, "the value of dealing with a prima donna in a very light-handed dilatory fashion." Einstein had departed from the house with a twinkle in his eye, saying, "Next autumn I will be on hand, punctually."[60]

Shortly afterward, the Einsteins bought a small house near the planned site for a future institute building. Albert could often be seen walking on the country roads, bent over in thought, answering a stranger's greeting, perhaps signing an autograph for a passerby. Sometimes he would agree to being photographed or exchange words with a fellow resident. He was altogether humble and unpretentious, endearing him to citizens of Princeton. In the afternoons he could usually be found in his study, which looked out over an expanse of garden. He traveled little, except for vacations in New England or northern New York.[61]

The first year of operations had met all of Flexner's expectations. He could not have been more enthusiastic about the first group of "workers" chosen by Veblen and his associates to do advanced study at the institute. From the first, an invitation to come to the institute was viewed as a mark of prestige. In all, twenty-three scholars came to Princeton the first year to work with the institute's mathematical faculty. The number increased steadily, reaching a high of fifty-eight in 1936. Nearly all of them were college teachers, some of them from Europe, whose "enthusiasm and gratitude," he told a trustee, "are very touching." For many "the idea of a year of leisure has turned them into boys." He expressed enthusiasm about his groundbreaking project: "We are doing something that has not hitherto been so easily possible for American scientists."[62]

While he had expected most of the workers (later called members) to be recent Ph.D.'s, only two of them had been recently in graduate school.

Some were already assistant or associate professors in distinguished universities. Every afternoon some sixty to seventy-five mathematicians came together in Fine Hall for tea and informal discussion. Seminars and lectures were quickly organized on a variety of topics. Flexner invited Fosdick to come down from New York to see "the happiness and release" in the faces of students and faculty. To William Henry Welch he wrote that he was reminded of the exciting early days at the Johns Hopkins School of Medicine. "I am called director," he told Welch, "but I am really a supernumerary, for all I do is to carry out the wishes of the mathematical group."[63]

Faculty life was informal and close. The Flexners and the Veblens, as well as colleagues from the Princeton faculty, gave dinner parties that brought the group closer together. At one such party Flexner described Einstein as "the unconscious lion of the evening" who "spoke with everybody and in the sweetest possible way."[64] Anne proved to be a much-liked hostess and guest at these faculty gatherings. Many of the early faculty and students looked back on this period of harmony and intellectual excitement as a golden era in the life of the institute.

Beneath the surface calm, however, lay a number of problems. Flexner found himself spending more and more time reassuring and placating the aging donors. From his experience with the Rockefellers he had assumed that the initial gift of the Bambergers would be followed by continuing support as the institute proved itself. Initially, there had been talk of as much as thirty million dollars. But Louis Bamberger, Flexner's primary contact in the family, was slow to make further commitments and, unlike the Rockefellers, frequently second-guessed Flexner's plans and actions.

Although Louis and Caroline withdrew from active involvement on the board in January 1933, their departure made Flexner's task more difficult. Now he was forced to journey frequently to South Orange to argue his case alone, without the support of the other trustees. Louis Bamberger continued to keep tight control over major decisions and to force Flexner into compromises that interfered with his plans. On staff appointments, salaries, pensions, and the faculty's role in self-government, Flexner often did not prevail. Bamberger had serious doubts, too, about Flexner's ideas for a program in economics, and he was slow to provide the funds needed to make the same brilliant start as in mathematics. In all their dealings, Flexner, completely loyal, supported his benefactors' wishes, rarely divulging even in private the differences between them.[65]

Because of this silence, faculty members were largely unaware of

Flexner's efforts to include them on the board of trustees. From the beginning, he had worked hard to incorporate the idea of faculty trustees in the institute's bylaws, as Beard had suggested. In one of his early memoranda he had proposed having as many as five voting faculty members on the fifteen-member board. He also urged the creation of a board committee on educational policy, half of whose members would be chosen by the faculty. Tactfully, Louis Bamberger and his allies foreclosed these options. In January 1932, any provision for faculty trustees was excluded. Instead, three members of the faculty would attend board meetings and give advice but would not vote. Flexner later convinced the board to restore the concept of voting faculty members, but it was clear that they were not to play any significant role.[66]

Louis Bamberger was simply unwilling to allow a strong faculty voice in institute affairs. He was sharply opposed to having formal consultations with the faculty in making appointments or determining overall policy. Disappointed but undaunted, Flexner persevered in the belief that the Bambergers would not long be active and that it was of paramount importance to preserve their resolve to give the institute the residue of their estate.

Ironically, as Flexner took full responsibility for the decisions, he came under fire from faculty members for not allowing them greater self-governance. Veblen, in particular, pressed for a clear commitment to the faculty's right to run its own affairs. "I think one of the surest ways to success and permanence of the Institute," he wrote, "would be to provide that it be ruled by the scholars who are its members."[67] Over the entire period of Flexner's tenure Veblen kept up a drumbeat of criticism of the director's decisions and sought to enlist others in his campaign. Flexner unintentionally made the situation worse by recommending Veblen as a faculty representative to the board.

It is curious that Flexner, who had depended so strongly on executive leadership in his previous career, allowed the institute to have such an ambiguous administrative structure. He was chided by Beard, as we have seen, for not taking a much stronger personal role in setting the framework of the institute. As Flexner tried to rationalize it, the institute was to be very small and members were to be world-class scholars and scientists. They would neither need nor welcome a more formal system of governance. Somewhat naively he spoke of a close group of cooperating scholars, free of the usual faculty politics, grateful for their unwonted freedom, who would themselves care for the simple routines connected with their work. As members of the board, furthermore, they would have an important voice in helping to determine policies and procedures. Their presence, he told trustee Percy Straus, who opposed allowing faculty members any role on the board, would help the institute avoid the conflicts and "absurdities" caused in most universities by separation of ruling boards from their faculties. No director of the institute, he said, should be able to accumulate autocratic power by dominating a lay board that did not understand the educational issues at stake. "I don't want to be Mussolini," he said, "but one could almost be if one were dealing with merely a lay board."[68]

Flexner genuinely wanted to elevate the status of faculty members in America. In setting high salaries for the first scholars and striving to establish the best possible working conditions, he believed that he was setting a precedent for the teaching profession. "The condition of the American professor and his family," he wrote in 1932, "is '*elend*' [wretched]." It was scarcely better than when he had first raised the issue with Franklin Mall in Munich twenty-two years before. "The prizes in America," he lamented, "are reserved for university presidents, which to my way of thinking is quite wrong." In the case of the institute, he said, "the Director . . . ought not to be substantially better off than the most distinguished figures on its staff." It must not follow the example of Harvard and Yale, he declared, of "putting up three millions worth of buildings . . . while there is not a single professor who is receiving a comfortable income." His objective, he said, was nothing less "than a complete revolution in the matter of salaries and retiring allowances."[69] Again, it was ironic that such benevolent views of the treatment of faculty members should ultimately play a role in his downfall.

All during these early years in Princeton, he continued to take a keen interest in educational projects and issues beyond the institute. Despite the heavy burden of launching a totally new learning enterprise, he wrote articles for major journals of opinion, spoke frequently to educational and business groups, advised on new projects, continued to fight old battles, and commented on current educational issues.

He followed his book on universities with articles in the *Atlantic Monthly*, calling for reducing the size of universities, minimizing their administrations, and returning graduate schools to their original mission of serious research and advanced learning. Too often, he wrote, the graduate school was merely a vocational school "training college graduates to be college and high-school teachers." So rapid had been the expansion of universities, he maintained, that they had not taken time to look critically at the many new activities they had taken on. Once committed, however, they had "justified their absurdities" by giving them such labels as "service" or "democracy"—labels that "merely [covered] a running sore." The difference between training and education was in danger of being lost. "One trains cooks, one trains plumbers, one trains bookkeepers, one trains businessmen; but one educates scholars, one educates philosophers, one educates economists, one educates physicians," he wrote.[70]

In another article based on his own experiences, he lauded the fruits of private philanthropy. A series of benefactors had been responsible for setting "higher standards in education, in public health, in the practice of medicine, in the development of art, and in social welfare." While the great crisis of the 1930s now made it necessary for government to play a much larger role, private support of these endeavors was still important. It was a mistake to see private and governmental effort as opposed. Too big a role for government—as in the regimes of "the Mussolinis, the Stalins, the Hitlers"—meant suppression of "everything that America values most highly." What was needed was a "middle way" between an all-powerful government and an unbridled laissez-faire economy. In the great human crisis of the time, when "democracies more or less inefficient" were said "to have had their day," Flexner asserted the contrary: democracy, with its necessary mixture of private and governmental initiatives, would emerge stronger from this difficult era.[71]

His interests took him in many directions. Between 1931 and 1935, he proposed the establishment of a school for gifted pupils in New York, arguing that outstanding intellect was all too often "poured into the gutter"; he wrote a laudatory introduction to a book on the honors program at Swarthmore College; he urged the Carnegie Foundation to undertake "without gloves" a critical survey of teacher training at places like Teachers College, Columbia University; and he continued to feud with officers at Yale and the University of Chicago about their deviations from full-time teaching in medicine.[72] Indeed, the extent and content of his correspondence with medical school deans and university presidents throughout these years was remarkable given that he no longer had an official role in supporting their programs. Many still regarded him as the reigning authority on all things pertaining to medical training and believed his support necessary in philanthropic circles.

None of his commitments caused Flexner more vexation than his membership on the board of trustees of Howard University, which began in 1930. In 1932, when he became the board's chairman, he was forced to address many disconcerting events. Since its founding in 1867, the university had grown steadily in stature, built a substantial physical plant, and attracted many of the nation's ablest students of color. Its support came principally from congressional appropriations and major foundations. In 1930, under its first black president, Mordecai W. Johnson, Howard's finances were reasonably stable and it was making some progress on a ten-year program of expansion.

But the university was wracked internally by dissent and controversy. Sharp differences existed among board members, between the administration and the faculty, and especially between the president and members of his own administration. Serious questions were being raised about the handling of finances and the accuracy of bookkeeping. Flexner was urged by Howard's benefactors to head the effort to "straighten things out." A leading board member, Jacob Billikopf, president of the Federation of Jewish Charities, assured him: "You have the respect, you have the unbounded admiration of everyone on the Board."[73]

At first he seemed to be making some headway. A key benefactor, Edwin Embree of the Rosenwald Foundation, who had known Flexner at the General Education Board, commended him for taking good fiscal measures, "clearing the situation of corruption and politics," and "getting some further recognition of honest intellectual standards." He met with Secretary of the Interior Harold Ickes, who recorded in his diary that Flexner seemed to have "a higher opinion" of the black board members than of the white.[74]

But the campus animosities were far more difficult to address. A number of the faculty members, including the well-known research zoologist Ernest E. Just, whose relationship with Flexner was sometimes rocky, were convinced that the president was slippery and dishonest and called for his downfall. By 1934, the entire faculty, it was said, "was in a frenzy about the future of the university."[75] By this time, Johnson was locked in feuds with the university's secretary, Emmett J. Scott, and its treasurer, Virginius D. Johnston, and was being accused of Communist leanings because of pro-Soviet remarks. The Soviet Union, Johnson was reported as saying, was having more success in helping the poor than the "capitalist" United States. To make matters worse, he was under investigation by a congressional committee for irregularities in university expenditures.

As chairman, Flexner was particularly concerned about the congressional charges. He met with Public Works Administration officials in June and reported that while they had "a most generous feeling of confidence" in the university, everyone at Howard needed to maintain a demeanor of "orderliness and goodwill" if that confidence were to continue. By October, Ickes had impounded one hundred thousand dollars in Public Works Administration funds and was demanding to see all the relevant records. The university's alumni association, Flexner reported to the board, was "gravely apprehensive" about Howard's "unsavory reputation" and deplored the lack of harmony in solving its problems. He met once more in December with Department of the Interior and Public Works Administration officials, again without success, in an effort to "straighten out finally all difficulties."[76]

Ickes then asked for a meeting with Flexner. What transpired at that meeting is unclear, but at a subsequent board meeting on February 8, 1935, the trustees failed to approve the actions, including the dismissal of Johnston, the treasurer, which Ickes and Flexner had apparently agreed upon. Ickes was subsequently quoted as saying that Johnston had made "such serious mistakes" that he would be "unwilling to deal with him in the future."[77]

The records are remarkably silent on the content of both Flexner's meeting with Ickes and the subsequent discussion among the trustees. Flexner's relationships with the board and with other constituencies of the university had meanwhile deteriorated. To a friend, Flexner wrote that there had been "a terrific explosion" on the board, "of such a character that I was convinced that my efforts had been practically in vain, and I therefore resigned." He was "terribly disappointed," he said, by the board members' "flaring up with savage hatred against one another."[78] Whatever the justice of his characterization of the situation, he was clearly relieved to be free of a seemingly insoluble set of problems.

By the time of this resignation, Flexner was deep into his preparations for opening the second and third schools of the Institute for Advanced Study. He had expected initially to start the program in economics soon after launching the School of Mathematics, but advice about advanced work in economics proved to be far more conflicting than in mathematics. Louis Bamberger, furthermore, was not convinced of the need for a program in economics and doubted the soundness of Flexner's approach. Further funding for the institute was now halting and unpredictable. The shortage of funds made worse his dealings with Veblen and other members of the mathematical faculty. Flexner had agreed to the appointment of a sixth mathematician, Marston Morse, who had wanted to leave Harvard for the institute. With his appointment the mathematical group was essentially complete.[79] Veblen then pushed hard for a new building, but the director, never impressed with the importance of bricks and mortar, was determined to move slowly in view of the urgent need to start putting together the other schools.

The institute had had a brilliant beginning. The appointments in mathematics, headed by Einstein, had been spectacular. The postdoctoral students had come from the strongest universities in America and Europe. The program's flexibility and small size made it the envy of scholars everywhere. The first visiting professor was mathematical physicist Paul Durac, who shared the Nobel Prize in Physics with Schrödinger in 1933. Princeton quickly became the home or temporary residence of some of the most renowned refugee scholars fleeing Nazism. Flexner understandably felt vindicated by the successful realization of his vision of a special place for truly accomplished scientists and scholars who would train the coming generation in research and advanced study.

He was once more at a peak of power and influence. Could he achieve the same auspicious beginning in the two new schools? He was nearing seventy years of age. His energy level, while still high, was no longer inexhaustible. He required more rest and sometimes complained of insomnia and indigestion. He became noticeably more irritable, and his vaunted equanimity was more frequently pierced. The summer months at Lake Ahmic became ever more precious. For the first time, he began to mention retirement in his exchanges with close friends. He let it be known that he had begun work on his memoirs. Then came the death of his brother Jacob in 1934, followed by that of Isadore two years later. Both deaths deeply affected him. In 1935 Simon retired after thirty-three years at the Rockefeller Institute.

In his own family, too, Flexner's children were drifting further away. Eleanor remained in New York to work in the theater, and Jean took up residence in Washington, where she was among the first employees of the Division of Labor Standards. Anne spent as much time in Princeton as she could but was often in New York. He told Eleanor that that was "unavoidable for the moment" but "yet a matter of very deep concern."[80]

Still, he wanted to finish the framework of the institute before he gave up the reins as director. There was much left to accomplish. Ahead lay four years of almost constant stress and conflict that rivaled anything he had experienced in his long and turbulent career.

12

Final Battles

Abraham Flexner's plans for the Institute for Advanced Study were deeply affected by the dismal economic conditions at home and the growing horrors abroad. At times he seemed paralyzed by the conflicting claims upon him. Fascinated by politics and international affairs from his youth, he found himself surrounded by refugee scholars, friends, and family members who were heavily involved in the growing crises. Each day brought visitors, letters, and telegrams telling him of some new crisis affecting old friends.

Both Jean and Eleanor talked to him of little else than the poverty and need they saw about them. Jean reported feeling overcome by "feelings of futility and inadequacy" and gave thought to quitting her job at the Labor Department and setting out on her own to experience the Depression. Like many disillusioned young people, she wanted to go to the Soviet Union, in her case with Harold Laski's daughter, but she became ill at the last moment.[1]

Eleanor was even more disturbed by the New Deal's failure to end the suffering and demoralization in the country. She was critical of the work she was doing in the commercial theater, finding it "paltry," "dull," and "money-minded." She wrote a book praising Clifford Odets, Irwin Shaw, and other "fellow-militants" who wrote about "people that really matter." Like them, she wanted to turn Broadway theater into "a genuine people's theatre." In 1936 she joined the Communist Party. "I think Fascism lies far closer to American temperament," she said, than most people realize. To her father's close friend, Tom Jones, she confided: "I have no love for Roosevelt, but if a reaction sweeps in the Republicans next fall, we shall have a perfectly awful reaction." By 1937, she was enlisting to help Mayor La Guardia win re-election in New York and raising money for the Spanish loyalists.[2]

264   Flexner's brothers all joined the campaign to rescue displaced refugees, especially scholars, from Nazi Germany. Bernard was in the forefront as

one of the principal organizers of the Emergency Committee in Aid of Displaced German Scholars. From 1933 to 1945, the committee, which included Abraham and received valuable help from Simon and Washington, was able to place nearly five hundred refugee scholars in teaching or research positions in American colleges and universities. Support came overwhelmingly from Jewish foundations, especially that of Julius Rosenwald, as well as from individuals. Positions for the displaced scholars were sought widely across the country to reduce the risk of an anti-Semitic reaction in any one community. The Institute for Advanced Study, under Flexner's leadership, accepted eleven of the committee-sponsored refugees, a number exceeded only by the number accepted into the much larger faculties of Harvard, Columbia, and New York University. The University in Exile, which found places for refugees in scores of universities across the country, placed far more.[3]

Beyond their work with the committee, the Flexners were busy counseling those who sought assistance and helping individual refugees. Jacob's daughter, Caroline, a special assistant to Governor Herbert H. Lehman of New York, worked to settle Jews in Argentina and Brazil. When Lehman became the head of the Office for Foreign Relief and Rehabilitation Operations, she helped find homes for 1,500 Poles who had fled the invading Nazis.[4] Trying to help the Jewish victims of the Nazi persecutions was very much a family enterprise.

Flexner himself was besieged by pleas for help throughout the Princeton years. "Daily I receive letters from distinguished Germans, mailed to me somehow or other, from Italy or Switzerland or Holland," he wrote in 1933, "telling me things [are] infinitely worse than anything that has appeared in the American or English press."[5] Often he journeyed to Washington on behalf of those trying to flee Germany.

He was irate at the actions of the Hitler regime. "Nothing crazier has happened in human history since the days of the French terror," he charged soon after Hitler's rise to power. The German university students supporting the Jewish persecutions "must all be mad," Flexner said. Why did not ordinary Germans *do* something? "That an intelligent nation should submit tamely to such a government," he wrote, "is worse than chaos." Even in despotic Russia, people had risked their lives for freedom against the czar, but the Germans were all "meek as lambs."[6] The Nazi terror was never far from his emotions, even as he fought to give form to the institute.

He and Oswald Veblen, also a member of the Emergency Committee, tried to find temporary positions for the refugees. Between 1933 and 1939 about a quarter of the visiting scholars at the institute—forty-five in all—were refugees from the storm in Europe. Among the many distinguished foreign visitors were Kurt Gödl, Wolfgang Pauli, Richard Courant, Enrico Fermi, Niels Bohr, and Max von Laue.[7]

Flexner tried to find a permanent position for Courant, until recently head of the renowned mathematical institute at Göttingen, and for Emily Noether, whom he described as not only "the most distinguished woman in the field of mathematics" but "one of the most distinguished of living mathematicians, quite regardless of sex." Courant was placed at New York University and Noether at Bryn Mawr College. He also found a temporary position for his friend Heinrich Poll. He and Simon were instrumental, too, in organizing a fund for the widow of the eminent biochemist Paul Ehrlich, who had found refuge in Switzerland.[8]

The volume of requests grew as the Nazi vice tightened around the Jews. "This last week," he wrote in 1938, "has been a hell on earth for everyone who has a heart. I have been overrun with letters and applications." He was upset by a statement by George Birkhoff in the *New York Times* objecting to the immigration of foreign mathematicians. "In this era of hate and prejudice," he wrote Birkhoff, "it seems to me of the utmost importance that no American should utter any opinion calculated to fan an anti-foreign feeling." In an address to the National Conference of Christians and Jews that fall, he asked, "What has this dreadful and unprecedented experience to teach us Americans?" The answer was "tolerance, tolerance, tolerance a thousand times over . . . The German terror should determine us not only to live but to let live."[9]

He was impatient with American policy. From as early as 1930 he had supported a united stand against the rise of the Nazis. He would not forgive Hoover or Roosevelt for their indifference to what was happening in Europe. Impatiently he urged Tom Jones, who was a close adviser to British prime ministers and was described as "one of the six most powerful men in Europe," to take a tougher line toward events in Germany.[10] Throughout the decade and into the war years, he used Jones to relay his opinions to the British government: Jones frequently sent Flexner's analyses of American opinion to the prime minister's attention.

"The world is surely mad," he wrote Jones after Hitler came to power. Once again he blamed the harshness of the Versailles Treaty for destroying the moderate parties in Germany. "What a world of contradictions," he sighed in 1936; "Great Britain sends a Jew, Lord Reading, to be Viceroy of India; France selects a Jew to be president of the council of ministers;

America chooses Jews to be governor of New York and Secretary of the Treasury . . . but across the Rhine a Jew is an outcast."[11]

The same year he strongly criticized Britain and America's weak response to Mussolini's seizure of Ethiopia. "It might be infinitely better," he advised Jones, "for England, France, and Russia to smash Hitler and Mussolini before they get so strong that it is going to take a four-year war . . . to do the job."[12]

When Jones accompanied David Lloyd George to see Hitler and the former prime minister called the dictator "the greatest living German," a furious Flexner shared his thoughts with Jones: "Lloyd George simply does not understand Germany and can never understand it through the medium of an interpreter after a couple of interviews with Hitler." It was a waste of time and energy "to talk to these lunatics." When the inevitable war came, he added, America would not "sit idly by if England [was] in real danger." A complacent speech by ambassador to Great Britain Joseph P. Kennedy he blasted as "the most isolationist utterance that has come from any American Ambassador in many years."[13]

When he learned that the "craven coward" Neville Chamberlain was preparing to go to Munich, he despaired of any hope for peace. "I had hoped that some way could be found to avoid war," but he confessed to Jones, "I am afraid that at the last minute war will be avoided." He likened the British and French "willingness to sell the Czechs 'down the river'" to a decision by Lincoln in 1861 to perpetuate slavery throughout the American union. Chamberlain's appeasement, he said, left him so "horribly moved and shocked" that he was "hardly able to sleep at night." "Don't think I am a bloodthirsty fool," he ended his outburst; "God knows I hate war," but sometimes, he said, there arises "a situation which [can] be solved in no other way."[14]

Flexner had little confidence in the administration in Washington. The election of 1932, he told Jones, "will not make the slightest difference," but "on the whole Roosevelt is the lesser of two evils." Neither Hoover nor Roosevelt, he wrote, "dares open his mouth on foreign affairs." After Roosevelt took office, Flexner found the President "extremely active" in comparison with Hoover but doubted whether he could "sit down and think" before acting. He did regard Frances Perkins, the new secretary of labor, as "first rate" and was proud of Jean's close, frequent, and prolonged contact with her. By 1935 he admitted that while he found Eleanor Roosevelt "an intolerable nuisance," her husband had "done a good deal of excellent work."[15]

The policy "of restoring prosperity by increasing governmental debts," however, was "a complete failure." His lifelong commitment to a Cleveland-style, laissez-faire framework of government was severely tested by the New Deal's spending policies: "If Keynes' theory that the government can spend a nation into prosperity were sound," he argued in 1936, "we should be having boom times, but . . . there is almost as much unemployment as there was." When Roosevelt moved to restructure the Supreme Court in 1937, Flexner found his proposals "outrageous" and confidently predicted that they would "either be voted down or talked to death in the Senate."[16]

As the president took a stronger line against the totalitarian regimes in his second term, Flexner found more to praise, although he felt Roosevelt was moving too slowly to avert a European war. If Roosevelt had been willing to risk his future, he might have been able to bring the democracies together "against any dictatorial combination," but by 1938, he believed, it was too late.[17]

After Roosevelt's death and victory in Europe, he softened his criticism. To the Oxford historian E.L. Woodward he wrote, "Roosevelt deserves all possible credit for bringing us into the war and for such far-seeing measures as lend-lease," but "he had great weaknesses as President—even though I voted for him four times." The last is highly doubtful. He may have voted for him in 1932 and 1944 but probably did not in 1936 or 1940.[18]

As he reached his seventieth birthday in 1936, Flexner admitted, "I am not quite equal to working at one hundred percent capacity." The troubles stirred up by Hitler and his own trials at the institute were taking a toll on him, he confided; they "consume all my time and wear out my strength."[19]

He worried constantly that too bold or public a stance in favor of the Jewish refugees would stir up anti-Semitism at Princeton. The university, after all, discriminated sharply against Jewish students—only 5 of 435 Princeton seniors were Jewish—and only a handful of its faculty members were Jews. Several of the trustees expressed to Flexner their fear that Princeton was basically anti-Semitic. Flexner felt that, under the circumstances, it made sense to work quietly and to call as little attention as possible to rescue efforts.[20]

He would be ready to step down as director by 1936, he made clear, but he wanted assurance that his plans for the institute would be continued under a sympathetic successor. He tried to persuade the faculty that he needed an "understudy," presumably Frank Aydelotte, to be ready to take over the reins, but the idea met strong resistance from Veblen and others who wanted a voice in naming the next director.[21]

In a polite letter of rejection, written principally by Veblen, the faculty was described as believing that such an appointment "would be unwise." Administration under Flexner had been reduced "to such a minimum" that no immediate help was needed, and the kind of successor needed— someone like Flexner himself—would not "be happy in the role of understudy." The letter concluded with expressions of concern for the director's health in "the severity of the winter weather in Princeton" and suggested that he "repeat regularly" the vacation that he had taken the previous winter.[22]

It was a masterpiece of deferential rejection and effectively blocked his hope for a gradual transfer of power to Aydelotte. He still intended to make Aydelotte his successor but was forced to move more slowly in planning his retirement. "It is high time I quit," he wrote the following year, but the board "will not hear of it." He repeated that he was "training a young fellow" to replace him and that someday he would "slip out unnoticed."[23]

It did not happen. Though he was to have his way in the choice of a successor, his path out of the institute was strewn with unpleasant recriminations and ugly confrontations. The first serious trouble came with the launching of the second and third schools—those for economics and politics, and humanistic studies—in the fall of 1935. Both schools opened with less fanfare and less financial support than the program in mathematics. Louis Bamberger made it clear that he was still skeptical about work in economics and that it could be dropped at any time.

In creating the School of Economics and Politics, Flexner relied heavily on two new trustees, Felix Frankfurter and the highly respected Wall Street economist Walter Stewart. Flexner had persuaded the two men to take the place of the retiring Bambergers. Flexner, in fact, hoped to attract Stewart to a faculty post, telling him he would hold a "vacant chair" for him. A quiet and retiring economic theorist, a pioneer in the use of statistics in governmental analysis, Stewart had been a professor and then adviser to both the Bank of England and the Federal Reserve Board. More conservative than Frankfurter, his views had greater influence on Flexner. Unlike Frankfurter, Stewart believed that monetary controls were important and should remain in the hands of the central bankers in the time of crisis.

Highly intelligent, quick-witted, and sharp-tongued, Frankfurter, a convert to Keynesianism, pushed for reform of some of America's most venerable institutions. In his view, the emphasis in the new school should be on historical economics rather than economic theory. He favored a close relationship between economics and the other social sciences. Economics and politics, he assured the board, were different from mathematics because they were "enmeshed in an emotional matrix." He ridiculed Flexner's concept of economics as a "clinical science" that, like medicine, combined scholarship and practical experience. "All talk about science," he told the board, "is misleading if we mean anything more than the temper of mind which seeks to be as objective and as disinterested as possible."[24]

Flexner and Frankfurter were able to agree on the school's first appointment, that of the Romanian-born political scientist David Mitrany, a close ally of Stewart's. But Mitrany, encouraged by Frankfurter, insisted that a national conference of social scientists be convened to advise on the further development of the school. Mitrany's demand annoyed Flexner; holding such a conference would mean surrendering his and the board's authority to an outside group.[25]

The real blowup came with Flexner's decision to appoint Winfield Riefler, a student of Stewart's and a well-regarded statistical economist at the Federal Reserve Board. With Riefler's appointment, Flexner told the warden of All Souls College at Oxford, "the School of Economics and Politics will be not merely an academic or theoretic affair, though, on the other hand, none of us wants it to represent day-to-day economic or political journalism."[26] The board quickly approved the appointment, but Frankfurter objected to Riefler's being paid two thousand dollars more than his colleagues in the school (the second appointment had gone to the ailing historian Edward Meade Earle, who was warmly recommended by his former Columbia colleague Charles Beard). The board supported Flexner in rejecting the idea of a uniform salary scale, while Frankfurter asked to be recorded as being against the disparity.

Flexner was caught in a dilemma. He would like to have kept all salaries at the very high level he had set for the first mathematicians, but the deteriorating financial situation and the Bambergers' reluctance to release further monies made it impossible. If he was to move ahead with the creation of the new schools, he desperately needed to cut costs in other areas. Furthermore, he knew that Riefler, who had turned down lucrative opportunities to join other institutions, expected further support for his researches. Instead of sharing his concerns about money frankly with Frankfurter, he kept silent in order not to provoke the Bambergers. To justify the salary differentials, he cited the practice of individual bargaining by faculty members in Germany and Britain.[27]

On returning to Cambridge, Frankfurter fired off an explosive letter to Riefler. He wanted Riefler to know, he said, that while he had voted for his appointment "with pleasure and hope," he had voted against the proposed salary "not because it was too high, but because it was higher than that given" to his colleagues in the school. "Inequality of treatment among men of substantially similar age and scholarly distinction," he lectured Riefler, was "inimical to the aims of a society of scholars."[28]

Flexner, on receiving a copy of the letter, was apoplectic. "My patience with you," he fumed, "is exhausted, and I shall write you with brutal candor." He called the Riefler letter "a piece of unmitigated impertinence." It "makes it absolutely impossible for you and me to collaborate in any enterprise whatsoever." Board meetings were "confidential affairs," and if every member acted as Frankfurter had, the result could be only total chaos. "Under no circumstances," he warned, could they both remain on the board: "They shall have to choose between us."[29]

The open hostilities provoked powerful reactions. A shocked Riefler threatened to withdraw and was only with difficulty persuaded to reconsider. Frankfurter stood firm and tried to enlist other board members to his cause. The Johns Hopkins anatomist Lewis Weed thanked Frankfurter for sending the exchange of letters with Flexner and suggested, "Perhaps we can go on stirring things up without being ejected." Frankfurter wrote also to Veblen, who was serving as a faculty trustee, saying that he supported the mathematician's effort to set a uniform salary of fifteen thousand dollars in the School of Mathematics. He tried, too, to convince Aydelotte of the correctness of his action, but the Swarthmore president would have none of it. He responded, "I should feel deeply injured if a member of my board in a similar situation took such action as you have taken."[30]

Flexner himself remained determined to force Frankfurter from the board. Most board members, appalled by Frankfurter's breach of confidence and circumvention of the director, supported Flexner. In March 1935, only a few years before his elevation to the Supreme Court, Frankfurter learned that he was persona non grata and that his retention on the board was impossible. With great reluctance, he agreed to resign.[31] It was a Pyrrhic victory for Flexner, who felt betrayed that even a few board and faculty members were willing to side with Frankfurter.

The School of Economics and Politics was now under way. The historian Earle's appointment was for one year at half-pay, while he was put on

sick leave to continue his slow recuperation. He later suffered a severe re-
lapse and did not actually begin work at the institute until the fall of 1937.
The appointment was the result of his warm friendship with Flexner and
probably had, as the institute's historian suggests, "a therapeutic design."[32]

The school thus opened with only two faculty members present and
without a clear plan of operation. To the board Flexner presented the unrealistic proposal that the three men might work together in "international politics and economics." But none of them was much interested in
working out a common program of teaching or research. Mitrany, in England when Riefler was appointed, was not sure that the school had been
properly organized. He was increasingly contentious in his dealings with
the director. Riefler, who had his own research agenda, was justifiably
worried about the institute's ability to finance his research. And Earle, a
historian interested in diplomacy and in military affairs, took no part at
all in the formation of the school.[33]

Unlike the School of Mathematics, the new venture was launched
under severe pressures. The quarrels with Frankfurter, the lack of agreement on how economics should be studied, the donors' suspicion about
the entire subject, and the growing financial malaise caused Flexner to
move less surefootedly than he had in mathematics. He now foresaw no
further commitments to the general endowment from the Bambergers, although they responded to special appeals on a case-by-case basis. His field
of maneuver was becoming ever more narrow.

To make matters worse, Flexner now faced a more querulous board,
not improved by the presence of Veblen. As a board member, Veblen vigorously championed the interests of his own school and paid scarce attention to the other schools. He repeatedly made the case for more money
and a separate building for mathematics; he favored, too, an economics
program that was rooted in mathematics; and he constantly pressed for a
larger faculty role in governance.

An exasperated Flexner argued that Veblen's behavior as a trustee jeop-
ardized the whole prospect of a faculty role in government. "I am trying
[an] experiment . . . against the judgment of nearly everyone whom I have
consulted," he wrote after one heated discussion, but "how far faculty
membership will be influenced," he warned, is "going to depend upon the
ability of those chosen to forget the particular faculty of which they are
members and to live with the Institute as a whole."[34] Blunt as Flexner's
warning was, there is little evidence that it affected Veblen's conduct at future meetings of the board.

The rift within the board grew more serious when Flexner moved ahead with his plans to create the School of Humanistic Studies. He was determined, he told the board, that before he laid down his duties, he would make at least a beginning in the humanities.[35] But several of the trustees, concerned about the growing financial pinch, wanted to put the School of Economics and Politics on a more secure basis before launching a third school. Still others, including Veblen, were seeking to acquire property and begin work on a building. For Flexner, a delay might rob him of the chance to complete the framework of the institute. He feared also that several outstanding scholars looking for positions would go elsewhere if he did not move.

At Princeton, he had the support of the powerful chairman of the Department of Art and Archaeology, Charles R. Morey, who saw in Flexner's future appointments a means of strengthening his own area of scholarship. He hoped to duplicate in his dealings with the institute what Veblen had done in mathematics. Morey made suggestions that reinforced Flexner's own priorities in making appointments to the new school. Because of his General Education Board experience, Flexner was more confident of his judgments in the humanities than in either mathematics or economics. He had long been cultivating a friendship with Greek epigraphist Benjamin Meritt, Basil Gildersleeve's successor at the Johns Hopkins University, and he had his eye, too, on eminent art historian Erwin Panofsky, who had just been dismissed by Hitler's education minister from the University of Hamburg.[36] Both men were on Morey's short list of candidates, and both were known to be considering other jobs.

Flexner decided to act, though he knew that finances were shaky. His presentation of Meritt and Panofsky for appointment at the April 1935 board meeting met stiff resistance, particularly from Percy Straus, a close friend of the Bambergers. Straus suggested that, given the expenses of the existing schools, a delay was in order. Flexner stood firm, saying that he was keeping a sharp eye on the budget and that the appointments would strengthen the institute's bonds to the university. He challenged the growing demand for property and a building: "The real greatness of the Institute depends and will forever depend not upon buildings but upon brains."[37]

Ominously, the vote to approve the director's recommendations was not unanimous. Louis Bamberger, disturbed at the growing acrimony, sided with Flexner, saying that the basic framework of the institute should be completed before the director retired. But he told Flexner that no further gifts would be forthcoming except to honor "present commitments."[38]

Flexner was able to persuade him that these commitments should include three more appointments to round out the School of Humanistic Studies. In January 1936, the donors contributed nearly a million dollars to finance these appointments and to buy 265 acres of property at a site known as Olden Farm.

The new appointments added luster to the humanities group. Foremost among them was the paleographer Elias Lowe, an Oxford scholar whom Flexner had met during his Rhodes lectures. Lowe was making a compilation of all known Latin manuscripts written over a nine-hundred-year period. Anxious to come to the institute, he had the warm backing of Morey and a chorus of distinguished American authorities. From German exile came Ernst Herzfeld, a widely respected expert in the archaeology and epigraphy of ancient Persia, who had found a temporary berth at the Oriental Institute in Chicago. And from a part-time position at Wellesley College came the young Princeton scholar W.A. Campbell, who was leading archaeological excavations at Antioch.

Another appointment was made to the School of Humanistic Studies in 1936 when Flexner recommended Hetty Goldman, another eminent archaeologist, who was in charge of excavations at Tarsus. Adding her to the faculty did not strain the budget. She was independently wealthy, and her research was supported by a private benefactor. The only woman among the early institute faculty, she sought only space to work and research assistance so that she could ready her work for publication.[39]

In a very short time, under unremitting pressure, Flexner had brought together a group of distinguished scholars in the humanities. The appointments were less contentious than those in economics and politics. To make the school a reality, however, he had had to cut corners, to pay smaller salaries than those in other schools, and to skimp on retirement benefits. Furthermore, the appointments lacked balance; they did not create a program embracing humanistic study as a whole.

The faculty members of the new school were largely interested in the archaeology of one or another Near Eastern civilization. Several came with expectations of institute support for scholarly journals or publications. Lacking a building of its own, the institute was forced to accept space at Princeton for the humanities faculty and to rent offices in homes and downtown buildings. No sense of community or common enterprise could develop under these conditions. Many of the faculty seemed better integrated into the work of Morey's department than into that of the institute. The early hope that the two new schools would create separate identities for themselves as the mathematicians' school had done began to fade. As Beatrice Stern rightly concluded in her history of these years, "an unhealthy situation now existed within the Institute."[40]

In Flexner's last years at the institute, he reaped the consequences of the years of constant improvisation. When the generous support initially mentioned by the donors failed to materialize, he had started to temporize, expecting that further endowment must inevitably come. He not only offered smaller salaries and retirement benefits, cut back on research assistance, and postponed talk of a separate building and grounds, but courted outside financial support, all in the belief that the expected monies would soon be transferred. But the Bambergers had not the deep reserve wealth of the Rockefellers. Even when they did finally agree to finance a building, they made no provision for its upkeep or maintenance. They did, however, continue to hold out the tantalizing prospect of generous funding to solve all of Flexner's problems. In the summer of 1937, Flexner told Simon that the Bambergers had "intimated" to him that they expected to "give the Institute more money than it would need for many years to come."[41]

But the problems continued to mount. Differences with Veblen grew sharper as the mathematician pressed not only for more space but for a separate building for mathematics. Tensions were growing between the mathematicians and their Princeton colleagues housed in the same building. "At the present moment," Flexner told Veblen in 1936, "the School of Mathematics is utilizing well nigh the entire income from the original endowment"; there was "no likelihood" that he would get more funds. His exasperation grew when Veblen pressed him to ask Princeton for more parking space close to Fine Hall. Parking, he admonished Veblen, was an "extremely trifling matter" for such high-level negotiation, especially since no faculty member had to walk more than three minutes from his car. Flexner himself, now in his seventieth year, walked much farther "even in bad weather" four times a day.[42]

The presence of faculty members, especially Veblen, at meetings of the trustees meant that these and other concerns, especially salary inequities and retirement benefits, were beginning to emerge openly at board meetings. Flexner was desperate, he told the board, to take steps to equalize salaries, but he worried about the effect of chronic faculty complaints on the donors. The Bambergers disliked controversy intensely and distrusted any faculty role in decision making.[43]

Flexner found himself disenchanted with the actuality of faculty participation in governance, even on the modest scale being practiced. He feared that "academic politics" were ruining his chances to work out a final accommodation with the donors. Would he have found more sympathy in the faculty if he had shared in confidence the state of his delicate negotiations with the Bambergers? Perhaps, but for him it was a matter of honor to protect the confidences of his benefactors. Besieged on all sides, the stage was set for the final battles that would lead to his departure from the institute in 1939. No one who has sat in an administrative chair will fail to understand his frustrations.

There were, to be sure, high moments in the midst of the discouragements. The institute was an undoubted success that claimed widespread attention among scholars. The world outside had no hint of the financial and personal strains that were disturbing the faculty and board. No one could dispute the brilliance of many of the appointments and the overall high quality of those assembled in Princeton. Flexner was hailed as an organizational wizard for the remarkable start he had made.

While some insisted that only the unique availability of scholars driven from Europe gave him his success, the truth was quite different. Only a minority of the first faculty were refugees from Nazism, and even these came to the institute only after rejecting other offers. Albert Einstein, for example, had his choice of at least a half-dozen distinguished positions when he accepted Flexner's offer to come to Princeton. With every new scholar who passed up offers from well-established institutions to accept Flexner's vision of a new kind of scholarly retreat, it became even clearer how powerful and appealing his ideas were.

By 1936 Flexner was turning down applications for appointment from such eminent figures as Bertrand Russell, who quietly asked to come to the institute "if there [was] a vacancy." That same year Harvard president James Conant spent three hours with him to learn about the institute. Conant told him that the founding of the institute was "the most important event in higher education in America since the establishment of the Johns Hopkins." It is small wonder that despite the rising frustrations, he was confident that his quiet persistence would ultimately succeed. Clearly, too, the board and the faculty believed, at least until the winter of 1938–39, that whatever their dissatisfactions, no one else was in a position to pick up the reins. "My only concern," trustee Herbert Maass told him, expressing a sentiment widely held at that time, "is that the program of expansion be enacted during the period of your own activities."[44]

And Flexner still did not give up his broader interests during these hard-pressed years. He wrote articles on educational issues, took stands on controversial subjects, kept up a wide correspondence, advised old friends in the universities and foundations, and read widely in history and current affairs. When M. Carey Thomas, long the president of Bryn Mawr College and Simon's sister-in-law, died in 1935, Flexner ranked her with Daniel Coit Gilman and Charles W. Eliot as an educational innovator and offered to write an account of her career and influence for *Science* magazine. "I should have a peculiar pleasure in doing something about her," he confided to Simon, "because I know she did not altogether approve of my views." He corresponded the same year with the pioneer cardiologist Sir Thomas Lewis, an old friend and supporter of his views on clinical medicine, concerning the latter's Huxley lecture on clinical science. "I wonder when university administrators are going to wake up," he wrote Lewis, that medical graduates "are of two types—those who . . . want to do something [i.e., become practitioners] and those who are animated by a . . . scientific interest in the study of disease."[45] When Aydelotte enlisted his support in a campaign against loyalty oaths for teachers in 1937, Flexner quickly responded, "Anything more ridiculous and absurd than requiring an oath of this kind of teachers it would be very hard to imagine."[46]

He carried out long discussions with friends about books he was reading. With Henry Pritchett, now living in California, he exchanged a number of letters about Douglas Southall Freeman's book *Lee's Lieutenants,* debating military strategy with him. He praised Anne Morrow Lindbergh's account of her flight across the Arctic and recommended it to Pritchett. "Though I have known her for some time," he said, "I had no idea that, timid and modest as she is, she possessed such literary and imaginative ability." His daughter Eleanor constantly pressed her liberal views upon him, insisting that he read a new book on Soviet medicine by Henry Sigerist, Welch's successor in the chair of medical history at the Johns Hopkins University. He found the book "most enthusiastic" but "uncritical"; "though the intention in regard to medicine is sound, Russia is too big and far too poorly supplied with hospitals and medical schools to realize its ideals for many, many years to come."[47]

He was greatly heartened when Raymond Fosdick, with whom he had again become close, was made president of the Rockefeller Foundation in 1936. Fosdick met with him several times, asked for his advice, and commissioned his help in preparing materials for a history of the General Education Board.[48] At Fosdick's request, Flexner sent Fosdick a thirty-six-page memorandum outlining his suggestions on foundation policy. It was characteristically Flexner: frank, specific, and in places eloquent. "A democracy," he wrote, "is a jealous type of society . . . envious of large fortunes and large privately directed enterprises." This placed limits on what a foundation could do.

Where were the resources of a foundation most beneficially applied? Without question they were most effective when used for education— "the cornerstone upon which democracy rests." No longer, to be sure, was foundation help as critical as it once had been in building secondary and rural education in the South, but it was still sorely needed in black education because of "the indifference of the South."

It was needed, too, in strengthening America's select private colleges and universities. They needed endowment rather than subsidies for "special departments" or support of the research of individual faculty members. These premier schools, suffering badly in the years of depression, were critical to the nation, he told Fosdick, "on account of their influence over the entire intellectual life of the country." He named Harvard, Princeton, Johns Hopkins, Columbia, Vanderbilt, Yale, the Massachusetts Institute of Technology, and the California Institute of Technology, as well as "the outstanding institutions for the education of women."

It was wrong, he lectured Fosdick, for foundations to give money for special topics and activities "in which their officers happened to be interested." "The tendency of foundations," he wrote, was "away from breadth in favor of specific performance, with the result that the usefulness of foundations has suffered accordingly." Nor did he like term grants that favored "mediocre men who turn out mediocre books within a specified time."[49]

He made the same argument in his speeches and articles. Education was becoming far too specialized, too preoccupied with research, too directed toward careers, he told a graduate convocation at Brown University. The greatest opportunities awaited those whose minds were "stored with the history and fruits of human experience," not those whose time in school was spent in preparing for a "particular niche." Chance favored "the prepared mind," he said, citing Pasteur, and pointed as exemplary William Henry Welch, who had not been told by any psychologist "precisely what he was fit for." Nor was a definite position waiting for Welch at the conclusion of his studies. It was not possible, he told the graduates, "to make special provision for every possible need that may develop in the course of human life." Specialization and vocationalism, he warned, were "crowding out . . . the great disciplines by which the human mind can actually be prepared for the opportunities and enjoyments of mature life."[50]

In a lecture at Bryn Mawr, he insisted similarly on "the usefulness of useless knowledge." He was pleading, he said, for the abolition of the word "use," and for the freeing of the human spirit. Who could predict the practical consequences of acquiring knowledge pursued for its own sake, as in Marconi's use of the theoretical work of Hertz and Maxwell in devising the radio? He held up the example of the Institute for Advanced Study as a place of undirected learning without routine, faculty meetings, committees, or a sizable administration. When asked by a visiting scholar what that scholar's duties at the institute would be, he had responded, he told the Bryn Mawr students, "You have no duties—only opportunities."[51]

Such idealized tributes to the power of liberal learning were happy diversions from the hard problems he faced at home. The sentiments were sincere enough, springing as they did from his deepest convictions about the value of education. Serious learning, he believed with an almost religious intensity, had the power to transform individual lives and society as a whole. From his earliest recollections, as recounted earlier, he had seen education as a means to improve the circumstances of his own life and that of his family. He believed that his own spectacular rise and that of Simon, in particular, were due solely to the chance they had been given to learn.

His heroes were those who created a new kind of advanced learning—Gilman, Eliot, and Welch—and he had only contempt for those who trivialized or commercialized the sacrament of learning. His own experience at Johns Hopkins, at his private school in Louisville, in founding the Lincoln School, in reorganizing medical learning, and now at the institute seemed to him proof of the soundness of these views.

But Flexner was becoming uncomfortably aware that the renowned scholars he had brought together in Princeton held interests other than serious intellectual effort. Some were preoccupied with the very concerns—rules, faculty meetings, administration—from which the institute was established to protect them. Some of the faculty, he discovered, were doing little serious work and resented being prodded to show evidence of their creativity. Beard, it seemed, had been right. Even those with the most exalted reputations showed a surprising amount of interest in how the institute was run. Naively, Flexner, who had never been a research scholar or an administrator, had expected that academic politics was beneath the dignity of such honored men. By the end of 1937 he knew otherwise. Financial pressures and faculty expectations weighed heavily upon him. He had had enough. He was searching for a way to retire with dignity, but only after making certain that all the programs were strong enough to survive.

To Flexner the key to completing the institute's framework was always the Bambergers. In the summer of 1937, they had thrown him what looked like a lifeline, with promises to finance both further appointments in economics and a building at Olden Farm, as well as raising his hopes of further endowment. These informal discussions, held at the Bambergers' waterfront cottage at Murray Bay, Canada, were not recorded, however, and the memory for detail of the aging donors was becoming unreliable.

By the following February, the monies for the expansion of the School of Economics and Politics and building construction had not been conveyed. Flexner embarked on a program of rigid economies that sharply affected existing programs. He moved to recover the monies unspent for stipends in the School of Mathematics, telling Veblen that in view of the budget deficit, they all had "to hew to the line." Money was needed, too, to begin the erection of a building—to be known as Fuld Hall for Bamberger's sister and brother-in-law—though the Bambergers had not yet committed a specific sum for its construction. He now regretted that he had ever agreed to begin the building project. In April the board's budget committee voted to make no further commitments to stipends for the following year.[52]

At a meeting a week later Flexner reminded the full board of how much had been done with so little. Despite a budget that was "incredibly small and an economic outlook that was dismal," he urged that the institute "proceed with courage and with faith in the future." He pleaded constantly with the Bambergers to authorize him to complete the program in economics, telling them, "I think of our problem day and night." Privately, Maass, a close associate of Louis Bamberger, informed him ominously, "Mr. Bamberger seems a bit hazy about what, if any, agreement he made with you" concerning the appointments in economics.[53]

But the director, on the basis of his discussions with the Bambergers, had already taken steps to complete the program in economics. He knew that trustee Walter Stewart had decided to take the "vacant chair" that Flexner had promised him, provided that two further appointments were authorized.[54] He was in close touch, too, with Henry Clay, economic adviser to the Bank of England, a friend of Stewart's, who seemed willing to come to the institute, until his wife refused to leave England. Stewart's other candidate was a colleague from the Federal Reserve Board, Robert B. Warren, who had worked with him at the Federal Reserve and in private investment.

All of these proposed appointments, curiously, reflected the practical, activist view of economics that Flexner had once rejected. Stewart and Riefler had won him over to a perspective closer to that of Beard and Frankfurter than to his own original thoughts. In notes he made in 1938 he observed: "I am convinced now more strongly than I ever was before of the soundness of taking men like Riefler and Stewart, who know theory and who have had practical experience, and putting them in a position . . . where they are free either to read and study . . . or to go out . . . to observe, on the spot, practical difficulties and problems."[55]

He now had Stewart's acceptance but no money to hire him. Faced with humiliation, he threw himself "with a great deal of emotion" on the good will of the Bambergers. "I need your faith once more," he told them. "I realize that I am no longer young, and it has not been easy to wait." To appoint Stewart and launch "probably the last field" that he would initiate, he urgently pleaded for their understanding and support. Stewart, he told them, was "the ablest person in Europe or America" to make real the promise of the new program, but time was short and the economist was considering other "tempting offers."[56]

At some time in the weeks following, the Bambergers relented and gave Flexner the assurances he needed. In October 1938, the trustees approved the appointments of Stewart and Warren at salaries equal to those of Einstein and Veblen. To a number of the trustees and especially to members of the faculty, aware of the institute's acute financial problems, the high salaries seemed reckless and the disparities sounded a note of alarm.

He tried to make the trustees understand his dilemma. The high salaries given Einstein, Veblen, and Weyl were predicated on a return to prosperity; if such a recovery had taken place, "we would have adhered rigidly to this standard," Flexner said. But prosperity had not returned. Indeed, things had gotten worse. He had been forced to suspend the salary and pension scale and pay only competitive rates; had he not, further development of the institute would have halted. If he had been forty instead of nearly seventy, he said, he might well have waited to begin the other schools. In addition, the Hitler regime was "throwing up on the academic market" persons who would never again be available. He had asked himself time and again whether to use the institute's "modest income" to begin the second and third schools, or to hew to the salary and pension standards set at the outset. "I decided that the future of the Institute would be safer and sounder," he told the board, "if my successor found in successful operation three schools."[57]

Flexner's last year was full of strife and disappointment. A sharp downturn in the economy increased the Bambergers' reluctance to make commitments. The faculty seethed over the new appointments, not only because of their high salaries but because of their lack of scholarly credentials. Further, Flexner had failed to consult about the appointments with Mitrany and Earle, neither of them economists, but both members of the School of Economics and Politics.

In the School of Mathematics, concern was growing that the size of offices in the new building would be reduced because of the shortage of funds. Flexner had warned Veblen in the summer of 1938 that it would be "necessary to reduce the size of studies." He had never believed, he told the mathematician, that they "could build on the scale" that Veblen had wanted "with the sum of money [they were] justified in putting into bricks and mortar."[58] Decisions about space plagued the director throughout the fall and winter.

More personally, Veblen felt insecure about the pension arrangements that had been made with him at the time of his appointment. He petitioned the board to insure the amounts promised beyond those contracted with the contributory Teachers Insurance and Annuity Association, but to no avail. Veblen clashed with Flexner, too, over his renewed demand for a larger faculty voice in educational decision making. Flexner insisted that such decisions should stay within the separate schools and that the institute was too small and too specialized for formal meetings of the whole faculty. He did relent somewhat at the January 1939 board meeting, saying he had "no objection" to the faculty coming together occasionally but that he opposed "any regular machinery" for such meetings.[59]

In February came another ominous confrontation. The director had agreed to meet with the members of all three schools to discuss the allocations of space in Fuld Hall. A few days earlier, the mathematicians had voted that faculty members moving to the new building should each have "a large study with an adjoining office" for assistants and that the space being vacated on the Princeton campus should be renovated for their continued use as lecture and seminar rooms. The space was needed, they said, in order to "continue without interruption our present relations with students and faculty of the university."[60] Flexner, disturbed by what he saw as inordinate demands, was determined to make certain that the faculty in the other schools had adequate space in the new building.

Why was it suddenly so pressing that the entire mathematical faculty and their assistants be moved en masse to Fuld Hall? Among other reasons, the mathematician James Alexander, apparently with Veblen's approval, cited the anti-Semitic climate at the university, which, he said, was harmful to the Jewish professors. To Flexner this was an explosive charge that threatened his long effort to cultivate good relations with the university. Whatever its truth, he believed that its repetition could only exacerbate tensions with the university. Angrily, he responded that the professor's remarks were "ill-advised" and that further meetings of the faculty would serve no purpose.[61] The meeting broke up in acrimony and without resolving the problems of space.

To Aydelotte, Flexner expressed his deep concern about the charges of anti-Semitism. Either "anti-Semitism or pro-Semitism," he said, was "unthinkable" at the high intellectual level of the institute. If it were even whispered that such charges were being made, the "doom of the Institute" would be sealed. That some anti-Semitic feeling existed at the university he did not doubt, but he believed that its "extent and strength" was not dangerous. To sacrifice the close cooperation that existed with the university because of such concerns, he warned, would be detrimental to all future plans. Some hostility to the institute existed at Princeton, but he attributed it to the early hiring of the university's mathematicians. He was relieved when Aydelotte told him that while anti-Semitism was rising in the country he thought that the institute would be "the last place to be affected by it."[62]

Events now moved rapidly. A discouraged Flexner seemed once more ready to retire. To board chairman Alanson Houghton he wrote, "We must begin to look about for someone who can step into my present post." In March, while he was absent from Princeton, the faculty held several informal meetings and concluded that Flexner should be asked to inform the board of the faculty members' "unanimous opinion" that they should be consulted about the choice of his successor. In a memorandum to Flexner, signed by Einstein, Goldman, and Marston Morse, they said that "a majority of the faculty" believed they should likewise be consulted on future faculty appointments. Flexner, worried about the Bambergers' probable reaction to such a document, told Einstein and Morse that he did not see how he could forward it. Privately, he believed that only Aydelotte, his own choice, would be acceptable to the donors. Einstein and Morse thereupon told several of the trustees, including Aydelotte, of their dilemma.[63] At the May board meeting, Flexner moved to contain the growing controversy by making clear that he would accept reappointment for another year. The trustees voted unanimously to reappoint him but offered none of the words of praise they had offered at similar moments in the past.

The lines were now sharply drawn. Two of the most influential trustees, Maass and Samuel Leidesdorf (the Bambergers' original emissaries to Flexner), were advised by Einstein and Earle that they believed that the director should retire. Veblen, as a trustee himself, took no part in these meetings but was an active participant in framing the faculty's strategy. The two trustees then met with Flexner and urged him to consider ending his service in the near future. After several weeks Flexner responded that he would have to give it further thought. He was ready to retire, he said, but reluctant to leave unresolved the financial crisis and the issue of the succession. He was also angry at the defection of Earle, whose presence at the institute was due solely to him, and particularly at Earle's role in seeking to force his resignation. In the case of Einstein, who normally had little interest in academic politics, Flexner apparently believed that the physicist was influenced by a warning from Veblen that continued deficit spending would imperil his pension benefits.[64]

It was a tense summer. Secret meetings, intrigues, and rising tempers marked the normally tranquil vacation months. Before Earle left for further tests at the tuberculosis sanitarium on Saranac Lake, the Flexners invited him to lunch. On the advice of Veblen, however, he declined and with the latter's help wrote the director a frank letter. "I have expressed to you my alarm on a number of points," he said: "your refusal to admit the presence of anti-Semitism in this community, your openly expressed contempt for fellow members of the faculty . . . your resistance to a measure of Faculty participation in vital decisions, your refusal to transmit to the Trustees a respectful modest request for such participation [and] your procedure in the most recent appointments in the School of Economics and Politics." Under the circumstances—"I know from bitter experience that you do not welcome criticism"—he could see no reason to meet with the director.[65]

The indictment was harsh. Earle could not have known the severe limitations under which Flexner worked—the maddening ambiguity of the donors, the institute's dependence on the university's good will, his earlier frustration in seeking a faculty voice in decision making. And Earle himself, together with his wife, had advised Flexner at the outset of the institute, "'Faculty government' would seem to us futile and ineffective . . . scholars should be let alone as much as possible . . . the ablest of them do not want to be bothered with self-government . . . they would much prefer to be relieved of administrative duties."[66] But Earle was surely right that Flexner had become querulous and short-tempered and had failed to understand the faculty's need to be consulted and assured of the institute's future.

By late June, Earle was assuring Veblen that the director was holding on "by the skin of his teeth." The two men agreed to keep in close touch and to keep others, particularly Einstein, informed. "I do not need to tell you," he told Veblen, "that allowing Abe to continue on any terms would be a major catastrophe." Did Veblen think it wise, he asked, that Einstein be asked to bring "further pressure" to bear? To Aydelotte he implied that Einstein would resign if Flexner did not go. For his part, Veblen was writing Aydelotte of the "bad effect on morale" of the "present tense and uncertain situation." Earle then wrote an "emphatic letter" to Maass, warning him that the continuing tension was "intolerable." He was concerned, he confided to Veblen, that his own life would be "pretty difficult" if Flexner were to stay on.[67]

At his summer camp in Canada an exhausted and ailing Flexner welcomed his ally Aydelotte for a week of conversation. While urging Flexner to retire, Aydelotte agreed that the director should not be forced out. Following Aydelotte's visit, Flexner wrote to Tom Jones that he intended to submit his resignation in October but that the date of its effectiveness would depend on the choice of a successor, "which is not going to be altogether a simple matter."[68] He also confided his plans to Simon and Bernard, telling the latter that "the foundations of the Institute" were "securely laid" and that he had "other tasks in view" to take up his time. "I am in no mood to struggle," he said, and "am strongly inclined to get out of the mess and to let my successor do with it what he pleases."

"With the exception of perhaps two men," he told Bernard, "everybody is, I believe, loyal to the Institute and clear as to its purpose." No purpose could be served by his staying on any longer. "I have no resentment," he added, "except insofar as a human disgust for Earle, which I shall, however, keep to myself." Simon urged him to handle the situation so that "no hard feelings" remained.[69]

After conversations with the Bambergers and their attorney, trustee John Hardin, Flexner was convinced that the appointment of Aydelotte as his successor was assured. No reason therefore remained for prolonging his service beyond the October board meeting. On August 12 he sent letters informing all the trustees of his decision to retire. A collective sign of relief, followed by gracious tributes, came from the faculty, especially those most involved in seeking his ouster. Veblen promptly expressed the hope that he would take the "deepest satisfaction at the extent to which the Institute" conformed to his "original plan." After a decent interval, Earle wrote, "Your name and spirit will always be associated with the Institute . . . you have created something unique in higher learning, not only in America but elsewhere, and have gathered together an unequaled group of scholars." On a personal note, he expressed his "profound gratitude" for his appointment and for Flexner's "never-failing . . . help, encouragement and affection" in "a trying period of illness and convalescence."[70]

For Panofsky, the tie to Flexner was "a uniquely personal relationship between an individual scholar and his superior," while Weyl praised his "kindness and flexibility" and asked himself "where [he] should have been without" Flexner.[71] Similar letters came from other members of the faculty.

The focus now turned to the question of succession. Aydelotte was the strong choice of both Flexner and the Bambergers, who made clear that their further support depended on an orderly succession. Aydelotte himself, who was privy to the dissatisfaction of some of the faculty, was sympathetic to their determination to play a role in the succession. A few days after Flexner's letter was sent, Veblen wrote Maass urging that steps be taken "immediately to choose a new director." Earle had already suggested to the trustee, he told Veblen, that all future directors should be chosen by a joint committee of faculty and trustees.[72]

Veblen and Earle were able to convince Aydelotte that a special board meeting should be called to begin the process, but Flexner vetoed the idea. It would create an impression of haste and pressure, Flexner responded, and he warned Aydelotte not to "under-estimate the fact that" he was "dealing with intriguers." He confessed to his old friend that he had been "a baby in their hands." "They wanted opportunities for scholarship, with high salaries," he said, "but they also wanted managerial and executive power." When they saw they could not get them through the director, Veblen and a few others "intrigued to get them indirectly."[73]

As it became clear that pressure was building for the swift appointment of Aydelotte, Earle told the Swarthmore president that they had "no objection" to him but felt that the proper procedure was still to choose the new director by a joint faculty-trustee committee.[74] It was not to be. Flexner was determined to retire with dignity, with no hint of pressure. Chairman Houghton, at Flexner's suggestion, met with Louis Bamberger and selected a committee of three reliable trustees. To appease the faculty, Flexner, at the urging of Riefler and Stewart, the other faculty trustees, told Houghton that it would be "in the interest of good feeling" for a committee member to consult individually with faculty members "to give them a sense of participation."[75] Houghton himself undertook the task.

All was now ready. At the October meeting, Flexner made his final report, the committee made its recommendations, and Aydelotte was appointed. No hint of controversy marred the proceedings. In his last words as director, Flexner reviewed his memorandum to the board of eight years before, emphasizing how closely he had followed its plans for the institute. He urged the trustees to remain flexible and to retain the "experimental character" of the enterprise. Houghton responded with high praise for his skill in realizing the "great and noble dream" of a company of scholars working together in complete freedom.[76]

A committee of trustees and faculty members was named to prepare resolutions to mark the director's retirement. At the next meeting, a statement signed by all of the faculty and trustees recorded their "permanent indebtedness" to him. "Whatever prestige the Institute enjoys or may enjoy in the future," the resolution read, "will be based upon the foundations established by Abraham Flexner."[77]

Another chapter was thus closed in Abraham Flexner's long and varied career. He had succeeded in creating one of the most innovative institutions in the history of American education. His original ideas had by and large proved sound. He had brought together in a very short time a unique gathering of scholars. He had kept the institute small, flexible, and open to new directions. Perhaps only the Rockefeller Institute, the Kaiser Wilhelm Gesellschaft, and the Collège de France, all created over a much longer period of time, were comparable in their structure and purpose. The *New York Times,* calling him "A Critic in Ordinary," described him as a "militant educator fighting for the higher things of life and especially for the education of the gifted." The institute, said the editorial writer, was the "constructive embodiment of his philosophy."[78]

In the years since 1940 only a handful of similar endeavors have been launched—the Center for Advanced Study in the Behavioral Sciences, the National Humanities Center, the Wissenschaftskolleg in Berlin, the Collegium Budapest, and perhaps a half-dozen other institutions—and all acknowledge their debt to the Institute for Advanced Study.[79] Unlike the institute at Princeton, the others have made no provision for a permanent faculty of resident scholars. None of the institutes has had the impact on advanced study that Flexner foresaw, primarily because universities themselves, under the spur of competition and governmental research incentives, have created a vast array of research institutes and programs since

1940. Still, the institute remains a prestigious and much-admired retreat for leading scholars and scientists.

For all his success, Flexner failed in important ways in what he attempted at Princeton. The institute appeared more stable than it actually was. He was not able to persuade the donors of the importance of secure funding of programs and appointments, and their close identification with the institute made it difficult to find other benefactors to make up the difference. The system of unequal salaries, unfunded pensions, and unendowed property, however justified by the circumstances, was a pernicious force in the life of the institute. Nor was Flexner able to create his much-desired sense of a total community among the faculty. The lack of a defining core of interest in the appointments to the Schools of Economics and Politics and Humanistic Studies, in particular, made their integration into the institute problematic at best. And he badly underestimated the role that academic politics would play in his community of brilliant scholars. He particularly misread the influence that Veblen, when teamed with Earle, could have in shaping faculty opinion.

Why had Flexner's generous intention toward faculty government turned out so badly? Initially, of course, when the number of faculty members was small, it made sense to have only informal arrangements. He missed the opportunity, as Beard had suggested, to lay down rules for future operations within the institute. Increasingly, as more faculty members were added, his time was spent in placating the donors and charting the future course of institute development. He had no experience in administrating an educational enterprise, while the newly appointed faculty all came from large universities with traditions of faculty consultation. The faculty effectively stymied his efforts to appoint a deputy who would become his successor. With advancing age, he became impatient about faculty concerns over space, parking, and relationships to Princeton University. The economic doldrums of the late thirties brought increased concerns about faculty pensions and future growth. In the period of crisis, Veblen was able to assert new leadership in faculty ranks and to persuade a number of them to join his effort to replace the leader. He was greatly aided by the politically skilled Earle. Flexner, beset by ill health and growing economic concerns, felt betrayed by those to whom he had personally been closest.

Contrary to impressions, Flexner had a close, even affectionate, relationship with most members of the faculty. He kept up friendships with most of the sixteen persons appointed during his tenure. Meritt and von

Neumann were his summer guests at Lake Ahmic; Panofsky and Weyl remained his good friends after he left Princeton; Einstein maintained a cordial relationship with him for the rest of his life; Riefler, Stewart, Warren, and Lowe were strong supporters even in the time of troubles; and the others, even Veblen and Earle, remained respectful and cordial in their contacts with him.

The final months took a terrible toll on his health and peace of mind. He was suddenly older, more impulsive, less inclined to weigh his actions deliberately. His family and friends were greatly concerned. "I have been working without interruption at a terrific pace since I was nineteen years of age," he told Tom Jones in an uncharacteristic admission of weariness. He had developed a chronic cough and sore throat and found work and travel difficult. "Now you should have a chance to recover your health and spirits," Simon counseled him, "and resume your regular sleeping habits." He urged him to leave Princeton and turn over responsibility as quickly as possible.[80]

In mid-October, he and Anne traveled south and became patients at the Johns Hopkins Hospital in an effort to recover their health. Gradually his outlook improved, and he began to make plans for the future. He was greatly heartened in February when Panofsky, on behalf of the institute faculty, presented him with a rare volume that had once belonged to Daniel Coit Gilman. It was inscribed: "To the First Director from the First Faculty." He told Bernard that he was "deeply stirred by this touching and beautiful act."[81]

What would he do now? For the second time in his life, he had "retired" from a high-pressure job, with no prospects for future employment. At age seventy-four, he was still not ready to surrender to age but was looking for "a substitute" to occupy him.[82] Already he had arranged for the use of an office at the Carnegie Corporation in New York. He would live for another twenty years, write four books, consult on numerous projects, refight old battles, keep up a lively interest in ongoing events, and remain a gadfly in the intellectual life of the nation. He did not go gently into the twilight years of his life.

13

"I Burn That I May Be of Use"

As the weariness and melancholy of the last months at Princeton began
to lift, Abraham Flexner started work once more on his autobiography.
His old enthusiasms, which had been dimmed during the long ordeal, returned. He made clear that he had no intention of giving up his active involvement in events around him. At age 74, he agreed to lead a drive to
raise six million dollars for Meharry Medical College, and he enlisted at
the same time in an effort to save the Lincoln School from amalgamation
with the Horace Mann School at Teachers College, Columbia.

The Lincoln campaign had started the year before when he urged parents and students at the school's commencement exercises to become "sol-
diers for a great cause" in resisting the move. His passionate call to action,
according to press reports, brought "bursts of applause" and a standing
ovation "which lasted for several minutes." The crusade to save the school's
independence, which consumed him for many months, was unsuccessful,
but the Meharry campaign, with the help of both Flexner and his old colleagues at the General Education Board, reached its goal.[1]

Writing his life story revived his spirits. He relived his triumphs and
glossed over his failures. Not a hint of the circumstances surrounding his
departure from the General Education Board or from the Institute for Advanced Studies can be found in its four hundred pages. Oswald Veblen
was effectively written out of his account of the institute, and Edward
Meade Earle is scarcely mentioned. His early support for faculty government is nowhere in evidence. None of his famous quarrels with Arthur
Dean Bevan, Frederick T. Gates, Felix Frankfurter, or Albert Einstein
found a place in the memoir.

The main events of his life are portrayed in casual anecdotes, as part of
a story of modest and almost accidental success. "I shall tell the story simply and unostentatiously," he had told Simon, for "I am struck by my lack
of originality. What I did was to take advantage of opportunity." Once
more he cited his luck in being sent to Johns Hopkins, the good fortune

of Anne's success, and the primary role of Gates, William Henry Welch, and Franklin Mall in his achievements in medicine. He had simply "grasped the skirts of circumstance" in his climb upward.[2]

As a portrayal of his life, this modest appraisal, of course, was manifestly a caricature. It ignored the passion, the conflict, the raw ambition, the careful calculation, the recurring despair, and the brilliant insights of his career. It undervalued his important accomplishments and downplayed the difficulty of achieving these successes. Historians have largely taken him at his word, however, in assigning him much too small a place in the history of education.

I Remember, published by Simon and Schuster in 1940, does provide insight into his deep sentimentality, his generosity of spirit, his love of family, his pride in achievement, his sense of humor, and his intense loyalties. He clearly aimed the book at a broad audience and not at the small circle who knew his work. He recounts with conviction the years of poverty in Louisville, the remarkable cohesion of his family, the intense years in Baltimore, his devotion to Anne and their children, and his loyalty to Daniel Coit Gilman, Henry Pritchett, Wallace Buttrick, and the Rockefellers. He writes of ideals, self-reliance, character, reverence for learning, and excellence. He came to realize, he said, that "America was still to be made" and "that this was a practical job."[3]

The book is fluently written, full of colorful portraits of people in his life, and straightforward. But it is at best incomplete—only the skeleton of a very full life. He concludes the memoir with a graceful vignette about the purpose of his life as he saw it. In his mind's eye as he was writing, he says, he saw the bookplate of Thomas Carlisle—a lighted candle with the words: "I burn that I may be of use."[4]

The book brought cheers from friends and reviewers. Simon was unusually enthusiastic, telling him that it was "a very remarkable document" in which he saw "a recurring pattern" in all his brother's undertakings— "a rare quickness of perception, an unusual power of acquisition of new things, a deep understanding of what was essential in them, and the ability to seek and find good advisers and learn from them." His had been an "extraordinary life" built on "natural gifts and hard work."[5]

A reviewer in the *New York Times* found the memoir remarkably modest and "not vainglorious" for so outstanding a career. Only between the lines, said the *Times* writer, could a personality be found—"warm, humanitarian, optimistic, loving that 'excellence' which is the key to a surpassingly useful career."[6]

Others commented on its "charming" style, its "restraint" and "understatement," and its reflection of "an active and useful life as a statesman of education." In the *Current Biography* for 1941, his old critic Hans Zinsser was quoted as saying: "Oh, Abraham Flexner! We have fought with you . . . have alternatively admired and disliked you, have applauded your wisdom and detested you for opinionatedness. But in just retrospect, layman as you are, we hail you as the father—or, better, the uncle of modern medical education in America."[7] Similar tributes came from colleagues across the spectrum of American learning.

His autobiography strengthened the view that his historic role in changing American education had been secondary and minor. Scholars have largely accepted the erroneous description of his many roles at face value. Many have cited the 1910 report on medical education, but few show signs of having read it carefully. His penetrating analysis of European education in 1912 and still-unmatched comparison of national systems of educating doctors in 1925 are largely unknown. Only a few scholars of higher education have studied his strong impact on primary and especially secondary education. And the story of his almost single-handed creation and shaping of the Institute for Advanced Study has never been told.

Nearly twenty years after the publication of *I Remember,* the editors of Simon and Schuster persuaded him to prepare a revised version of the book—reduced in size, without illustrations, and with five chapters on the years after 1940. Flexner did not live to see its publication, but his daughters were disappointed that the book did not match in popularity the earlier edition.

Flexner continued to keep an active schedule, as he had for more than fifty years. He maintained a warm interest in the affairs of the Institute for Advanced Study, followed the war in Europe with passionate concern, and kept up a steady stream of correspondence with leaders in education, medicine, and philanthropy.

He began a close friendship with the historian Allan Nevins at Columbia, who, knowing of his connection with the Rockefellers, had sent him the galley proofs of his biography of John D. Rockefeller. Nevins's treatment of the Rockefeller philanthropies he found "too vague," and he advised him to stress the "elasticity and flexibility" of the oilman's charitable enterprises and to make clear that once "having accumulated this vast fortune," he had no other reasonable way to "get rid of it." Important, too, was the "absolute objectivity" of both father and son in never interfering once a gift had been made.[8] Over the next twenty years Nevins and Flexner became very close, trading manuscripts, exchanging visits (including a number of Nevins family visits to Lake Ahmic), and sharing family occasions. No one would be closer to Flexner in the last years of his life.

With the completion of the 1940 autobiography, he plunged into the writing of a long-promised biography of Pritchett. His former chief had died in 1939, and Pritchett's wife, Eva, urged him to get started on the task. He worked each day at offices provided for him at the Carnegie Corporation, where Pritchett had so long presided over the Carnegie enterprises. Writing the biography of Pritchett took Flexner two years. Eva had carefully maintained her husband's correspondence and "a great variety of material," most importantly a personal memoir that Pritchett had left behind. Flexner was in touch with a number of persons who had known Pritchett and was able to use the extensive files of correspondence at both the Carnegie Corporation and the Carnegie Foundation for the Advancement of Teaching.

The final work is a fulsome tribute to his mentor's life. Uncharacteristically for Flexner, it is largely uncritical, makes extensive use of long quotations, and strives, not altogether successfully, to avoid a tone of adulation. Straightforwardly the book traces the formative influences of Pritchett's life—the years of study in Germany, his career as an astronomer, his leadership of the Coast and Geodetic Survey, his presidency of the Massachusetts Institute of Technology—before focusing on the crucial quarter-century in which he led the foundation. He rightly gives Pritchett considerable credit for beginning the movement for college pensions and for the pioneering surveys of professional schools, including those by Flexner, which set national standards. "He was a reformer in every field in which he entered," Flexner wrote, "and a reformer who never lost his good temper and who never displayed bitterness in disappointment."

In memory, he almost certainly saw his mentor the same way that he wanted to be remembered—as a "veritable statesman of education who took all of its functions into view."[9] Not a notable biography, *Henry S. Pritchett* nevertheless kept alive the memory of one of the most creative educators of his time.

After "having paid part of the debt" he owed to Pritchett, he turned with enthusiasm to another hero in his pantheon of educational leaders, Daniel Coit Gilman. The first Johns Hopkins president, he explained to Tom Jones, was "by all odds the greatest of American university presidents."[10] Because an earlier biography by Fabian Franklin had dealt with

Gilman's entire career, Flexner chose to concentrate on his years at the Johns Hopkins helm.

In Flexner's view, Gilman was "the creator of the American type of university," the most important educator of the nineteenth century. "No other American of his day," he wrote, "had a comparable . . . knowledge of coming educational change or experience with innovation." When "abundant resources" and "a clean slate" were suddenly given to him in Baltimore, Gilman "knew precisely what he wanted to do." Unlike his contemporaries, he had the vision and the courage to build a place of truly advanced learning, where research was a fundamental and overriding concern. No other educator, in his experience, "ever wrought such a miracle as Gilman performed, first in the faculty of arts and sciences, later in the Medical School."[11]

More even than his life of Pritchett, the Gilman biography was a work of heartfelt piety. "Those who know something of my work long after Gilman's day," he wrote in his autobiography, "will recognize Gilman's influence in all I have done or tried to do." Only Gilman's attitude toward women seemed to surprise him. "It had not occurred to me," he told Florence Sabin, "that his opposition to the admission of women to the University was due to his fear that women would not measure up to men." Gilman would learn, he advised, that their presence "actually purified and elevated" life at Johns Hopkins.[12]

Throughout the writing of the two biographies, Flexner was mightily distracted by the ominous events in Europe. The outbreak of war in September 1939 made even more emotional his ties to lifelong friends in Germany, Britain, and other European countries. "We are almost as much preoccupied with the war," he wrote Tom Jones, "as if we were living in Great Britain." "What I really want to do," he said in June 1940, "is to knock forty years off my age, shoulder my musket, and participate in the European war."[13]

He turned against Charles Lindbergh when the aviator became active in the campaign to avert war. "I am sorry about Lindbergh for he has ruined his whole life," he wrote in 1941. "He is a nice boy whom I know well, but he is uneducated and was completely taken in" by the Nazis. "After the kidnapping of his child he sought my advice—a Jew. When he wished to be sure of the safety of his family, he sought the hospitality and quiet of Great Britain." But now he had no regard for his British or Jewish friends.[14]

Flexner applauded Roosevelt's decision to send fifty destroyers to

Britain even if it "stretched the Constitution," and he felt "exalted" by the lend-lease bill, regretting only that the vote was not unanimous.[15]

Despite his retirement from Princeton, the stream of refugees and would-be refugees continued unabated: "A great proportion . . . come to me," he wrote. Frequently he traveled to Washington to do what he could to help them.[16]

In December 1940, Flexner made "a hemispheric broadcast" by radio on the American way of life, in which he expressed regret "that Democracy [had] not come to prevail in the relations between the colored man and the white man [nor] in the relations between men and women." He called for a "militant" extension of freedom.[17]

The following May he wrote to Secretary of State Cordell Hull, offering to come to Washington as a volunteer "in any capacity."[18] The war, it seemed, was making him more energetic and outspoken in his political views.

After Pearl Harbor, Flexner was anxious but confident that the tide would turn against the Axis powers. "We will lose . . . in these early stages," he told Jones, but "within less than a year we shall be turning out ships and planes and guns and ammunitions and we will have an overwhelming army and navy." The country was united as never before behind the president, who had "undivided and ungrudging popular and congressional support."[19]

His attention turned to conditions after the war, especially in education and social relations. "We are a generation behind England in our social legislation," he told Jones in 1943, and racial and religious prejudice would have to be addressed. "Here and there antisemitism exists in spots," he wrote; and "there is some antiCatholic prejudice in certain sections particularly in the South." The South was, in his assessment, "very far from having done its duty by the Negro."[20]

He saw dangers to the humanities in the wartime emphasis on "mechanism, utility, and science." He urged his friend Benjamin Meritt not to be drawn too deeply into the war effort. He was particularly struck, he told Meritt, by the efforts of Henry Sigerist, Welch's successor in the chair of medical history at Johns Hopkins, to keep alive cultural studies; "they are going to have a tough time in competition with pure and applied science" after the war, he said. He called Sigerist "the only man who . . . seems to realize the chaos which . . . characterizes our institutions of learning." Universities would have to be rebuilt at war's end, "just as Hamburg" would "be rebuilt."[21]

He turned down an invitation to join a group planning for postwar education in Germany and Japan. Such an effort, he said, was both "ignorant" and "arrogant," since those involved knew "absolutely nothing" about education in these countries. Unless the "spiritual and intellectual forces in these countries" themselves undertook the task, the outlook would be "hopeless."[22]

At the end of the war came a series of personal and family events that shook him badly and left him more isolated than ever before. In rapid succession his brother Bernard died in 1945, followed by Simon in 1946, and his sister Mary the following year. His younger brother, Washington, had died during the war, leaving him and his other sister Gertrude as the two surviving siblings of the original nine children.

Bernard, he knew, was hailed in death as "a great American Jew" for his work on behalf of Palestine and the wartime refugees. Abraham mourned his loss but was even more stricken by the death of Simon. "I did not feel that I could feel anything as keenly as I feel Simon's death," he told his longtime secretary, Esther Bailey. "For sixty years he and I have been close . . . Our lives would have been very different but for our influence upon one another."[23]

The greatest blow of all, however, was the rapid deterioration of Anne's mental condition. She became increasingly forgetful and unable to cope with the ordinary tasks of life. He later recounted how "from a faultless memory she changed to forgetfulness." She misplaced things, became restless, and was unable to write. A neurologist told him that she had "a hardening of the cerebral blood vessels" for which there was no cure. He hired a day nurse, then a night nurse, and finally a weekend nurse. "She is utterly unaware of what is happening to her," he wrote her sister. They stayed in their old apartment on Seventy-Second Street until 1947, when conditions became intolerable. He was forced to keep his door locked at night in order to get any sleep. She was now "absolutely incoherent" but he resisted her being moved to an institution. "You can imagine how profoundly I am distressed," he wrote to Tom Jones.[24] Finally, in April, the decision was made to take her to a sanitarium in Providence, Rhode Island. While Jean and Eleanor went periodically to see their mother, he was never able to do so.

To some it may seem strange that Abraham, who had been so close to Anne for half a century, should seem so remote in her hour of need. He responded as he did for several reasons: he was deeply hurt by Anne's estrangement from him as her disease developed, unable to grasp the fact that his close companion no longer recognized him, and interested in preserving his instinct for life and continued achievements. He listened attentively to Jean's and Eleanor's description of her life at the renowned Providence retreat, and he rejoiced at the news that she seemed not unhappy and occasionally played the piano. So close did he feel to the woman who had shared his life for so long, however, he could not contemplate spending time with someone who saw him as a total stranger. He must have deeply mourned her passing from his life while regretting his weakness at not being able to offer her any comfort in her isolated existence.

Flexner was shattered by Anne's departure. "I cannot read now," he said, "with Anne in the sanitarium and my sister, Mary, dying of cirrhosis of the liver." With the help of Jean and Paul, he disposed of the furnishings in the apartment they had shared so long and moved into a residential hotel just east of Central Park. He later confided that he had had a breakdown himself when Anne was sent to Providence. He grew very close to the Nevins family during the months of crisis as they brought him into their lives and gave him encouragement. Jean and Eleanor, as well as Bailey and other friends, did all they could to help him keep his balance, but he said it was "the most terrible trial" that he had ever had to endure.[25]

At age 81, he began a new life. From his two-room suite at the Hotel Adams, he journeyed each day to an office made available to him by the Rosenwald family on Fifth Avenue at Forty-Fourth Street. Bailey, who had nominally retired in 1941, returned to help with secretarial work, along with Marie Eischseler, a vivacious younger woman who had begun working for him in Princeton. The two women remained close to him for the rest of his life. They were treated as members of his family, joining him for meals, accompanying him to the theater or opera, and spending the summers at Lake Ahmic. They were "a great comfort" to him, he said, for he had not yet solved "the problem of living alone and enjoying it." While in New York, Eischseler completed a master's degree at Columbia University. At his suggestion she chose a topic in comparative literature that enabled her to spend a term in Paris at the Sorbonne.[26] The following summer he joined her on a tour of southern Italy.

It was Eischseler who, seeing his loneliness, suggested that he begin taking classes at Columbia University. Knowing his love for Shakespeare, she told him of a course taught by Professor Oscar Campbell, the author of a well-regarded book called *The Living Shakespeare*. According to Nevins, the appearance of Flexner on the Morningside Heights campus "electrified" students and faculty. When he enrolled in a course in the history of art, the instructor, Everard Upjohn, asked Nevins: "Not Dr. Flexner from the Institute for Advanced Study? The man who brought Panofsky and Herzfeld and all those other celebrities to Princeton? He doesn't want to take *my* course!" Soon he was taking courses in Chaucer and in Russian history and culture. He began giving an annual party for the staff of the Russian Institute and included George Kennan, who regularly made the journey from Princeton. He attended a seminar given by Claude Bowers, former ambassador to Chile, who brought him to the faculty club before class, where they were frequently joined by Nevins, Dean Harry Carman, journalism professor Louis Starr, and others.[27]

Most stimulating to Flexner were the seminars of Allan Nevins on such specialized topics as the bibliography of American history. He found the experience to be "a most satisfying intellectual treat." In the seminars, he wrote, he came to know and befriend a dozen young men and women who were training to be historians. The evenings at Columbia were an important part of his emotional recovery. "When I first began attending your lectures," he told Nevins later, "I was trying to relieve loneliness. I little dreamt that I was starting the most intimate and congenial friendship of my life; for you and Mary are (or better have become) parts of my daily existence." And Eischseler, who was also a good friend of Nevins's, had "been all that a daughter could be," Flexner said.[28]

Aside from reading and attending classes at Columbia, he kept up his interest in music, theater, and opera. On his desk in his hotel apartment, a young relative remembered seeing two inscribed photographs: one of Einstein, the other of Arturo Toscanini, the latter signed "to my dearest friend." He was regularly at the Metropolitan Opera, frequently attended recitals at Carnegie Hall, never failed to see performances of Gilbert and Sullivan, went to the theater, and was fond of ballet. Such musical comedies as *Brigadoon* and *My Fair Lady* he found "enchanting."

Much of his time at home was spent in reading, especially history, biography, and literature. He became fascinated with the civil war diaries of Gideon Welles and George Templeton Strong, the reminiscences of Carl Schurz, and the Sandburg and Charnwood lives of Abraham Lincoln. He was impressed by Arthur M. Schlesinger Jr.'s *The Crisis of the Old Order,* the first volume of a biography of Franklin D. Roosevelt. He reread much of Shakespeare and Dickens as well as the poetry of Wordsworth and Milton. He found a new interest in English history and biography, which he discussed avidly with Tom Jones.[29]

With the help of Eischseler and Bailey he continued to go each summer to Lake Ahmic, where frequent guests—the Tom Jones family, Allan and Mary Nevins, the E.L. Woodwards, the violinist Efrem Zimbalist, his old friends the William R. Boyds from Iowa, John von Neumann, Benjamin Meritt, and others—came and went. A younger member of the family who was there in 1951 remembered that there were long talks at each meal and that no radios were allowed.[30]

Flexner remained skeptical about whether radio and later television were good influences on American life. "Between radio and television," he wrote, "education is becoming too passive, and I think the results are apparent in the American college."[31] This was in 1954!

But his principal salvation in these years was work. Daily, he made his way to his downtown office, wrote or dictated for several hours, received callers, lunched with friends, and gave advice to organizations and individuals. He became friends with a new generation of philanthropic executives: Paul Hoffman of the Ford Foundation, John Gardner of the Carnegie Foundation, Dean Rusk of the Rockefeller Foundation, John Barrett of the Bollingen Foundation, and Paul Mellon, who consulted him on a number of his charitable gifts.

Regularly he scolded the foundations for their neglect of the humanities and their failure to take greater risks in the management of their funds. He remained harshly critical of the giving of small grants to individuals rather than to universities as a whole. Philanthropy was now reduced, he wrote, to "a confusingly long list of tiny disconnected, one-year grants." Such grants could do little to advance scholarship. "Their main effect is to keep the recipients on their knees, holding out their hats from year to year."[32]

In 1948 he determined to write a book on the modern foundation. For more than three years he gathered material, met with foundation leaders, and debated with others about charitable giving. The resulting book, *Funds and Foundations*, published by Harper in 1952, was a highly critical account of recent directions of policy in all the major foundations. The General Education Board had since his departure given hundreds of individual grants to universities all over the country, largely for small scientific projects. But how was it possible, he asked, "for any group of men to administer intelligently funds so freely distributed to agencies, the competence of which no man and no group of men could possibly judge?"[33]

In the Rockefeller Foundation and the Carnegie Corporation, the same "dreary pattern" could be found year after year. Nearly all of the grants had gone to science, medicine, or engineering—what of the humanities?

Most urgently needed, he argued, was a new foundation committed to humanistic studies. "If the proper study of mankind is man, the proper study of man is the literature that he has created."[34]

Tirelessly he worked to interest those commanding great wealth in a new venture in the humanities. When Dean Rusk became president of the Rockefeller Foundation in 1952, Flexner did his best to persuade him to invest more in humanistic study. He wrote, too, to Alan Waterman, director of the newly created National Science Foundation, endeavoring to persuade him that scientists in particular should take the lead in seeking "abundant support" for the humanities "as an essential part of the development of superior human beings." Waterman responded by asking for a meeting, saying that he agreed that "in a very real sense" all learning was humanistic learning.[35]

He received support for his crusade from his old friends Milton Winternitz and Alan Gregg. "What an opportunity to start again," Winternitz wrote from Yale after reading the book on foundations. Gregg told him not to be dismayed, that he was having more influence than he realized. "Your own direct and personal contribution," he said, "still acts as the vector for the energies of able young men neither you nor I know."[36]

For a while Flexner believed that he was at the point of a breakthrough in creating a new program in the humanities. To Tom Jones he wrote mysteriously that he was working on "one of the most important tasks" that he had "ever undertaken." "I can't give you the details, for the whole thing may collapse." With Simon dead and Anne in an institution, he now had no one with whom he shared his most intimate hopes and plans. Again, in 1952, he told Jones, "I am making no promises, but there is a possibility that a foundation for the humanities is in the making."[37]

He was referring to conversations he had had with the philanthropist Paul Mellon, who was much impressed with Flexner's book on foundations. Later that year he confided to Jones that Mellon was considering "the possibility of utilizing the unspent portion of his father's [Andrew Mellon's] estate—something like $40,000,000—to establish a foundation for the encouragement of humanistic studies." The matter was now "before the trustees," and, despite "legal technicalities," action was expected soon.

Mellon made approval of the plan conditional, Flexner told Jones, on the 86-year-old Flexner's "starting the thing and training" a successor. A few days later Mellon asked him for suggestions of those who might serve on the board of trustees. Flexner promptly arranged luncheons for Mellon with each of those he named: Allan Nevins, Caryl Haskins of the Carnegie Institution, and Gordon Wasson of J.P. Morgan and Company.[38]

In early 1953 Mellon asked him for a detailed proposal to present to the trustees, who apparently still had reservations. Flexner prepared a seventeen-page single-spaced memorandum on the purpose of "a foundation for humanistic and related studies." In it he described an organization that would be "flexible," would be bold in design, and would always take the initiative in making grants and not simply respond to outside proposals. At the helm of the small staff would be a director "of the very highest caliber." He described the fields of the humanities that should be included—the visual arts, music and drama, literature, history, linguistics, law, geography, and philosophy—and then outlined a number of "action programs" that might stimulate a revival of the humanities: the history and philosophy of science, the processes of human communication, world population problems, the place of humanistic study in American life, the structure and process of ideation, and adult education in the liberal arts. To the historian George Sarton he wrote, "If ever I have a chance to use my influence in behalf of a humanistic development, the history of science will be one of the first things with which I should occupy myself."[39]

It was a remarkably innovative and well-written proposal. It clearly intrigued Mellon. For whatever reason, however, Mellon was not able to bring the negotiations to closure. Throughout the 1950s the two men continued to meet regularly and to exchange ideas and memoranda. As late as 1957, when Flexner was past ninety years old, he told Nevins, "I have been told very confidentially that there is some chance for the idea of a foundation for the humanities."[40]

Eventually, Mellon decided, at least for the moment, against a separate foundation and in favor of an enlarged Bollingen Foundation, another Mellon philanthropy largely devoted to humanistic enterprises.[41] Flexner, however, never gave up on the idea of a vast new enterprise in the humanities that would counterbalance the support going to medicine and the sciences. Incredibly, he clung to the belief that if such a venture were launched, he would lead it. He may have misread the signals from Mellon, but his immense self-confidence, still visible at ninety-one, told him it was still possible.

In other ways, the old warrior continued to struggle to influence the course of educational development. For some years after leaving Princeton he continued to advise and help his successor. He attended board meetings, recommended new trustees, criticized Frank Aydelotte's efforts

to make peace with Veblen, and intervened several times at Aydelotte's behest with the Bambergers. Aydelotte found himself in much the same
plight as Flexner had once been, cutting salaries and lamenting the lack
of endowment. In time Flexner fell out with his former ally and faulted
the trustees for not consulting him in 1947 in choosing J. Robert Oppenheimer as Aydelotte's successor.[42]

He did stay in touch with a number of his old institute colleagues. In
1944 von Neumann asked him to review and comment upon his manuscript on game theory. Five years later Meritt, seeking further aid for excavations in Greece, asked for Flexner's help and for his file on the Agora.
Seeing the documents, Meritt recalled, "How much we all owe you . . .
we could never have excavated the Agora without your intercession."[43]

He had his hand in a dozen other enterprises as well. As a member of
a committee planning a medical school for Israel, he rendered "valiant
service," according to its chairman, who wrote that "the deeds of Flexner
shine brightly out of the darkness" of the new nation's dark days. In 1948,
Nevins enlisted him in an effort to persuade the new president of Columbia, Dwight D. Eisenhower, to make a thorough review of the curriculum. "I have a feeling that Eisenhower is groping for guidance," said
Nevins, and "if you would be willing to take charge of such an operation
. . . you could perform a great service." Flexner was willing to help but
doubted the university's willingness to reorganize, and he questioned
Nevins closely about the attitude of the trustees and faculty toward him.
Had President Butler's long-time enmity toward him rubbed off on the
current trustees?[44] Butler had just retired as president after more than
forty years of service. Although the Carnegie Corporation agreed to support the study, Nevins was not able to win approval for the Flexner initiative.

The historian was more successful in getting Flexner's support for creating an archive in oral history at Columbia. He was able to use Flexner's
extensive contacts with foundations and donors, especially the Rosen-
walds, to launch the first such enterprise in the nation.[45]

In 1949, Johns Hopkins, for which he had done so much, awarded
Flexner an honorary degree, and the following year the university invited
him to give the principal address at the centennial celebration of the birth
of William Henry Welch.[46]

Flexner's interest in politics and events abroad never wavered. Through
Tom Jones he was invited to Washington in 1948 to discuss American politics with the new British ambassador, Sir Oliver Franks. Flexner expressed

his views on public affairs increasingly bluntly in these postwar years. "We are all Socialists these days," he said, "but I cannot swallow Russian communism." He complained of the Truman administration's "hysterical" fear of the Soviet Union and the danger of radical subversion at home. "There is just about as much danger of a Russian-inspired revolution over here," he said, "as there was in England at the time of the general strike."[47]

He was incensed at Senator McCarthy's campaign against subversives. He called the Wisconsin senator "a jackass who . . . has distinguished himself by his baseless and outrageous attacks." He would have been even more upset had he known that his daughter Jean was the subject of a loyalty investigation. In a formal letter she was charged, as she explained it, with "being unfit for further federal employment . . . on grounds of association with suspect characters." The foremost of these "characters," she said, "appears to be my sister Eleanor!" She was eventually cleared after getting testimonials to her character and loyalty from Frances Perkins, Tom Jones, E.L. Woodward, Herbert Lehman, and others. Her father, she told Jones, must be protected "from the shock of hearing about this."[48]

By 1952 Flexner was completely disillusioned with the political climate in Washington. "We shall have to go back to Harding and General Grant," he wrote, "to match the tone of public life in our national capital today." In the political campaign that year he strongly supported Adlai Stevenson over Dwight Eisenhower. When the latter was elected Flexner became an unremitting critic of the president's actions: his failure to crack down on McCarthy, his appointment of John Foster Dulles as secretary of state ("absolutely incomprehensible"), the Dixon-Yates contract with the Tennessee Valley Authority, the support of the French in Indo-China. By the time of the next election, he was convinced that Stevenson would prevail and he urged Nevins, who was working for the Illinois governor, to call the candidate's attention to George Kennan for secretary of state.[49]

He continued to reach out for new social and intellectual contacts. He invited the Spanish historian and diplomat Salvador de Madariago to lunch. He struck up a correspondence with the art critic Bernard Berenson, who had praised the book on foundations. The eighty-nine-year-old Berenson urged him to visit Italy for discussions since it would be easier for the "younger" Flexner (eighty-seven years old) to "come and stay" with him. He enjoyed the company of the classicist Gilbert Highet and his novelist wife, Helen MacInnes. He described a dinner party with the Highets at which the hosts played duets of Bach, Ravel, and other composers on their two grand pianos.[50] When Highet sent him his latest book, *The Art of Teaching* (1951), Flexner told him it was "a better book" than it had been when he had read it in proof. He then added candidly, "It does not seem to me a really important book because of flaws due . . . to limited experience." Highet did not really understand that "the teacher who does not know that concentration must be taught is beyond help."

From his own experience, Flexner told Highet, "the awakening of the pupil's interest" was necessary for learning. To awaken that interest, he had learned sixty years before, many avenues were open, all dependent on the teacher, but none of them on "reading about it or being taught about it." Nor was he any friend of teachers' colleges "in the form they [had] assumed."

He questioned, too, Highet's treatment of bedside teaching in medicine. Bedside teaching, he said, matters because "it has consequences. It destroys planned lecture presentation of clinical subjects, for the patient determines the subject." It was why effective clinical teachers gave so few systematic lectures.[51] Although now in his mid-eighties, the old schoolmaster was still vitally interested in how children and adults learn.

As he neared his ninetieth birthday, he was shaken by new losses among those closest to him. In Aberystwyth, Wales, the death of his old comrade Tom Jones brought to an end a transatlantic friendship that Jones once described as the closest of his life. Across the years of depression, war, and turmoil, the two men had traded visits, become part of one another's families, and written hundreds of letters that form a running commentary on the notable events of the previous quarter-century. The last summer of the Welshman's life was spent quietly with his friend on the shores of Lake Ahmic.

Closer to home, shortly before Jones's death, word came to him of the unexpected death of Anne at her sanctuary in Providence. "The effect of Anne's passing on me," he wrote, "was somewhat unexpected." For eight years he had not seen her; he was told by Jean and Eleanor that her condition was virtually unchanged. He could not bring himself to see her in her memoryless existence. But with the news of her death, Flexner said, "The flood of memories was almost too much for me, and for a week I did little or nothing."[52]

She was buried in her uncle's plot in the Cave Hill Cemetery in Louisville, a place she had loved as a child. Her family offered to reserve the neighboring plot for Flexner, and he gladly accepted: "When the time comes the urn with my ashes may be deposited beside [hers]." He visited the grave the following year on his last visit to Louisville, where he was given an honorary degree by the University of Louisville. He also spent time at the Jewish cemetery on Preston Street, where his parents and other family members were buried.[53]

He saw no reason to celebrate his ninetieth birthday. Friends and relatives commented that he was unusually quiet in the months after Anne's death. Jean told an interviewer that when conversations became animated he would be silent. This silence was unprecedented; she had never before seen him "in a conversation that he did not dominate."[54] Still, his health remained remarkably good. He swam in the summer, and he continued to go to his office, sometimes on foot, five days a week. His ninetieth year brought a series of honors, awards, and public recognitions that lifted his spirits somewhat.

Foremost among them was the presentation of the Frank Lahey Award for his contributions to medicine. Sponsored by the American Medical Association, the Association of American Medical Colleges, and the National Fund for Medical Education, the award had been given previously to Dwight D. Eisenhower and Herbert Hoover. Before him on the night of April 23, 1956, sat more than three hundred national leaders in education, government, philanthropy, and medicine, including most of the deans of America's medical schools, in the great ballroom of the Waldorf-Astoria Hotel. Although in his ninetieth year, he stood erect and spoke clearly.

It was a night of triumph. As he approached the podium, reaching into the inside pocket of his tuxedo for his remarks, the crowd jumped to its feet and applauded, remained standing, and applauded some more. Some in the audience were longtime friends and admirers, and some were old enemies, but most were too young to have known him in his days of glory. To most he was a legend, the man who, in the words that night of H.G. Weiskotten, chairman of the American Medical Association's Council on Medical Education and Hospitals, had "made the greatest single contribution that [had] ever been made to the advancement of medical education in America."

The evening was full of nostalgic reminiscence. The president of the Carnegie Corporation, John W. Gardner (a future secretary of Health, Education, and Welfare in the Lyndon Johnson administration), recounted the story of how Abraham Flexner, then an obscure schoolmaster from Louisville, came to undertake the most famous study ever made of American medical schools. Gardner explained how his predecessor, Henry Pritchett, had made the "brilliant stroke" of seeing Flexner's potential and how the schoolmaster's "penetrating mind, his stubborn regard for facts, his courage, and his capacity to communicate his ideas" ensured that the undertaking would succeed.

He was followed by Dean Rusk, president of the Rockefeller Foundation, who was to serve as secretary of state under Presidents Kennedy and Johnson. Rusk described the fifteen momentous years that Flexner had spent at Rockefeller's General Education Board. In that post, he said, Flexner had arguably exerted more direct influence over the course of medical and other educational affairs in America than any person in history. The qualities that Rusk saw as crucial in Flexner's ascent to power were "a burning ambition for excellence . . . the deep sympathy which expresses itself in candor—and not mere courtesy—contempt for pretense and fraud; a deep respect for an able mind wherever it is found; patience and persistence in the approach to perfection."

When Flexner spoke, he characteristically refused all credit for the great reforms that the others had praised. The real heroes in medical education, he said, were William Henry Welch, who created a new kind of medical school at Johns Hopkins, and Henry Pritchett, the Carnegie Foundation chief who had seen the great need for national standards in all the professions. He praised, too, Frederick T. Gates, who had seen the survey of medical schools as not just a criticism but a program of action.[55]

Most of the nation's metropolitan newspapers carried editorials praising his long life. The Chicago Medical College established a scholarship in his name. Allan Nevins wrote a piece entitled "Flexner at 90 Charts a New Course" for the *New York Times Magazine.* In it Nevins stressed his friend's continuing crusade for a foundation in the humanities, which would "correct the distortion" that threatened to lead to "a lopsided America." In the *New York Times,* education correspondent Benjamin Fine reported that "this intellectual giant," whose impact on America's schools and universities had been so large, was spending his birthday at his office from "early in the morning . . . until late afternoon."[56]

The years alone in New York were about to end. After a final year of daily work at his office and a last summer at Lake Ahmic he was prevailed upon by his daughters, concerned about his growing frailty, to give up his independent life. Jean bought a small house for him near her in Falls Church, Virginia, and he moved in on November 1, 1957. Eischseler volunteered to accompany him and to take charge of housekeeping. When his longtime cook at Lake Ahmic learned of his plans, she too agreed to come. "If everyone goes to Washington," she was reported as saying, "I go to Washington."[57]

He described the next two years of his life as pleasant: "We go to concerts frequently, to art galleries occasionally, and I have a considerable number of callers." He enjoyed drives in the country, kept up his steady reading, and looked forward to the visits of Allan Nevins and other old friends. He was particularly interested in Eleanor's forthcoming book on the history of the women's rights movement in the United States. She talked often with him about it, and he lived long enough to read the first favorable reviews. The book, *Century of Struggle,* published by Harvard University Press in 1959, was an instant success and would sell more than a hundred thousand copies. The last visitor to the little house in Falls Church was the faithful Allan Nevins, who spent several hours with him on the night before his death on September 21, 1959.[58]

He died an esteemed figure in American life. Tributes poured in from scores of old friends and those whose lives he had touched. The American Medical Association devoted an unprecedented memorial issue to his life and accomplishments. In *Science,* John Gardner wrote of his "razor-edged mind, fierce integrity, limitless courage, and the capacity to express himself clearly and vividly." No one ever called the imperious Flexner, said Gardner, "comfortable as an old shoe." He had spent his life fighting "a holy war against slackness, triviality, and educational quackery." A writer in the *Washington Post* described him as "the severest critic and the best friend American medicine ever had." In the view of the *New York Times,* which carried his picture and news of his death on the front page, "no other American of his generation" had done more for "the welfare of his country and [for] humanity in general." The *Cleveland Plain Dealer*'s opinion was that the nation was fortunate that his parents had chosen to come to America more than a century before. A small newspaper in upstate New York opined that he had had "a greater impact" on all Americans' lives "than any ten popular celebrities." In Great Britain, a writer in *Lancet* said that Flexner's ideas were important in making British medical education something to "be proud" of.[59]

His life had been full of remarkable, even historic, achievements. From a modest, severely limited background, with little formal education, for twenty years the mainstay of a large family, he had gone on to change forever the education of physicians, left decisive marks on public education, and created a new kind of postdoctoral learning. Throughout, he had remained publicly modest, refusing all credit for his achievements, attributing to others or to chance what had been his greatest contributions. Whatever his private ego and sense of pride, he disowned again and again the leadership role he had played across the spectrum of American and European education.

He was fundamentally a deeply gifted human being, warm-hearted, decent, and dedicated to his causes and extended family. He was the last American whose interests and activities embraced the entire range of learning, from kindergarten to postgraduate study. He was an innovator possessed of unusual imagination and thick-skinned when it came to criticism. He had powerful executive skills and an unusual talent for writing. He moved easily across the boundaries of power between government, business, academia, and philanthropy. He raised more money for education than any individual of his time or since. And his prescriptions for greater flexibility and experimentation in medical education; for more modern public schools with higher standards; and for world-class institutions of advanced learning have largely been heeded.

Had he lived longer, he would surely have supported efforts to broaden the public's access to good medicine. In his most active years, the demand for medical service was far less important as a public issue than efforts to improve the supply. Medical costs were still quite low, and improvements in training seemed far more important. Health insurance was just emerging as a national issue as Flexner joined the General Education Board. At that time, after observing British efforts to develop a national system of health insurance, he said that if Americans were to benefit from improved medical services, medical care for the nation as a whole might "in part at least have to be borne by society as a whole." As it was, it was interesting, he reflected, that "strongly individualistic" Britain was leading "in a more comprehensive organization of medical service." A few years later, critics of public health insurance assumed that Flexner was behind schemes to broaden health coverage. A leading New York physician charged in 1917 that compulsory health insurance "was part of a vicious conspiracy, hatched by Abraham Flexner." Still later, in the 1930s, he excoriated the doctors who, "by their opposition to medical insurance," were making "something far more drastic probable in the long run." In actuality, Flexner's efforts were concentrated almost entirely on the supply side of medical economics, but his private sympathies were clearly on the side of those battling for reform in demand.[60]

The questions he raised about how Americans learn are with us still. No issue is more earnestly debated in our time than the need for higher standards in our schools and a serious academic core of learning for all children. The number of young people enrolled in an academic, as opposed to a general or vocational, curriculum has risen spectacularly in recent years.[61] The respect for learning that characterized Flexner's version of educational progressivism has gained new support. His challenge to liberal arts colleges—that they need to sharpen their focus—still resonates. His criticisms of a number of university practices apply with equal force today. And few are the discussions of medical education in our time that fail to mention his name.

It had been a long journey from the streets of post–Civil War Louisville. No one living in 1959 could remember the obscure immigrant couple with their nine children, the tight-knit Jewish community around them, the old temple on Sixth Street and Broadway, the disorderly neighborhood streets, the open, muddy river, the stiff and crowded classrooms, and the small private libraries that had nurtured him growing up. In him and his siblings his parents had invested all their hopes for education and success in the new country. In their children's accomplishments, the parents' own lives had indeed been justified. He had left the city with Anne fifty-four years before and gone on to build a spectacularly powerful career. Now his ashes were returned to his native earth to rest beside Anne's in the city where it had all begun.

Notes

INTRODUCTION

1. Kenneth M. Ludmerer, "Curriculum Reform, 2000: An Analysis," in *The Education of Medical Students: Ten Stories of Curriculum Change*, ed. Association of American Medical Colleges and the Milbank Memorial Fund (New York: Milbank Memorial Fund, 2000), 20.

2. Jacques Barzun, "Trim the College?—A Utopia!" *Chronicle of Higher Education* 22 June 2001, B24.

3. Abraham Flexner, *Medical Education in the United States and Canada*, Bulletin no. 4 (New York: Carnegie Foundation for the Advancement of Teaching, 1910), 216–17.

4. Thomas N. Bonner, *Medicine in Chicago 1850–1950: A Chapter in the Social and Intellectual Development of a City* (Madison, Wisc.: American History Research Center, 1957), 115.

5. Thomas N. Bonner, *The Kansas Doctor: A Century of Pioneering* (Lawrence: University of Kansas Press, 1959), 148.

6. Kenneth R. Manning, *Black Apollo of Science: The Life of Ernest Everett Just* (New York: Oxford University Press, 1983), 303.

7. Henry James to Abraham Flexner, n.d., Abraham Flexner Papers, Library of Congress.

8. Darwin H. Stapleton, Director, Rockefeller Archive Center, letter to author, 23 April 2001. For Flexner's similarity to other leaders in Britain and America who moved across intellectual boundaries, see the writings of Daniel M. Fox, e.g., his *Health Policies, Health Politics* (Princeton: Princeton University Press, 1986).

CHAPTER 1: "OUR CHILDREN WILL JUSTIFY US"

1. Abraham Flexner, *I Remember* (New York: Simon and Schuster, 1940), 12–13 (hereafter, all references to this book will be in abbreviated form).

2. Guido Kisch, *In Search of Freedom: A History of American Jews in Czechoslovakia* (London: Edward Goldston & Son, 1949), 183.

3. Herman Landau, *Adath Louisville: The Story of a Jewish Community* (Louisville: privately printed, 1981), 25; Leo Loeb, letter to author, 14 September 2001.

4. Esther Flexner, "Father," 1, Simon Flexner Papers, American Philosophical Society (APS). See also Simon's unpublished autobiography at the APS.

5. E. Flexner, "Memories of my Youth," 1–2, Simon Flexner Papers.

6. E. Flexner, "Father," 1.

7. E. Flexner, "Memories," 3–4.

311

8. E. Flexner, "Father," 1–3.

9. Ibid., 3; A. Flexner, *I Remember,* 5.

10. E. Flexner, "Memories," 6–8.

11. James T. Flexner, *An American Saga: The Story of Helen Thomas and Simon Flexner* (New York: Fordham University Press, 1993), 17 (hereafter, all references to this book will be in abbreviated form).

12. Ibid., 18; E. Flexner, "Father," 6.

13. A. Flexner, *I Remember,* 6.

14. Jacob Flexner, "Memoirs of My Mother," 1–2, Bernard Flexner Papers, Mudd Library, Princeton, N.J.

15. Simon Flexner, "Notes on Migrations of My Father—Morris Flexner," 3–4, Simon Flexner Papers.

16. A. Flexner, *I Remember,* 14, 36.

17. Ibid., 13; J. T. Flexner, *American Saga,* 7.

18. A. Flexner, *I Remember,* 8; J. T. Flexner, *American Saga,* 21–23; J. Flexner, "Memories," 3–4.

19. A. Flexner, *I Remember,* 17; Marion B. Lucas, *A History of Blacks in Kentucky,* 2 vols. (Frankfort: Kentucky Historical Society, 1992), I:196.

20. *Encyclopedia Britannica,* 1883, 23; Sam Adkins and M.R. Holtzman, *The First Hundred Years: The Story of Louisville Male High School* (Louisville: Alumni of Louisville Male High School, 1910), 15. George H. Yates, *Two Hundred Years at the Falls of the Ohio* (Louisville: Filson Club, 1987), 98–118; Lucas, *History of Blacks,* I:246–48; Thomas C. Venable, "A History of Negro Education in Kentucky" (master's thesis, Western Kentucky University, 1952), 100; Blaine Hudson, Department of African-American Studies, University of Louisville, telephone interview by author, 30 July 1997; George D. Wilson, "A Century of Negro Education in Louisville, Kentucky," Works Progress Administration Project, Louisville Municipal College, [1937].

21. Lucas, *History of Blacks,* I:247; John E. Kleber, ed., *The Encyclopedia of Louisville* (Lexington, Ky.: University Press of Kentucky, 2001), 16. A. Flexner, *I Remember,* 20.

22. Landau, *Adath Louisville,* 26.

23. J. T. Flexner, *American Saga,* 45.

24. Bernard Flexner to Alfred E. Cohn, 23 February 1927, Bernard Flexner Papers, Mudd Library; A. Flexner, *I Remember,* 13–14.

25. B. Flexner to Cohn, 23 February 1927; J. T. Flexner, *American Saga,* 47.

26. Abraham Flexner to Samuel Dorfman, 3 January 1944, Abraham Flexner Papers, Library of Congress.

27. Susan E. Tifft and Alex S. Jones, "The Family: How Being Jewish Shaped the Dynasty That Runs the *Times,*" *New Yorker,* 11 April 1999, 45–46; David A. Hollinger, *Science, Jews, and Secular Culture* (Princeton: Princeton University Press, 1996), 19–24; Abraham Flexner to Anne Flexner, [1913], Abraham Flexner Papers.

28. Bernard Flexner, "Random Notes of Bernard Flexner," 2, Bernard Flexner Papers, Mudd Library; Jacob Flexner, "A Vanishing Profession," *Atlantic Monthly* 148 (1931):16.

29. Abraham Flexner to Eleanor Flexner, 3 October 1924, Abraham Flexner Papers; A. Flexner, *I Remember,* 15.

30. J. Flexner, "Memoirs," 8–9.

31. J. T. Flexner, *American Saga,* 37–38.

32. A. Flexner, *I Remember,* 20–22.

33. Ibid., 28–35.

34. Ibid., 25; Hambleton Tapp and James C. Klotter, *Kentucky: Decades of Discord, 1865–1900* (Frankfort: Kentucky Historical Society, 1977), 189.

35. Ibid., 191; A. Flexner, *I Remember,* 25–27; Theodore R. Sizer, *Secondary Schools at the Turn of the Century* (New Haven: Yale University Press, 1964), 18–29; Sam Adams and M.R. Holtzman, *The First Hundred Years: The Story of Louisville Male High School* (Louisville: Alumni of Louisville Male High School, 1910), 12–13, 32, 34.

36. Louisville Male High School, Academic Records, 1873–85, Filson Club, Louisville, Ky.

37. J. Flexner, "Memoirs," 11; A. Flexner, *I Remember,* 44.

38. A. Flexner, *I Remember,* 44.

39. Ibid., 44–46.

40. Ibid., 42.

CHAPTER 2: A UNIVERSITY LIKE NO OTHER

1. A. Flexner, *I Remember,* 52–59.

2. Cyrus Adler, *I Have Considered the Days* (Philadelphia: Jewish Publication Society of America, 1941), 64; interview with Dr. Abraham Flexner, December 1954, 33, Oral History Project, Columbia University.

3. Hugh Hawkins, *Pioneer: A History of the Johns Hopkins University, 1873–1889* (Ithaca: Cornell University Press, 1960), 239, 255.

4. Application of Abraham Flexner, 13 May 1884, Special Collections, Eisenhower Library, Johns Hopkins University; A. Flexner, *I Remember,* 52–55; Johns Hopkins University, *Register,* 1884, 23.

5. Hawkins, *Pioneer,* 244–45.

6. A. Flexner, *I Remember,* 53–55.

7. Fabian Franklin, *The Life of Daniel Coit Gilman* (New York: Dodd, Mead, 1910), 228; Josiah Royce, "Present Ideals of American University Life," *Scribner's Magazine* 10 (1891):383–84.

8. Hawkins, *Pioneer,* 265.

9. A. Flexner, *I Remember,* 49–59. Hawkins's evaluation of the atmosphere at Johns Hopkins is in a private letter to the author, 3 August 2001.

10. Transcript of Abraham Flexner, 1884–1885, Special Collections, Eisenhower Library; A. Flexner, *I Remember,* 60.

11. Transcript of Abraham Flexner, 1885–1886, Special Collections, Eisenhower Library; Robert E. Cyphers, Registrar, to Professor David J. King, 11 November 1974, Registrar's Office, Johns Hopkins University, answering a query from Professor King; Ronald F. Movrich, "Before the Gates of Excellence: Abraham Flexner and Education, 1866–1918" (Ph.D. diss., University of California, Berkeley, 1981), 59.

12. A. Flexner, *I Remember,* 62.

13. Application of Abraham Flexner, 13 May 1884, Special Collections, Eisenhower Library; A. Flexner, *I Remember,* 66; Abraham Flexner to D. C. Gilman, 3 June 1886, Special Collections, Eisenhower Library.

14. Ron Chernow, *Titan: The Life of John D. Rockefeller Sr.* (New York: Random House, 1998), 22–24.

15. A. Flexner, *I Remember,* 56.

16. Information about the Flexner family assembled by Harry Rosenberg (grandson of Gertrude) of Chicago; *Louisville City Directory* (Louisville, 1886).

17. Abraham Flexner to Daniel C. Gilman, 12 June 1886, newspaper clipping dated 1887, both in Special Collections, Eisenhower Library.

18. A. Flexner, *I Remember,* 69–70.

19. Ibid., 70.

20. Ibid., 72; n.d. newspaper clipping, 1887, Special Collections, Eisenhower Library.

21. Ibid., 74.

22. Abraham Flexner, "The Ultimate Importance of the Kindergarten Idea," *Kindergarten* (Chicago) 3 (1889):199–201.

23. *Nation,* 43 (1888):149, 249–50, 312–13, 395, 476.

24. *Nation,* 49 (1889):410; 50 (1890):412–13; 51 (1891):11, 292–93; 56 (1893):158; 57 (1895): 171–72.

25. Abraham Flexner to Mr. Ball, Registrar, 9 November 1889, Special Collections, Eisenhower Library; Abraham Flexner to Daniel C. Gilman, 11 January 1892, Special Collections, Eisenhower Library.

CHAPTER 3: MR. FLEXNER'S SCHOOL

1. James T. Flexner, "My Father, Simon Flexner," in *Institute to University: A Seventy-Fifth Anniversary Colloquium* (New York: Rockefeller University, 1977), 8; Saul Benison, "Simon Flexner: The Evolution of a Career in Medical Science," *Institute to University,* 14–15.

2. A. Flexner, "William Henry Welch," *Bulletin of the History of Medicine* 87 (suppl.) (1950):48; J. T. Flexner, *American Saga,* 108–15, 130–34; "The Reminiscences of Abraham Flexner," 1970, Oral History Research Office, Columbia University, 3.

3. J. T. Flexner, *American Saga,* 137.

4. Simon Flexner to Abraham Flexner, 1 June 1930, Abraham Flexner Papers, Library of Congress.

5. Abraham Flexner to Simon Flexner, 9 December 1890, 30 January 1892, Simon Flexner Papers, American Philosophical Society.

6. Abraham Flexner to Simon Flexner, 22 February, 20 March, 1 December 1892, 14 November 1895, Simon Flexner Papers.

7. J. T. Flexner, *American Saga,* 120.

8. Abraham Flexner to Simon Flexner, 1 December 1890, Simon Flexner Papers.

9. *Caron's Directory* (Louisville), 1890–97.

10. Ibid., 1893; Abraham Flexner to Simon Flexner, 21 January 1891, 6 February 1892, Simon Flexner Papers.

11. Abraham Flexner to Simon Flexner, 10 May 1892, Simon Flexner Papers. In his autobiography and other writings, Flexner dates the beginning of his private school in 1890, but this is clearly in error. He continued to be listed on the faculty of the high school through 1891–92, and his correspondence shows that he opened his private classes in the fall of 1892.

12. Abraham Flexner to Simon Flexner, 1 September, 10 September, 24 September 1892, Simon Flexner Papers.

13. Abraham Flexner to Simon Flexner, 1 December 1892, 10 February 1894, Simon Flexner Papers.

14. *Louisville Courier-Journal,* 18 February 1940.

15. *Mr. Flexner's School* [1902], 22. Copies of these rare catalogs are found in the Bernard Flexner Papers, Mudd Library, Princeton, N.J.; U.S. Commissioner of Education, *Reports,* 1893–1906; "Profile," *New Yorker,* 22 November 1930, 31.

16. A. Flexner, *I Remember,* 81.

17. Diane Ravitch, *Left Back: A Century of Failed School Reforms* (New York: Simon & Schuster, 2000), 30–43; Hugh Hawkins, *Between Harvard and America: The Educational Leadership of Charles W. Eliot* (New York: Oxford University Press, 1972), 231–35.

18. Charles W. Eliot to Abraham Flexner, 26 November 1899, Abraham Flexner Papers.

19. A. Flexner, *I Remember,* 81–82; "A Freshman at Nineteen," *Educational Review,* 18 (1899):358.

20. Abraham Flexner, "The Preparatory School," *Atlantic Monthly* 94 (1904):373.

21. *Mr. Flexner's School* [1895], 5–10.

22. A. Flexner, *I Remember,* 75–76.

23. *Mr. Flexner's School* [1897], 6; Abraham Flexner to Simon Flexner, 9 March 1904, Simon Flexner Papers.

24. *Mr. Flexner's School* [1897], 5–6; *Mr. Flexner's School* [1892], 21–22.

25. John Dewey, *The School and Society* (New York: McClure, Phillips, 1900), 25, 39, 51, 119.

26. Abraham Flexner, "The Religious Training of Children," *International Journal of Ethics* 7 (1897):319–22.

27. Abraham Flexner to Simon Flexner, n.d. [1899]; Abraham Flexner to Simon Flexner, n.d. [Christmas 1901], Simon Flexner Papers; Abraham Flexner to John Dewey, 19 October 1949, Abraham Flexner Papers.

28. This discussion owes much to Ronald F. Movrich, "Before the Gates of Excellence: Abraham Flexner and Education, 1866–1918" (Ph.D. diss., University of California, Berkeley, 1981), 66–74.

29. A. Flexner, "Preparatory School," 374–77.

30. A. Flexner, "Freshman at Nineteen," 353–58.

31. A. Flexner, "Preparatory School," 376; A. Flexner, "Religious Training of Children," 318.

32. Abraham Flexner to Joshua Glasser, 29 March 1943, Abraham Flexner Papers. Glasser was the son-in-law of Abraham's brother Washington.

33. Abraham Flexner to Simon Flexner, 16 May 1892, 17 February 1893, n.d. [1893], Simon Flexner Papers.

34. J. T. Flexner, *American Saga,* 257–58.

35. Abraham Flexner to Simon Flexner, 17 January, 10 February 1894, Simon Flexner Papers.

36. Abraham Flexner to Simon Flexner, n.d. [1895], 26 July [1895], Simon Flexner Papers.

37. Abraham Flexner to Simon Flexner, 12 September 1896, Simon Flexner Papers.

38. Simon Flexner to Bernard and Mary Flexner, 19 June 1939, Bernard Flexner Papers, Mudd Library; Abraham Flexner to Simon Flexner, n.d. [1897], Simon Flexner Papers.

39. Abraham Flexner to Simon Flexner, n.d. [1897?], Simon Flexner Papers.

40. Ibid.

CHAPTER 4: BREAKING FREE

1. Abraham Flexner to Simon Flexner, 18 November 1890, 15 April 1891, 26 November 1891, 14 January 1892, 3 April 1892, 9 April 1892, 10 May 1892, n.d. [1892], Simon Flexner Papers, American Philosophical Society.

2. Abraham Flexner to Simon Flexner, 22 October 1894, Simon Flexner Papers.

3. Abraham Flexner to Rush Rhees, 19 June 1925, General Education Board Files, Rockefeller Archive Center, Sleepy Hollow, N.Y.; A. Flexner, *I Remember,* 87.

4. J. T. Flexner, *American Saga,* 372; information supplied by Harry Rosenberg of Chicago, a grandnephew; A. Flexner, *I Remember,* 83.

5. A. Flexner, *I Remember,* 89; J. T. Flexner, *American Saga,* 373; Jean Flexner Lewinson, interview by author, Westboro, Mass., 18 November 1995.

6. Abraham Flexner to Simon Flexner, n.d. [1899], 21 June 1899, Simon Flexner Papers.

7. Abraham Flexner to Simon Flexner, 20 June 1900, 12 December 1901, 13 December 1901, 27 September 1902, 4 November 1902, 28 April 1903, Simon Flexner Papers.

8. Abraham Flexner to Simon Flexner, 26 February, 21 June, 4 November 1902, Simon Flexner Papers.

9. Jean Flexner Lewinson, "A Family Memoir, 1899–1989," 11–12, MS. in author's possession; Abraham Flexner to Simon Flexner, 28 September 1902, Simon Flexner Papers; Eleanor Flexner, interview by Jacqueline Van Voris, 8 January 1977, 32, MS., Eleanor Flexner Papers, Schlesinger Library, Radcliffe College.

10. Brooks Atkinson, *Broadway* (New York: Macmillan, 1971), 33; Abraham Flexner to Simon Flexner, 20 June 1900, Simon Flexner Papers. See also Archie Binns, *Mrs. Fiske of the American Theatre* (New York: Crown, 1955).

11. J. T. Flexner, *American Saga,* 376–77; *New York Daily Tribune,* 25 September 1901.

12. Alice Hegan Rice, *Mrs. Wiggs of the Cabbage Patch* (Mattituck, N.Y.: American House, 1991), introduction by W.F. Axton, iv–vii; Alice Hegan Rice, *The Inky Way* (New York: Appleton-Century, 1940), 172–77.

13. J. T. Flexner, *American Saga,* 379; Abraham Flexner to Simon Flexner, 9 March 1904, Simon Flexner Papers.

14. "Journal of Anne Crawford Flexner with Notes for Plays, Daily Entries, Financial Records, etc., 1903," entry for 1 January, Eleanor Flexner Papers; Abraham Flexner to Simon Flexner, 29 May 1904, Simon Flexner Papers.

15. Abraham Flexner to Simon Flexner, 28 September 1904, Simon Flexner Papers.

16. Abraham Flexner to Simon Flexner, 4 November 1902, 27 November 1904, Simon Flexner Papers.

17. Abraham Flexner to Simon Flexner, 2 July 1905, Simon Flexner Papers.

18. Lewinson, "Family Memoir," 12; Abraham Flexner to Simon Flexner, 28 September 1905, Simon Flexner Papers.

19. Abraham Flexner to Simon Flexner, 3 November, 10 December 1905, 1 August 1906, Simon Flexner Papers.

20. A. Flexner to S. Flexner, 10 December 1905, Simon Flexner Papers.

21. A. Flexner, *I Remember*, 101.

22. Ibid., 102; Abraham Flexner to Simon Flexner, 10 December 1905, 11 March 1906, Simon Flexner Papers.

23. A. Flexner, *I Remember*, 101; Abraham Flexner to Simon Flexner, 2 January 1906, Simon Flexner Papers; Transcript of Abraham Flexner, 1905–06, Registrar's Office, Harvard University.

24. A. Flexner to S. Flexner, 11 March 1906, Simon Flexner Papers; Lewinson, "Family Memoir," 12.

25. Abraham Flexner to Simon Flexner, 1 August 1906, Simon Flexner Papers; A. Flexner, *I Remember*, 102.

26. Nicholas Murray Butler, *Across the Busy Years*, 2 vols. (New York: Scribner's, 1939–40), I:122; A. Flexner, *I Remember*, 107; Abraham Flexner to Simon Flexner, 4 November 1906, Simon Flexner Papers.

27. Quoted from a contemporary letter in A. Flexner, *I Remember*, 107; A. Flexner to S. Flexner, 4 November 1906, Simon Flexner Papers.

28. Abraham Flexner to Simon Flexner, 2 November 1906, Simon Flexner Papers; student notebooks, Berlin, Abraham Flexner Papers, Box 25.

29. Lewinson, "Family Memoir," 14. Abraham Flexner to Simon Flexner, 4 November 1906, 4 February, 3 March 1907, Simon Flexner Papers; A. Flexner, *I Remember*, 1906.

30. A. Flexner to S. Flexner, 4 February 1907, Simon Flexner Papers; A. Flexner, *I Remember*, 106.

31. A. Flexner to S. Flexner, 2 November 1906, Simon Flexner Papers.

32. Ric Burns and James Sanders, *New York: An Illustrated History* (New York: Knopf, 1999), 231, 245.

33. Lewinson, "Family Memoir," 15–16.

34. Ibid., 17.

35. *Nation* 85 (1907):278.

36. Abraham Flexner, *The American College: A Criticism* (New York: Century, 1908), 32.

37. Ibid., 70–89.

38. Abraham Flexner to Simon Flexner, 28 September 1904, Simon Flexner Papers.

39. A. Flexner, *American College*, 120–21, 139, 173, 180–83, 193–200.

40. Ibid., 216–34; *Educational Review* 36 (1908):513–15; Abraham Flexner to Hermann Weyl, 21 March 1944, Abraham Flexner Papers.

41. Abraham Flexner to Simon Flexner, September 1908, Simon Flexner Papers; Ellen C. Lagemann, *Private Power for the Public Good: A History of the Carnegie Foundation for the Advancement of Teaching* (Middletown, Conn.: Wesleyan University Press, 1983), 59–61; Abraham Flexner to William R. Boyd, 28 September 1935. Boyd was a regent of the University of Iowa. I am indebted to Ronald F. Movrich's dissertation, "Before the Gates of Excellence: Abraham Flexner and Education, 1866–1918" (Ph.D. diss., University of California, Berkeley, 1981), 93, for calling my attention to the Boyd letter.

42. In a letter to the historian Allan Nevins, Flexner wrote in 1949: "Dr. Butler for some reason never liked me and, though I had never spoken to him or he to me, he was op-

posed to Pritchett's choice of me to do the medical report." Abraham Flexner to Allan
Nevins, 11 July 1949, Allan Nevins Papers, Rare Book and Manuscript Library, Columbia University.

43. Abraham Flexner, *Henry S. Pritchett: A Biography* (New York: Columbia University
Press, 1943), 109–10; Howard J. Savage, *Fruit of an Impulse: Forty-Five Years of the
Carnegie Foundation, 1905–1950* (New York: Harcourt, Brace, 1953), 105; Abraham
Flexner to David Starr Jordan, 2 November 1908, David Starr Jordan Papers, Special
Collections, Stanford University Libraries; Abraham Flexner to Simon Flexner, 17 No-
vember 1908, Simon Flexner Papers; Henry S. Pritchett to Abraham Flexner, 2 De-
cember 1908, Henry S. Pritchett Papers, Library of Congress.

CHAPTER 5: A LEGEND IS BORN

1. *New York Times,* 24 July 1910, magazine section; *World's Work* 22 (1911):1441–42; *Collier's* 45 (1910):16; *Harper's Weekly* 54 (1910).

2. Simon Flexner to Abraham Flexner, 6 June 1910, Simon Flexner Record Group, box
2, folder 4, Rockefeller Archive Center, Sleepy Hollow, N.Y.; Abraham Flexner to
Anne Flexner, 8 October 1910, Abraham Flexner Papers, Library of Congress.

3. Abraham Flexner, "Medical Education in America," *Atlantic Monthly* 105 (1910):799.

4. Benjamin Michailovsky, "Some Points in Medical Education Considered from the
Standpoint of the Students," *Medical Record* 73 (1908):18.

5. Abraham Flexner, "A Layman's View of Osteopathy," *JAMA* 62 (1914):1831.

6. Frank Billings, "Medical Education in the United States," *JAMA* 40 (1903):1272; Abra-
ham Flexner, *Medical Education in the United States and Canada*, Bulletin no. 4 (New
York: Carnegie Foundation for the Advancement of Teaching, 1910), 35, 216; Abraham
Flexner, "Medical Colleges," *World's Work* 21 (1911):14241.

7. Donald Fleming, *William H. Welch and the Rise of American Medicine* (Baltimore: Johns
Hopkins University Press, 1954), 174; Howard J. Savage, *Fruit of an Impulse: Forty-Five
Years of the Carnegie Foundation, 1905–1950* (New York: Harcourt, Brace, 1953), 106;
George W. Corner, *Two Centuries of Medicine: A History of the School of Medicine, University of Pennsylvania* (Philadelphia: J. B. Lippincott, 1965), 221, 229; Paul Starr, *The Social Transformation of American Medicine* (New York: Basil Books, 1982), 120. I reviewed
historical writing on the Flexner Report in "Abraham Flexner and the Historians," *Journal of the History of Medicine and Allied Sciences* 45 (1990):3–10.

8. Kenneth M. Ludmerer, *Learning to Heal: The Development of American Medical Education* (New York: Basic Books, 1985), 78. The quotation about a random patient is attributed to Lawrence J. Henderson, a biochemist at Harvard. See Gert H. Brieger,
"The Flexner Report: Revised or Revisited?" *Medical Heritage* 1 (1985):32.

9. Henry K. Beecher and Mark D. Altshule, *Medicine at Harvard: The First Three Hundred Years* (Hanover; N.H.: University Press of New England, 1977), 95.

10. Arthur D. Bevan, "Medical Education in the United States: The Need for a Uniform
Standard," *JAMA* 51 (1908):567; American Medical Association, Proceedings, June
3–7, 1907, 10, AMA Library, Chicago; Arthur Bevan, "Cooperation in Medical Education and Medical Service," *JAMA* 90 (1928):1173.

11. Council on Medical Education, Minutes of the Business Meeting, 28 December 1908,
AMA Library.

12. "Scheme for a Projected Report on Medical Education in the United States and Canada," Abraham Flexner Papers.

13. Ibid., 1.

14. Council on Medical Education, Minutes, 28 December 1908, AMA Archives.

15. Henry S. Pritchett to Cyrus Adler, 22 January 1909; Henry S. Pritchett to Jerome Greene and William T. Councilman, 22 January 1909; William T. Councilman to Henry S. Pritchett, 26 January 1909, all Henry S. Pritchett Papers, Library of Congress.

16. A. Flexner, *Medical Education in the United States and Canada,* 280; A. Flexner, *I Remember,* 114.

17. Abraham Flexner to Jean Flexner, 18 November 1917, Abraham Flexner Papers.

18. A. Flexner, *I Remember,* 115; Abraham Flexner to Philip H. Sachzer, New York Post-Graduate Medical School, 26 March 1956, Abraham Flexner Papers.

19. Report of the Council on Medical Education of the American Medical Association to the House of Delegates, 6 June 1910, AMA Archives; "The Committee of One Hundred to Prepare a Standard Medical Curriculum," *JAMA* 51 (1908):1886–88; A. Flexner, *Medical Education in the United States and Canada,* 325–26.

20. I follow here the careful compilation of Ronald F. Movrich, "Before the Gates of Excellence: Abraham Flexner and Education, 1866–1918" (Ph.D. diss., University of California, Berkeley, 1981), table 41, 128.

21. A. Flexner, *I Remember,* 121.

22. Brieger, "Flexner Report," 27.

23. A. Flexner, *Medical Education in the United States and Canada,* 187, 190, 205, 216, 227, 235, 256, 304, 306, 319.

24. Abraham Flexner to Henry S. Pritchett, 17 April, 4 November 1909, and Anson Phelps Stokes to Abraham Flexner, 24 June 1910, Abraham Flexner Papers; Ellen C. Cangi, "Principles before Practice: The Reform of Medical Education in Cincinnati before and after the Flexner Report" (Ph.D. diss., University of Cincinnati, 1983), 184.

25. Edwin Mims, *Chancellor Kirkland of Vanderbilt* (Nashville: Vanderbilt University Press, 1940), 201; "A Report of the Medical Department of Washington University [1909]," MS., Abraham Flexner Papers.

26. Donna B. Munger, "Robert Brookings and the Flexner Report," *Journal of the History of Medicine and Allied Sciences* 23 (1968):360; Henry S. Pritchett to David Houston, 20 November 1909, David Houston to Henry S. Pritchett, 22 November 1909, Marjorie F. Grisham, Notes on Carnegie Foundation files, Archives, Washington University School of Medicine (the Carnegie Foundation files for this period are currently unavailable and presumed lost; they were last used by scholars before their transfer to Columbia University c. 1990); John F. Fulton, *Harvey Cushing: A Biography* (Springfield, Ill.: Charles C Thomas, 1986), 306. At the meeting, Brookings "unfolded his plans to Johns Hopkinize the Medical Department of the Washington University."

27. Abraham Flexner to H. S. Wilgus, 4 January 1909, Bentley Library, University of Michigan; Abraham Flexner to Henry S. Pritchett, 2 March 1909, John G. Bowman to Abraham Flexner, 2 March 1909, Abraham Flexner to Allan Nevins, 19 November 1953, all in Abraham Flexner Papers; Abraham Flexner, "The Problem of College Ped-

agogy," *Atlantic Monthly* 103 (1909):838–44; Abraham Flexner, "Adjusting the College to American Life," *Science* 29 (1909):361–72.

28. Abraham Flexner to Simon Flexner, [1909], Simon Flexner Papers, American Philosophical Society.

29. Jean Flexner Lewinson, "A Family Memoir, 1899–1989," 16–21, MS. in author's possession.

30. Abraham Flexner to Simon Flexner, n.d. [1909], 30 July 1909, Simon Flexner Papers.

31. A. Flexner, *Medical Education in the United States and Canada,* 53, emphasis in original; Ludmerer, *Learning to Heal,* 63–71.

32. A. Flexner, *Medical Education in the United States and Canada,* 55–56, 105.

33. Ibid., 91–102.

34. Ibid., 20, 26, 154.

35. Ludmerer, *Learning to Heal,* 180–81.

36. A. Flexner, *Medical Education in the United States and Canada,* 42–43.

37. Ibid., 169.

38. Ibid., 49, 150–53.

39. Abraham Flexner to Gilbert Highet, 5 August 1950, Rare Book and Manuscript Library, Columbia University.

40. A. Flexner, *Medical Education in the United States and Canada,* 178–81.

41. Ibid., 155; A. Flexner, *I Remember,* 106.

42. Abraham Flexner, "Aristocratic and Democratic Education," *Atlantic Monthly* 108 (1911):386–95.

43. Carnegie Foundation for the Advancement of Teaching, Minutes of the Executive Committee, 5 May 1910, 13–14, Butler Library, Columbia University; A. Flexner, "Medical Education in America," 797–804; A. Flexner, "The Plethora of Doctors," *Atlantic Monthly* 106 (1910):20–25; A. Flexner, "Medical Education in the United States and Canada," *Science* 32 (1910):41–50; A. Flexner, "Fewer and Better Doctors," *American Review of Reviews* 42 (1910):203–10; Charles W. Eliot to Andrew Carnegie, 7 June 1910, Abraham Flexner Papers.

44. Ludmerer, *Learning to Heal,* 180–81.

45. Simon Flexner and James T. Flexner, *William Henry Welch and the Heroic Age of American Medicine* (New York: Viking Press, 1941), 500, n. 8.

46. Henry S. Pritchett to Charles W. Eliot, 9 June 1910, Henry S. Pritchett Papers; "Summary of Reactions to the Flexner Report," *Charlotte Medical Journal,* 1910, reprinted in *Charlotte Medical Journal* 56 (1995):537; James G. Burrow, *Organized Medicine in the Progressive Era: The Move toward Monopoly* (Baltimore: Johns Hopkins University Press), 1977, 45; Carleton B. Chapman, "The Flexner Report," *Daedalus* 104 (1974): 109.

47. J. T. Flexner, *American Saga,* 382.

48. Abraham Flexner to Anne Flexner, 27 November 1910, Abraham Flexner Papers.

CHAPTER 6: MASTER OF THE SURVEY

1. Jean Flexner Lewinson, "A Family Memoir, 1899–1989," 23, MS. in author's possession; A. Flexner, *I Remember,* 133.

2. Lewinson, "Family Memoir," 22.

3. Abraham Flexner to Simon Flexner, 23 July 1910, Simon Flexner Papers, American Philosophical Society.

4. A. Flexner, *I Remember,* 135–36; Abraham Flexner to Henry S. Pritchett, 22 November 1910, Abraham Flexner Papers, Library of Congress.

5. Abraham Flexner to Anne Flexner, 8 October 1910, Abraham Flexner Papers; Henry Miller, "Fifty Years after Flexner," *Lancet,* 24 September 1966, 648.

6. George Haines IV, *Essays on German Influence upon English Education and Science, 1850–1919* (Hamden, Conn.: Aichon Books, 1969), 151–52; Peter Alster, *The Reluctant Patron: Science and the State in Britain, 1850–1920* (Oxford: Berg, 1987); Harvey Cushing, *The Life of Sir William Osler* (London: Oxford University Press, 1940), 876.

7. This discussion follows in part my "Abraham Flexner as Critic of British and Continental Medical Education," *Medical History* 33 (1989):472–79.

8. Abraham Flexner to Henry Pritchett, 21 October, 9 November 1910, Abraham Flexner Papers.

9. Royal Commission on University Education in London, *Reports,* 5 vols. (London: His Majesty's Stationery Office, 1910–12), 3:2, 6; Abraham Flexner to Simon Flexner, 12 November 1910, 22 April 1935, Simon Flexner Papers.

10. Royal Commission on University Education, *Reports,* 5:21–25; Abraham Flexner to Henry S. Pritchett, 13 November 1910, Abraham Flexner Papers.

11. *Nature* 92 (1913–14):270–71; Royal Commission on University Education in London, *Final Report* (London: His Majesty's Stationery Office, 1913), 121.

12. A. Flexner, *I Remember,* 144; Simon Flexner to Abraham Flexner, 23 November 1910, Simon Flexner Papers; M. Carey Thomas to Abraham Flexner, 26 September 1913, Abraham Flexner Papers.

13. Abraham Flexner, *Medical Education in Europe,* Bulletin no. 6 (New York: Carnegie Foundation for the Advancement of Teaching, 1912), 50.

14. Ibid., 142–43.

15. Ibid., 15, 113, 122, 144.

16. Ibid., 8, 84, 89.

17. Abraham Flexner to Henry Pritchett, 22 November 1910, Abraham Flexner Papers.

18. Abraham Flexner to Simon Flexner, 6 September 1910, Simon Flexner Papers.

19. Abraham Flexner to Anne Flexner, 27 November 1910, Abraham Flexner Papers.

20. A. Flexner, *I Remember,* 174–76.

21. Abraham Flexner to Anne Flexner, 8 October 1910, Abraham Flexner Papers.

22. Abraham Flexner to Henry S. Pritchett, 18 July, 15 August 1911, Abraham Flexner Papers; Abraham Flexner to Simon Flexner, 6 September 1910, Simon Flexner Papers.

23. Abraham Flexner to A. Lawrence Lowell, 16 October 1911, A. Lawrence Lowell Papers, Harvard University Archives, Pusey Library. Other letters in the Flexner-Lowell exchange are Flexner to Lowell, 13 October 1911 and 18 October 1911, and Lowell to Flexner, 14 October 1911 and 17 October 1911, A. Lawrence Lowell Papers.

24. Abraham Flexner to Franklin Paine Mall, 29 July 1911, Simon Flexner Papers. For some unknown reason, the Mall-Flexner correspondence of 1911 is part of his brother's papers. Perhaps Simon asked for them when he was working on his biography of William Henry Welch.

25. Simon Flexner to Abraham Flexner, 14 August 1911, Simon Flexner Papers.

26. Howard J. Savage to Abraham Flexner, 18 July 1924, Clyde Furst to Abraham Flexner, 19 July 1912, Abraham Flexner Papers.

27. Frederick T. Gates, "The Memoirs of Frederick T. Gates," *American Heritage* 6 (1955):73.

28. Frederick T. Gates to William H. Welch, 6 January, 10 January, 30 January 1911, William Henry Welch Papers, Alan M. Chesney Archives, Johns Hopkins University.

29. Simon Flexner to Abraham Flexner, 17 February 1911, Abraham Flexner to Franklin Paine Mall, 14 February 1911, Simon Flexner Papers.

30. Franklin Paine Mall to Lewellys Barker, 3 August 1902, Lewellys Barker Papers, Alan M. Chesney Archives. The best account of the development of the full-time plan is by W. Bruce Fye, "The Origin of the Full-Time Faculty System," *JAMA* 265 (1991): 1555–62.

31. Florence R. Sabin, *Franklin Paine Mall: The Story of a Mind* (Baltimore: Johns Hopkins Press, 1934), 261.

32. Abraham Flexner, "The Johns Hopkins School," 17–23, MS., Abraham Flexner Papers.

33. Ibid., 36; Steven C. Wheatley, *The Politics of Philanthropy: Abraham Flexner and Medical Education* (Madison: University of Wisconsin Press, 1988), 63.

34. Abraham Flexner to Anne Flexner, 2 April 1911, Abraham Flexner Papers.

35. William Osler to Ira Remsen, 1 September 1911, Abraham Flexner to William Osler, 6 October 1911, William Osler Papers, Osler Library, McGill University, Montreal; Abraham Flexner to Franklin Paine Mall, 26 September 1911, Simon Flexner Papers.

36. Simon Flexner and James T. Flexner, *William Henry Welch and the Heroic Age of American Medicine* (New York: Viking Press, 1941), 310.

37. Abraham Flexner to Simon Flexner, 8 June, 28 August 1911, Simon Flexner Papers; Lewellys Barker to Abraham Flexner, 7 March 1911, Abraham Flexner Papers.

38. Abraham Flexner to Simon Flexner, 16 June, 23 August, 14 September 1911, Simon Flexner Papers.

39. A. McGehee Harvey, *Science at the Bedside: Clinical Research in American Medicine, 1905–1945* (Baltimore: Johns Hopkins University Press, 1981), 139; Howard S. Berliner, *A System of Scientific Medicine: Philanthropic Foundations in the Flexner Era* (New York: Tavistock, 1985), 159.

40. S. Flexner and J. T. Flexner, *Welch,* 324; Arthur D. Bevan to Henry S. Pritchett, 10 January 1912, Abraham Flexner Papers; Harvey, *Science at the Bedside,* 183.

41. Peter Collier and David Horowitz, *The Rockefellers: An American Dynasty* (New York: Holt, Rinehart and Winston, 1976), 106.

42. A. Flexner, *I Remember,* 186; John D. Rockefeller Jr. to Abraham Flexner, 9 February 1911, Office of the Messrs. Rockefeller General Files, Rockefeller Archive Center, Sleepy Hollow, N.Y.

43. Henry S. Pritchett to Abraham Flexner, 23 October 1911, Abraham Flexner Papers; A. Flexner, *I Remember,* 187.

44. Abraham Flexner to Anne Flexner, 27 November 1910, Abraham Flexner Papers.

45. Abraham Flexner to Anne Flexner, 12 January 1912, Abraham Flexner Papers.

46. A. Flexner, *I Remember,* 187–90.

47. Abraham Flexner, *Prostitution in Europe* (New York: Century, 1914), 3–31.

48. Ibid., 39–57.

49. Horton A. Johnson, "The Other Flexner Report: How Abraham Flexner Was Diverted from Medical Schools to Brothels," *Pharos,* spring 1986, 11.

50. Abraham Flexner to Anne Flexner, 28 January 1912, Abraham Flexner Papers.

51. A. Flexner, *I Remember,* 193–94.

52. Abraham Flexner to Anne Flexner, 11 March, 5 May 1912, Abraham Flexner Papers; John D. Rockefeller Jr. to Abraham Flexner, 3 March 1912, 4 April 1912, 18 July 1913, Office of the Messrs. Rockefeller General Files.

53. Abraham Flexner to Anne Flexner, 10 January, 11 February, 25 February 1912, telegram, 28 February 1912, Abraham Flexner Papers.

54. Abraham Flexner to Anne Flexner, 6 March, 12 April, [May] 1912, Abraham Flexner Papers.

55. A. Flexner, *Prostitution in Europe,* 159–61, 216–17, 344.

56. Ibid., 395, 401.

57. Raymond B. Fosdick to Abraham Flexner, 1 June 1918, 10 June 1918, Office of the Messrs. Rockefeller General Files; review of *Prostitution in Europe, American Journal of Sociology* 23 (1917–18):126; "Civilization Must Fling Down the Gauntlet," *Journal of Social Hygiene* 22 (1936):420.

58. Abraham Flexner to Simon Flexner, 18 May 1912, Simon Flexner Papers.

59. Abraham Flexner to Simon Flexner, 20 September, 28 October, 1 November 1911, Simon Flexner Papers; Abraham Flexner to Sir William McCormick, 14 November 1912, Abraham Flexner Papers.

60. Abraham Flexner to Simon Flexner, 1 November 1912, Simon Flexner Papers.

CHAPTER 7: A SECURE BERTH—AT LAST

1. A. Flexner, *I Remember,* 75.

2. Frederick T. Gates, "A System of Higher Education," [1906], 1, MS., Francis Countway Library of Medicine, Harvard University.

3. Steven Wheatley, *The Politics of Philanthropy: Abraham Flexner and Medical Education* (Madison: University of Wisconsin Press, 1988), 20.

4. A. Flexner, *I Remember,* 214.

5. Abraham Flexner to Jean Flexner, 21 November 1913, 17 February 1914, Abraham Flexner Papers, Library of Congress.

6. Abraham Flexner to Jackson Davis, J.H. Dillard, H.B. Frissill, John Hope, et al., 9 November 1915, Abraham Flexner Papers; "Conference of the General Education Board of the Rockefeller Foundation on 'Negro Education,'" 29 November 1915, Rockefeller Archive Center, Special Collections, Series VII, Reports, Sleepy Hollow, N.Y. See, too, the perceptive account by Eric Anderson and Alfred A. Moss Jr. in *Dangerous Donations: Northern Philanthropy and Southern Black Education, 1902–1930* (Columbia: University of Missouri, 1999), esp. 86–95.

7. Frederick T. Gates to Charles W. Eliot, 15 January 1914, Charles W. Eliot Papers, Harvard University Archives, Pusey Library.

8. Abraham Flexner to Jean Flexner, 19 October 1919, Abraham Flexner Papers.

9. Abraham Flexner to Wallace Buttrick, 1 May 1919, General Education Board Files; Abraham Flexner to Charles W. Eliot, 22 November 1920, Charles W. Eliot Papers; Abraham Flexner to Anne Flexner, n.d. [1916], Abraham Flexner Papers.

10. Abraham Flexner, *Medical Education in the United States and Canada*, Bulletin no. 4 (New York: Carnegie Foundation for the Advancement of Teaching, 1910), 178–79.

11. Abraham Flexner to M. Carey Thomas, 5 October 1911, Simon Flexner Papers, American Philosophical Society; Abraham Flexner to Robert W. Lovett, 6 December 1918, General Education Board Files, Rockefeller Archive Center; Abraham Flexner to Jean Flexner, 6 November 1921, Abraham Flexner Papers.

12. Eleanor Flexner, interview by Jacqueline Van Voris, 8 January 1977, 86, MS., Eleanor Flexner Papers, Schlesinger Library, Radcliffe College; *New York Post*, 13 January 1917; *New Orleans Times Picayune*, 25 February 1917.

13. Abraham Flexner to Jean Flexner, 10 May 1920, Abraham Flexner Papers.

14. Anne Flexner to Abraham Flexner, 15 June 1914, Abraham Flexner to Anne Flexner, 5 June 1915, Abraham Flexner Papers.

15. Abraham Flexner to Anne Flexner, n.d. [1915], 11 April 1916, Abraham Flexner Papers.

16. Abraham Flexner to Jean Flexner, 28 October 1917, 17 November 1917, Abraham Flexner Papers.

17. Abraham Flexner to Simon Flexner, 11 September 1913, and n.d. [1913], Simon Flexner Papers; Abraham Flexner to Anne Flexner, 6 March 1916, Abraham Flexner Papers; Abraham Flexner to Jacob Flexner, 3 September 1918, Simon Flexner Papers.

18. Abraham Flexner to Simon Flexner, 29 November 1912, Simon Flexner Papers.

19. Abraham Flexner to Henry S. Pritchett, 3 December 1915, 14 July 1916, 25 October 1918, Abraham Flexner Papers.

20. Abraham Flexner, "Upbuilding American Education: The National Work of the General Education Board," *Independent*, 9 August 1915, 188–91.

21. Wallace Buttrick to Abraham Flexner, 31 July 1915, George Vincent to Abraham Flexner, 15 July 1916, Abraham Flexner Papers.

22. A. Flexner, *I Remember*, 245.

23. Abraham Flexner and Frank P. Bachman, *Public Education in Maryland* (New York: General Education Board, 1916); M. Bates Stephens to Wallace Buttrick, 18 April 1916, Charles W. Eliot Papers, Harvard University Archives, Pusey Library.

24. Simon Flexner to Abraham Flexner, 8 February 1917, Abraham Flexner to Simon Flexner, 13 February 1917, Simon Flexner Papers.

25. Raymond B. Fosdick, *Adventure in Giving: The Story of the General Education Board* (New York: Harper & Row, 1962), 118–19.

26. Abraham Flexner to Frank P. Bachman, 5 February 1919, General Education Board Files.

27. Lawrence A. Cremin, *The Transformation of the School: Progressivism in American Education, 1876–1957* (New York: Knopf, 1962), 155.

28. Ronald D. Cohen and Raymond A. Mohl, *The Paradox of Progressive Education: The Gary Plan and Urban Schooling* (Port Washington, N.Y.: National University Publications, 1979), 7–8.

29. "Topics for Investigation by the General Education Board," 17 June 1915, General Education Board Files; Abraham Flexner to William Wirt, 23 June 1915, General Education Board Files; Cremin, *Transformation of the School*, 157.

30. Sol Cohen, *Progressivism and Urban School Reform: The Public Education Association of New York City 1895–1954* (New York: Teachers College, 1964), 87–90.

31. Abraham Flexner to Charles Judd, 2 October 1915, General Education Board Files. The fullest description of Flexner's role in the Gary survey is in Ronald F. Movrich, "Before the Gates of Excellence: Abraham Flexner and Education, 1866–1918" (Ph.D. diss., University of California, Berkeley, 1981), 158–201.

32. Abraham Flexner to Leonard Ayres, 16 September 1915, General Education Board Files; A. Flexner, *I Remember,* 254.

33. Cohen and Mohl, *Paradox of Progressive Education,* 41–46; Federation of Neighborhood Associations of the Public Schools, "Our Garyized Children: Why Do I Not Want My Child to Go to a Gary School?" [1916], Office of the Messrs. Rockefeller General Files, Rockefeller Archive Center.

34. Cohen and Mohl, *Paradox of Progressive Education,* 47, 50–51; Cohen, *Progressive and Urban School Reform,* 96.

35. "The Universal Spider," Office of the Messrs. Rockefeller General Files.

36. John D. Rockefeller to the Rev. John Zeiter, 1 June 1917, Office of the Messrs. Rockefeller General Files; Abraham Flexner to Anne Flexner, 10 April 1916, Abraham Flexner Papers.

37. Abraham Flexner to Anne Flexner, 10 March 1916, Abraham Flexner to Jean Flexner, 15 May 1915, Abraham Flexner Papers.

38. Movrich, "Before the Gates of Excellence," 199–200.

39. Abraham Flexner and Frank P. Bachman, *The Gary Schools* (New York: General Education Board, 1918), 47, 196–98, 202–6.

40. Franklin Parker, "Abraham Flexner, 1866–1959," *History of Education* 2 (1962):205–6.

41. Minutes, General Education Board, October 1914, Rockefeller Archive Center.

42. Charles W. Eliot to Abraham Flexner, 23 June 1915, General Education Board Files.

43. Abraham Flexner to Anne Flexner, 9 July 1915, Abraham Flexner Papers; Minutes, General Education Board, 1915–16, Rockefeller Archive Center, 36–37.

44. Abraham Flexner to Anne Flexner, 9 July 1915, 12 July 1915, Abraham Flexner Papers.

45. Frederick T. Gates to John D. Rockefeller Jr., 9 August 1915, copy in Simon Flexner Papers.

46. John D. Rockefeller Jr. to Abraham Flexner, 21 January 1916, Frederick T. Gates to Abraham Flexner, 18 August 1916, General Education Board Files.

47. Abraham Flexner, "A Modern School," *American Review of Reviews* 53 (1916):465–74. The report was later reprinted in his *A Modern College and a Modern School* (Garden City, N.Y.: Doubleday, 1923).

48. A. Flexner, "A Modern School," 2–7, 22–26, MS., General Education Board Files. Emphasis in original.

49. Abraham Flexner to Jean Flexner, 5 May 1915, Abraham Flexner Papers.

50. A. Flexner, "A Modern School," 11–21.

51. "Report on the Modern School," [May 1916], 2, MS., General Education Board Files.

52. Fosdick, *Adventure in Giving,* 216–19.

53. Charles W. Eliot to Abraham Flexner, 2 February 1918, Abraham Flexner Papers; Cremin, *Transformation of the School,* 280–86.

54. General Education Board, *Review and Final Report, 1902–1964* (New York: General Education Board, 1964), 45–46.

55. Abraham Flexner to Charles W. Eliot, 30 October 1917, Charles W. Eliot Papers.

56. Peter Collins and David Horowitz, *The Rockefellers: An American Dynasty* (New York: Holt, Rinehart and Winston, 1976), 192; James T. Flexner, *Maverick's Progress: An Autobiography* (New York: Fordham University Press, 1996), 98; Eleanor Flexner, interview by Jacqueline Van Voris, 8 November 1977, 10, 87, MS., Eleanor Flexner Papers.

57. Cremin, *Transformation of the School,* 286–88; Charles P. Howland to Abraham Flexner, 15 December 1919, General Education Board Files; Abraham Flexner to J. D. Rockefeller, Jr., 11 December 1919, General Education Board Files.

58. Movrich, "Before the Gates of Excellence," 149–51; *New York Times,* 8 July 1917; Walter F. McDuffee to George Vincent, 27 July 1918, General Education Board Files; George Vincent to Abraham Flexner, 3 June 1918, General Education Board Files.

59. A. Flexner, *I Remember,* 252.

60. Abraham Flexner to Simon Flexner, 2 November 1918, Simon Flexner Papers. Emphasis in original.

61. Abraham Flexner, "Parents and Schools," *Atlantic Monthly* 118 (1916):26–27. Emphasis in original.

62. Abraham Flexner, "Education as Mental Discipline," *Atlantic Monthly* 118 (1916): 452–64; Abraham Flexner to Simon Flexner, 3 July 1916, Simon Flexner Papers.

63. Abraham Flexner to A. Lawrence Lowell, 17 November 1916, A. Lawrence Lowell Papers, Harvard University Archives, Pusey Library.

64. Robert E. Kohler, *Partners in Science: Foundations and Natural Scientists, 1900–1945* (Chicago: University of Chicago Press, 1991), 47, 80–81; Abraham Flexner to A. Lawrence Lowell, 16 November 1918, A. Lawrence Lowell Papers; Fosdick, *Adventure in Giving,* 318; Paul Hanus, *Adventuring in Education* (Cambridge: Harvard University Press), 224–25.

65. Abraham Flexner, "Is Social Work a Profession?" *Proceedings of the National Conference of Charities and Corrections* 42 (1915):576–90.

66. Abraham Flexner to trustee George Rublee, Report, 21 February 1913. I am much indebted to Mark D. Desjardins, who sent me a copy of the Flexner report on Groton, as well as a chapter from his forthcoming dissertation on the history of the Groton School.

67. Abraham Flexner to Anne Flexner, 7 October 1916, Abraham Flexner Papers.

68. Wallace Buttrick to Abraham Flexner, 9 December 1921, Abraham Flexner Papers; John D. Rockefeller Jr. to Abraham Flexner, 4 March 1918, Office of the Messrs. Rockefeller General Files; Abraham Flexner to Simon Flexner, 29 September 1918, Simon Flexner Papers.

69. Fosdick, *Adventure in Giving,* 151; oral interview with Alan Gregg, 2 April 1956, National Library of Medicine, Bethesda, Md.

70. Fosdick, *Adventure in Giving,* 14; Wallace Buttrick to Charles W. Eliot, 9 March 1920, 12 December, 15 December 1921, Charles W. Eliot Papers.

71. Abraham Flexner to Anne Flexner, 10 August 1913, Abraham Flexner Papers.

72. Abraham Flexner to Simon Flexner, 20 January 1919, Simon Flexner Papers; Abraham Flexner to Anne Flexner, 15 December 1918, Abraham Flexner Papers. This account closely follows Jean Flexner Lewinson, "A Family Memoir, 1899–1989," 26–27, MS. in author's possession.

73. Lewinson, "Family Memoir," 27.

74. A. Flexner, *I Remember,* 277; "Medical Education 1898–1927," Memorandum in Box 11, Abraham Flexner Papers.

CHAPTER 8: AT THE PINNACLE

1. Abraham Flexner, *Medical Education in the United States and Canada,* Bulletin no. 4 (New York: Carnegie Foundation for the Advancement of Teaching, 1910), appendix. Author's estimate of expenditures in 1920.

2. Abraham Flexner to Jean Flexner, 8 May 1921, Abraham Flexner Papers, Library of Congress.

3. A. Flexner, *Medical Education in the United States and Canada,* 143–55.

4. Abraham Flexner to Anne Flexner, 23 October 1913, Abraham Flexner Papers.

5. Abraham Flexner, "The English Side of Medical Education," *Atlantic Monthly* 116 (1915):529–30; Abraham Flexner, "The German Side of Medical Education," *Atlantic Monthly* 112 (1913):654–62.

6. Steven Wheatley, *The Politics of Philanthropy: Abraham Flexner and Medical Education* (Madison: University of Wisconsin Press, 1988), 46.

7. Abraham Flexner to J. Whitridge Williams, 15 July 1913, General Education Board Files, Rockefeller Archive Center, Sleepy Hollow, N.Y.; Wallace Buttrick to William Henry Welch, 29 October 1913, William Henry Welch to Wallace Buttrick, 19 June 1914, William Henry Welch Papers, Alan M. Chesney Archives, Johns Hopkins University.

8. Charles A. Richmond to Abraham Flexner, 28 December 1914, Abraham Flexner to Charles A. Richmond, 4 January 1915, General Education Board Files.

9. Marjorie Fox, "History of Washington University School of Medicine," 7–8, MS., Washington University School of Medicine Archive. Other good accounts of the reorganization at Washington University may be found in Kenneth M. Ludmerer, "Reform of Medical Education at Washington University," *Journal of the History of Medicine and Advanced Sciences* 35 (1980):149–73; Donna B. Munger, "Robert Brookings and the Flexner Report," *Journal of the History of Medicine and Advanced Sciences,* 23 (1968):356–71; Eugene L. Opie, "Adoption of Standards of the Best Medical Schools of Western Europe by Those in the United States," *Perspectives in Biology and Medicine* 13 (1970):309–42; and Ralph E. Morrow, *Washington University in St. Louis* (St. Louis: Missouri Historical Society Press, 1996), 195–227.

10. G. Canby Robinson, *Adventures in Medical Education* (Cambridge: Harvard University Press, 1957), 14–20; Abraham Flexner to P.A. Shaffer, 6 November 1916, General Education Board Files.

11. Fox, "History," 16.

12. William H. Welch, "Recent Improvements in Medical Education," in *The Dedication of the New Buildings of Washington University Medical School* (St. Louis: Washington University, 1915), 38.

13. A. Flexner, *Medical Education in the United States and Canada,* 200; A. Flexner, *I Remember,* 258; Abraham Flexner, *The General Education Board: An Account of Its Activities, 1902–1914* (New York: General Education Board, 1915), 171; "Appropriations Made by the General Education Board to Medical Schools (White) from 1902 to December 29, 1924," Frederick T. Gates Papers, Rockefeller Archive Center.

14. Abraham Flexner to Milton Winternitz, 1 May 1930, Abraham Flexner Papers; A. Flexner, *I Remember,* 260.

15. Arthur Dean Bevan to Abraham Flexner, 9 January 1912, Arthur Dean Bevan to Henry S. Pritchett, 10 January 1912, Abraham Flexner Papers.

16. Abraham Flexner to Henry S. Pritchett, 5 December 1913, Abraham Flexner Papers.

17. Abraham Flexner to George Dock, 20 February 1914, Abraham Flexner Papers. This was a letter to be read at the council meeting, which Flexner could not attend, but Bevan blocked its presentation.

18. Kenneth M. Ludmerer, *Learning to Heal* (New York: Basic Books, 1985), 246–47; Abraham Flexner to Henry S. Pritchett, 26 March 1914, Abraham Flexner Papers. Ludmerer was able to use letters from the now-missing files of the Carnegie Foundation Archives to describe the clash between Bevan and Flexner.

19. A. Flexner, *Medical Education in the United States and Canada,* 240.

20. Henry A. Christian to Wallace Buttrick, 28 March 1913, with attached application, General Education Board Files.

21. Wallace Buttrick to Henry A. Christian, 25 May 1913, General Education Board Files; Abraham Flexner to Henry A. Christian, 26 June 1913, Harvard University Archives, Pusey Library.

22. A. Lawrence Lowell to Jerome Greene, 27 October 1913, A. Lawrence Lowell Papers, Harvard University Archives, Pusey Library; Councilman to Abraham Flexner, 28 October 1913, General Education Board Files.

23. Henry A. Christian to Charles W. Eliot, 1 November 1913, Countway Library of Medicine, Harvard Medical School; Jerome Greene to A. Lawrence Lowell, 15 October, 25 October, 28 October 1913, A. Lawrence Lowell Papers.

24. A. Lawrence Lowell to Jerome Greene, 30 October, 15 November 1913, A. Lawrence Lowell Papers.

25. David Edsall to A. Lawrence Lowell, 30 March 1913, A. Lawrence Lowell Papers.

26. A. Lawrence Lowell to Abraham Flexner, 19 January, 14 April 1914, Abraham Flexner to A. Lawrence Lowell, 1 May 1914, General Education Board Files.

27. Abraham Flexner to Simon Flexner, 10 November 1915, Simon Flexner Papers, American Philosophical Society; Wheatley, *Politics of Philanthropy,* 75–77.

28. William S. Thayer to Charles W. Eliot, 3 October 1916, Charles W. Eliot Papers, Harvard University Archives. Emphasis in original.

29. "Provisional memorandum about aid for the Harvard Medical School from the General Education Board, 22 December 1916," General Education Board Files; Wheatley, *Politics of Philanthropy,* 80.

30. Wallace Buttrick to Charles W. Eliot, 26 December 1916, Charles W. Eliot Papers; "Comments on Dr. Eliot's Memorandum," 30 January 1917, General Education Board Files. Emphasis in original.

31. Charles W. Eliot to Wallace Buttrick, 18 April, 24 April 1917, Charles W. Eliot Papers; A. Lawrence Lowell to William S. Thayer, 5 May 1917, A. Lawrence Lowell Papers; quoted in Wheatley, *Politics of Philanthropy,* 82.

32. "Extract from letter of F. T. Gates to Drs. Goodspeed and Harper, 19 January 1898," Abraham Flexner Papers.

33. Henry Pratt Judson to Abraham Flexner, 2 January 1915, General Education Board Files.

34. Abraham Flexner, "A Plan for the Development of Medical Education in Chicago, July 1916," MS., Henry Pratt Judson Papers, University of Chicago Archives.

35. Henry Pratt Judson to Abraham Flexner, 2 January 1915, Abraham Flexner Papers; "Comments on Dr. Bevan's Address before the American Medical Association, Boston, 25 June 1921," MS., General Education Board Files.

36. A. Flexner, "Comments on Dr. Bevan's Address."

37. I owe much in this and the following paragraph to *Albert* R. Lamb, *The Presbyterian Hospital and the Columbia-Presbyterian Medical Center, 1868–1942* (New York: Columbia University Press, 1955), 125–62, and Wheatley, *Politics of Philanthropy,* 90–97.

38. John D. Rockefeller Jr. to Abraham Flexner, 30 January 1917, General Education Board Files.

39. Abraham Flexner, "Memorandum on Columbia University and Medical Education," [1917], Abraham Flexner Papers.

40. Henry S. Pritchett to Abraham Flexner, 7 May 1918, Abraham Flexner Papers.

41. Abraham Flexner to Simon Flexner, 27 October 1918, Simon Flexner Papers.

42. Henry S. Pritchett to Abraham Flexner, 19 May 1919, 23 December 1920, Abraham Flexner Papers; Theodore C. Janeway, "Outside Professional Engagements by Members of Professional Faculties," *Educational Review* 56 (1918):209; Theodore C. Janeway to Samuel Lambert, 3 December 1917, Alan M. Chesney Archives.

43. David Edsall to Abraham Flexner, 3 August 1919, Countway Library, Harvard University School of Medicine, Boston.

44. A. McGehee Harvey, *Science at the Bedside: Clinical Research in American Medicine, 1905–1945* (Baltimore: Johns Hopkins University Press, 1981), 183.

45. Abraham Flexner, "Memorandum regarding Mr. Rockefeller's Gift to Be Devoted to the Improvement of Medical Education in the United States," [October, 1919], MS., 5; "Medical Education in the United States: A Program, [June, 1919], MS., 3–10, General Education Board Files; N.P. Colwell to Abraham Flexner, 9 October 1919, General Education Board Files.

46. Abraham Flexner, "Memorandum," 3–5; Abraham Flexner, "Medical Education in the United States: A Program," [June 1919], MS., 4–5, General Education Board Files.

47. A. Flexner, *I Remember,* 281–82.

48. Abraham Flexner, "Memorandum on Medical Education," [1920], MS., General Education Board Files.

49. Ibid., 1.

50. James H. Kirkland, "A Statement by J. H. Kirkland, Chancellor, Vanderbilt University," MS., James H. Kirkland Papers, Vanderbilt University Archive; A. Flexner, *Medical Education in the United States and Canada,* 308; Paul K. Conkin, *Gone with the*

Ivy: A Biography of Vanderbilt University (Knoxville: University of Tennessee Press, 1985), 207; Abraham Flexner and Wallace Buttrick to James H. Kirkland, 15 December 1914, James H. Kirkland Papers.

51. Edwin Mims, *Chancellor Kirkland of Vanderbilt* (Nashville: Vanderbilt University Press, 1940), 218; Abraham Flexner, memorandum marked "Confidential" (April–May 1919), 7 November 1919, MSS., Chancellor's Office Files, Vanderbilt University Archive.

52. James H. Kirkland to Abraham Flexner, 4 November 1920, Chancellor's Office Files; Conkin, *Gone with the Ivy,* 270.

53. Mims, *Chancellor Kirkland,* 229.

54. Abraham Flexner to James H. Kirkland, 27 May 1921, Chancellor's Office Files; Timothy C. Jacobson, *Making Medical Doctors: Science and Medicine at Vanderbilt since Flexner* (Tuscaloosa: University of Alabama Press, 1987), 121; Bernard Flexner to James H. Kirkland, 13 November 1927, Chancellor's Office files, Vanderbilt University Archive.

55. Charles Dabney to Abraham Flexner, 14 July 1913, General Education Board Files. Emphasis in original.

56. Christian Holmes to Abraham Flexner, 8 January 1919, Abraham Flexner to Christian Holmes, 19 July 1919, Telegram, Abraham Flexner to Frederick C. Hicks, 5 November 1920, George Heuer to Board of Directors, University of Cincinnati, 6 August 1922, all General Education Board Files; Ellen C. Cangi, "Abraham Flexner's Philanthropy: The Full-Time System in the Department of Surgery at the University of Cincinnati College of Medicine, 1910–1930," *Bulletin of the History of Medicine* 56 (1982):167–68. A full account of the developments in Cincinnati is in Ellen C. Cangi, "Principles before Practice: The Reform of Medical Education in Cincinnati before and after the Flexner Report, 1870–1930" (Ph.D. diss., University of Cincinnati, 1983).

57. Abraham Flexner, "Memorandum re Cornell Medical School," 24 February 1927, MS., General Education Board Files.

58. Abraham Flexner to Anne Flexner, 6 February 1920, Abraham Flexner Papers; A. Flexner, *I Remember,* 288.

59. "Memorandum: Proposed School of Medicine and Dentistry—University of Rochester," [1920], MS., General Education Board Files.

60. Abraham Flexner, "Rochester Speech," 11 June 1920, MS., University of Rochester Archive, Rush Rhees Library; *Rochester Democrat and Chronicle* clipping; Abraham Flexner to Rush Rhees, 24 February 1920, General Education Board Files.

61. Rush Rhees to George H. Whipple, 21 October 1920, George H. Whipple to Rush Rhees, 8 November 1920, General Education Board Files; oral interview with George H. Whipple, 6 June 1972, Edward G. Miner Library, University of Rochester School of Medicine and Dentistry.

62. Rush Rhees to Abraham Flexner, 16 October 1922, University of Rochester Archive; Abraham Flexner to William S. McCann, 26 January 1925, General Education Board Files; Carl W. Ackerman, *George Eastman* (Boston: Houghton Mifflin, 1930), 484–87.

63. Henry S. Pritchett to Abraham Flexner, 28 July 1920, Henry S. Pritchett to Wallace Buttrick, 7 February 1921, General Education Board Files.

64. A. Flexner, *I Remember,* 291.

65. Abraham Flexner, "Medical Department, University of Iowa, Iowa City, Iowa, visited December 8 and 9, 1920," MS., General Education Board Files.

66. Abraham Flexner to L. W. Dean, 15 May 1922, General Education Board Files.

67. Henry S. Pritchett to Abraham Flexner, 31 October 1921, Abraham Flexner to Henry S. Pritchett, 1 November 1921, Boyd to Abraham Flexner, 28 November 1921, General Education Board Files.

68. Raymond B. Fosdick, "Rockefeller Foundation: Source Material," Rockefeller Archive Center.

69. Raymond B. Fosdick, *Adventure in Giving: The Story of the General Education Board* (New York: Harper & Row, 1962), 167; Frederick T. Gates, "Suggestions regarding Policy in Medicine for the General Education Board and the Rockefeller Foundation Covering the Present and the Next Generation," MS., copy in David Edsall Papers, Countway Library of Medicine, Harvard Medical School. Emphasis in original.

70. General Education Board Minutes, 10/12–14/22, 99–100, Rockefeller Archive Center.

71. Frederick T. Gates to Abraham Flexner, 2 December 1922, General Education Board Files; Lee Anderson, "'A Great Victory': Abraham Flexner and the New Medical Campus at the University of Iowa," *Annals of Iowa* 51 (1992):251. See, too, the same author's *Internal Medicine and the Structures of Modern Medical Science: The University of Iowa, 1870–1990* (Ames: Iowa State University Press, 1996).

72. Charles Thwing to Abraham Flexner, 16 December 1913, and enclosure, General Education Board Files; Charles Thwing to Abraham Flexner, 25 May 1915, Case Western Reserve Archives, Cleveland. For a full account of Flexner's role at Western Reserve, see Darwin H. Stapleton, "Abraham Flexner, Rockefeller Philanthropy and the Western Reserve School of Medicine," *Ohio History* 101 (1992):100–113.

73. Abraham Flexner, "Memorandum re Cornell Medical School," 17 February 1920, MS., General Education Board Files. Three years later a tentative agreement, approved by Flexner, was reached: "Memorandum of the Possible Establishment of a Hospital and Medical Education Centre in New York City," 16 July 1923, General Education Board Files; Abraham Flexner to Simon Flexner, 29 September 1918, Simon Flexner Papers.

74. Abraham Flexner to President P. I. Campbell, 27 May 1921, Abraham Flexner to President George Norlin, 28 May 1922, General Education Board Files.

75. Wheatley, *Politics of Philanthropy,* ix.

76. Wallace Buttrick to Ray Lyman Wilbur, 15 December 1921, General Education Board Files.

77. Alan Gregg, oral interview, 2 April 1956, Oral History Project, Butler Library, Columbia University; Fosdick, *Adventure in Giving,* 321.

78. The action to revise medical contracts in regard to full-time came at a meeting of the Executive Committee, General Education Board, 30 September 1925 (Rockefeller Archive Center); Abraham Flexner to Graham Lusk, 5 December 1919, Simon Flexner Papers; Abraham Flexner to Charles W. Eliot, 2 May 1921, Charles W. Eliot Papers; Abraham Flexner to Anne Flexner, 6 December 1920, Abraham Flexner Papers.

79. Fosdick, *Adventure in Giving,* 226–27.

CHAPTER 9: A FALL FROM OLYMPUS

1. Eleanor Flexner, interview by Jacqueline Van Voris, 8 January, 15 January 1977, 88–89, MS., Eleanor Flexner Papers, Schlesinger Library, Radcliffe College; Miriam F. Maderer, letter to author, 2 December 1997. Miriam Maderer is the daughter of Flexner's younger brother, Washington.

2. Jean Flexner Lewinson, "A Family Memoir, 1899–1989," 27–33, MS. in author's possession.

3. "The Reminiscences of Abraham Flexner," 27, Oral History Project, Columbia University; Lewinson, "Family Memoir," 35–39.

4. Abraham Flexner to Jean Flexner, 3 July 1918, 6 April 1919, 8 February 1920, 10 May 1921, Abraham Flexner Papers, Library of Congress.

5. Abraham Flexner to Jean Flexner, 24 January 1922, Abraham Flexner Papers.

6. Lewinson, "Family Memoir," 44–45; Abraham Flexner to Jean Flexner, 11 September 1922, Abraham Flexner Papers.

7. Eleanor Flexner, interview by Jacqueline Van Voris, 6, 10, 15, 32, 34, 85–88; Abraham Flexner to Anne Flexner, 22 May 1924, Abraham Flexner Papers. Emphasis in original.

8. Elmer Bendiner, "Simon Flexner: His 'Rock' Was for the Ages," *Hospital Practice,* 15 (April 1988), 213.

9. Saul Benison, "Simon Flexner: The Evolution of a Career in Medical Science," in *Institute to University: A Seventy-Fifth Anniversary Colloquium, June 8, 1976* (New York: Rockefeller University, 1976), 29–30; Raymond B. Fosdick, "Simon Flexner," in *Memorial Meeting for Simon Flexner* (New York: Rockefeller Institute for Medical Research, 1946), 26–27.

10. Bernard Flexner to Dr. Alfred Cohn, 23 February 1927, Bernard Flexner Papers, Mudd Library, Princeton, N.J.

11. Bernard Flexner to Mary Flexner, 5 January, 16 January 1919, Bernard Flexner Papers, Mudd Library; Minutes, Board of Directors, Palestine Economic Corporation, 8 May 1945, Temple Adath Archive, Louisville, Ky.

12. Abraham Flexner to Dr. Morris Jastrow, 14 January 1919, Morris Jastrow Papers, American Jewish Archives, Cincinnati.

13. *Louisville Courier-Journal,* 18 February 1927.

14. Transcript of interview with Florence Hind, 119, Oral History Project, Butler Library, Columbia University.

15. Daniel M. Fox, "Abraham Flexner's Unpublished Report: Foundations and Medical Education, 1909–1928," *Bulletin of the History of Medicine* 54 (1980):480.

16. A. Flexner, *I Remember,* 399, 402.

17. Raymond B. Fosdick, Adventure in Giving: The Story of the General Education Board (New York: Harper & Row, 1962), 226–32; Abraham Flexner to Charles Howland, 13 April 1927, General Education Board Files, Rockefeller Archive Center, Sleepy Hollow, N.Y.

18. Alan Gregg, transcript of oral interview, 2 April 1956, 121, National Library of Medicine, Bethesda, Md.

19. Abraham Flexner to Jean Flexner, 23 March 1922, Abraham Flexner to Anne Flexner, 28 March, 31 March 1922, Abraham Flexner Papers; Abraham Flexner to Simon Flexner, 9 July 1922, Simon Flexner Papers, American Philosophical Society.

20. Abraham Flexner to Richard Pearce, 9 July 1922, Alanson Houghton to Abraham Flexner, 10 July 1922, Simon Flexner Papers; Gregg, transcript of oral interview, 121.

21. Abraham Flexner to Jean Flexner, 27 October, 13 November, 18 November, 1 December 1918, Abraham Flexner Papers.

22. Abraham Flexner to Jean Flexner, 20 November 1918, 2 April 1922, Abraham Flexner Papers; Abraham Flexner to Simon Flexner, 9 July 1922, Simon Flexner Papers.

23. Abraham Flexner to Jean Flexner, 3 March 1918; Abraham Flexner to Eleanor Flexner, 10 November 1923, Abraham Flexner Papers. Emphasis in original.

24. Abraham Flexner to Jean Flexner, 11 January 1920. Emphasis in original.

25. Abraham Flexner, *Medical Education: A Comparative Study* (New York: Macmillan, 1925), vii.

26. Abraham Flexner to Anne Flexner, 11 January 1921, 8 February 1922, Abraham Flexner Papers. For the influence of Flexner on Newman, see W. F. Bynum, "Sir George Newman and the American Way," *Clio Medica*, 1995, 3037–50.

27. Abraham Flexner to Anne Flexner, 26 March 1922, Abraham Flexner Papers.

28. Abraham Flexner, "Medical Education, 1909–1924," *Educational Record*, April 1924, 3–19.

29. A. Flexner, *Medical Education: A Comparative Study*, 19–58.

30. Ibid., 178–79, 183. Emphasis in original.

31. Ibid., 238, 256.

32. *La presse medicale* 8 (October 1927):1261–62; William Henry Welch to Abraham Flexner, 10 August 1927, Abraham Flexner Papers; *Lancet*, 28 March 1925, 667–68; *New York Times Book Review*, 12 July 1925.

33. Raymond B. Fosdick to Wickliffe Rose, 22 September 1925, General Education Board Files; Lewis Weed to Abraham Flexner, 27 May 1924, Lewis Weed Papers, Alan M. Chesney Archives, Johns Hopkins University; Henry S. Pritchett to Abraham Flexner, 9 July 1924, Abraham Flexner Papers.

34. Abraham Flexner, "The German Side of Medical Education," *Atlantic Monthly* 112 (1913):658; Abraham Flexner to Harvey Cushing, 4 April 1921, General Education Board Files.

35. A. Flexner, *Medical Education: A Comparative Study*, 137–51; Abraham Flexner to David Edsall, 20 March 1924, Countway Library of Medicine, Harvard Medical School, Boston; Abraham Flexner to Simon Flexner, 15 April 1925, Simon Flexner Papers; "Proposal for Revision of Curriculum," 5 April 1925, Lewis Weed Papers.

36. Aaron M. Moore to Abraham Flexner, 22 May 1918, General Education Board Files.

37. Abraham Flexner to Henry S. Pritchett, 25 April 1921, Abraham Flexner Papers; Abraham Flexner to Nathan P. Colwell, 29 May 1918, General Education Board Files.

38. John J. Mullowney, *American Gives a Chance* (Tampa: Tribune Press, 1940), 87.

39. James Summerville, *Educating Black Doctors: A History of Meharry Medical College* (Tuscaloosa: University of Alabama Press, 1983), 64.

40. Marlene Y. Macleish, "Medical Education in Black Colleges and Universities in the United States of America" (Ed.D. diss., Harvard University, 1978), 162; Fosdick, *Adventure in Giving*, 179.

41. Abraham Flexner to Julius Rosenwald, 16 June 1919, General Education Board Files; Abraham Flexner to William Henry Welch, David Edsall, and Victor Vaughn, 7 July 1919, Abraham Flexner Papers. It is of some interest that a major influence on Rosenwald was Rabbi Emil Hirsch, now of Chicago, who had a similar influence on Flexner in Louisville.

42. Abraham Flexner to William Henry Welch, David Edsall, and Victor Vaughn, 26 December 1919, David Edsall to Abraham Flexner, 29 December 1919, General Education Board Files.

43. Abraham Flexner to Julius Rosenwald, 15 August 1919; Julius Rosenwald to Abraham Flexner, 18 August 1919, General Education Board Files.

44. Abraham Flexner to Wallace Buttrick, 27 April 1921, General Education Board Files.

45. Abraham Flexner to William C. Graves (Rosenwald's assistant), 2 September 1920, David Edsall to Abraham Flexner, 7 May 1920, General Education Board Files.

46. Kenneth R. Manning, *Black Apollo of Science: The Life of Ernest Everett Just* (New York: Oxford University Press, 1983), 125, 303.

47. H. A. Hitchcock, registrar, to Abraham Flexner, 16 July 1919, General Education Board Files; John Mullowney, *An Autobiography* (Miami: Florida Press, 1940), 400; MacLeish, "Medical Education in Black Colleges and Universities," 167; Fosdick, *Adventure in Giving*, 308.

48. Abraham Flexner to Julius Rosenwald, 28 November 1925, Julius Rosenwald Papers, University of Chicago.

49. Wickliffe Rose diary, 3 March 1921, Rockefeller Archive Center; Fosdick, *Adventure in Giving*, 308; Abraham Flexner to Richard B. Dillehunt, 26 January 1925, General Education Board Files.

50. Raymond Paul, "Distribution of Physicians in the U.S.," *Journal of the American Medical Association* 84 (1925):1026.

51. Lewis Mayers and Leonard V. Harrison, *The Distribution of Physicians in the United States* (New York: General Education Board, 1924), 47–48.

52. Abraham Flexner to Anne Flexner, 1 March, 4 March 1925, Abraham Flexner Papers.

53. Henry S. Pritchett to Abraham Flexner, 9 July 1924, Abraham Flexner Papers.

54. Abraham Flexner, "Purpose in the American College," *School and Society* 22 (1925): 729–36.

55. Frank Aydelotte to Abraham Flexner, 22 September 1925, Flexner File, Frank Aydelotte Papers, Swarthmore College.

56. Abraham Flexner, *A Modern College and a Modern School* (Garden City, N.Y.: Doubleday, 1923), xv–xvi; Abraham Flexner, "The University in American Life," *Atlantic Monthly* 149 (1932):626; Abraham Flexner, "A Modern University," *Atlantic Monthly* 136 (1925):530.

57. Raymond B. Fosdick to John D. Rockefeller Jr., 15 November 1922, copy in Bernard Flexner Papers, Mudd Library.

58. Abraham Flexner, "A Proposal to Establish an American University," [November 1922], MS., Abraham Flexner Papers. Emphasis in original.

59. George Vincent to Abraham Flexner, 22 November 1922, Frank Aydelotte Papers.

60. A. Flexner, "A Modern University"; General Education Board, *Annual Report,* 1924–25, 5–6.

61. Fosdick, *Adventure in Giving,* 233; Abraham Flexner, "The Humanities," [1924], MS., copy in Benjamin D. Meritt Papers, American Philosophical Society; Abraham Flexner to Simon Flexner, 18 May 1925, Simon Flexner Papers.

62. Frank Aydelotte to Abraham Flexner, 21 February 1939, Frank Aydelotte Papers.

63. Frances Blanshard, *Frank Aydelotte of Swarthmore* (Middletown, Conn.: Wesleyan University Press, 1970), 209.

64. I have relied heavily in this paragraph on an unpublished chapter by Joel Colton and Malcolm Richardson from their forthcoming book, *The Humanities and "The Well-Being of Mankind": The Humanities at the Rockefeller Foundation since 1928.* I am grateful to the authors for sending me a copy of the chapter "Origins and Early Stages: The Humanities at the General Education Board and the Foundation, 1913–1929."

65. Fosdick, *Adventure in Giving,* 235.

66. A. Lawrence Lowell to Abraham Flexner, 16 March 1928, A. Lawrence Lowell Papers, Harvard University Archives, Pusey Library; telegram from Abraham Flexner in Minutes, board of trustees, University of Chicago, 9 June 1927, Regenstein Library, University of Chicago; Fosdick, *Adventure in Giving,* 236.

67. Abraham Flexner to William Henry Welch, 28 April 1925, William Henry Welch Papers, Alan M. Chesney Archives, Johns Hopkins University; Lewis Weed to Abraham Flexner, 21 May 1925, Lewis Weed Papers; Abraham Flexner to Wickliffe Rose, 30 August 1927, General Education Board Files.

68. A. Flexner, *Medical Education: A Comparative Study,* 11–12.

69. A. Flexner, *I Remember,* 324–26.

70. Fosdick, *Adventure in Giving,* 237.

71. A. Flexner, *I Remember,* 329–31.

72. Raymond B. Fosdick, *John D. Rockefeller, Jr.: A Portrait* (New York: Harper, 1956), 367; Louis E. Lord, *A History of the American School of Classical Studies at Athens, 1882–1942* (Cambridge: Harvard University Press, 1947), 194–95; Colton and Richardson, *Humanities and "The Well-Being of Mankind,"* 16; Fosdick, *Adventure in Giving,* 236.

73. Fosdick to W. W. Brierley, 25 April 1927, Raymond B. Fosdick Papers, Mudd Library, Princeton University; Fosdick, *John D. Rockefeller, Jr.,* 396–97; A. Flexner, *I Remember,* 322.

74. Abraham Flexner to Robert S. Brookings, [1927], Abraham Flexner Papers.

75. Abraham Flexner to Simon Flexner, 20 July, 1 August 1925, Simon Flexner Papers.

76. John D. Rockefeller Jr. to Frank S. Staley, 6 March 1925, Office of the Messrs. Rockefeller General Files, Rockefeller Archive Center; [Flexner], "Comments on Mr. Staley's Chart," 1 October 1925, MS., Office of the Messrs. Rockefeller General Files.

77. Edwin Embree, MS., no title, n.d., Edwin Embree Papers, Rockefeller Archive Center.

78. Robert E. Kohler, "A Policy for the Advancement of Science: The Rockefeller Foundation, 1924–29," *Minerva* 16 (1978):489.

79. Ibid., 497–99.

80. Abraham Flexner, "Memorandum regarding General Education Board," 4 January 1927, General Education Board Files.

81. Wilder Penfield, *The Difficult Art of Giving: The Epic of Alan Gregg* (Boston: Little, Brown, 1967), 202; Alan Gregg to Raymond B. Fosdick, 24 July 1926, Alan Gregg Papers, National Library of Medicine, Bethesda, Md.

82. Milton Winternitz to Abraham Flexner, 2 February 1923, Milton Winternitz Papers, Yale Medical School Archives; Ilza Veith and Franklin C. McLean, *Medicine at the University of Chicago, 1927–1952* (Chicago: University of Chicago Press, 1952), 23–24; Franklin C. McLean to Hans Zinsser, 25 November 1931, Franklin C. McLean Papers, Department of Special Collections, Regenstein Library, University of Chicago; James H. Kirkland to Abraham Flexner, 31 December 1923, James H. Kirkland Papers, Heard Library, Vanderbilt University; Abraham Flexner to James H. Kirkland, 2 January 1924, James H. Kirkland Papers; Albert R. Lamb, *The Presbyterian Hospital and the Columbia-Presbyterian Medical Center, 1868–1943* (New York: Columbia University Press, 1955), 196–224; R. B. Fosdick, "Source Material: Hist. 1, V.20," 5148–82, History Collection, Rockefeller Archive Center; Edward C. Atwater, "A Modest but Good Institution," in *To Each His Farthest Star: University of Rochester Medical Center, 1925–1975* (Rochester: University of Rochester Medical Center, 1975), 13. For a thorough discussion of the demise of strict full-time that is highly critical of Flexner see Michael S. Lepore, *Death of the Clinician* (Springfield, Ill.: Charles C Thomas, 1982).

83. David Edsall to Richard Pearce, 5 April 1927, David Edsall Papers, Countway Medical Library, Boston.

84. Francis W. Peabody, *Doctor and Patient* (New York: Macmillan, 1930), 95.

85. Hans Zinsser, "The Perils of Magnanimity: A Problem in American Education," *Atlantic Monthly,* February 1927, 247–49.

86. Abraham Flexner to Franklin C. McLean, 26 January 1927, Franklin C. McLean Papers, Regenstein Library, University of Chicago.

87. Frederick Gates, "The General Education Board," [1925], MS., Frederick T. Gates Papers, Rockefeller Archive Center; Alan Gregg to Abraham Flexner, 30 June 1924, General Education Board Files; Anson Phelps Stokes to Abraham Flexner, 19 March 1924, General Education Board Files; Abraham Flexner to Simon Flexner, 22 April 1925, Simon Flexner Papers; Henry S. Pritchett to Abraham Flexner, 23 December 1920, Simon Flexner Papers.

88. Steven C. Wheatley, *The Politics of Philanthropy: Abraham Flexner and Medical Education* (Madison: University of Wisconsin Press, 1988), 138–39.

89. George Vincent, "Memorandum on Policy and Organization," 29 January 1927, MS., Rockefeller Foundation Files, Rockefeller Archive Center.

90. Raymond B. Fosdick to John D. Rockefeller Jr., 10 November 1927, Rockefeller Foundation Files.

91. Raymond B. Fosdick to John D. Rockefeller Jr., 21 February 1928, Rockefeller Foundation Files.

92. Abraham Flexner to Anne Flexner, 16 December, 17 December 1925, Abraham Flexner Papers; Eleanor Flexner, interview by Jacqueline Van Voris, 8 January 1977, 91–92, MS., Eleanor Flexner Papers, Schlesinger Library, Radcliffe College.

93. Jean Flexner Lewinson, "A Family Memoir, 1899–1989," 48–54, MS. in author's possession; Paul Lewinson, *Race, Class, and Party—A History of Negro Suffrage and White Politics in the South* (New York: Oxford University Press, 1932).

94. Abraham Flexner, "Memo," 29 March 1928, Abraham Flexner Papers.

95. Abraham Flexner to Anne Flexner, 4 April 1928, Abraham Flexner Papers.

96. Abraham Flexner to Simon Flexner, 29 April, 29 December 1928, Simon Flexner Papers; Abraham Flexner to Anne Flexner, 31 March, 6 April 1928, Abraham Flexner Papers.

97. Abraham Flexner to Raymond B. Fosdick, 19 April 1928, copy in Bernard Flexner Papers, Mudd Library; Abraham Flexner, "To My Friends," 28 May 1928, Abraham Flexner Papers.

98. *New York Times,* 20 May, 28 May 1928; *New York World,* 26 May 1928; "Statement by W. W. Brierley, Secretary of the General Education Board, 27 May 1928," copy in Bernard Flexner Papers, Mudd Library.

CHAPTER 10: PHOENIX RISING

1. Steven C. Wheatley, "Abraham Flexner and the Politics of Educational Reform," *History of Higher Education Annual* 8 (1988):45.

2. John D. Rockefeller Jr. to Abraham Flexner, 9 April 1928, Abraham Flexner Papers, Library of Congress.

3. Steven C. Wheatley, *The Politics of Philanthropy: Abraham Flexner and Medical Education* (Madison: University of Wisconsin Press, 1988), ix, 170; Warren Weaver, *U.S. Philanthropic Foundations: Their History, Structure, Management, and Record* (New York: Harper & Row, 1967), 111; Editorial, *New York Times,* 28 May 1928.

4. Simon Flexner to Abraham Flexner, 31 May 1928, Simon Flexner Papers, American Philosophical Society; Raymond B. Fosdick to John D. Rockefeller, 6 June 1928, copy in Bernard Flexner Papers, Mudd Library, Princeton University.

5. Alfred E. Cohn to Abraham Flexner, 6 June 1928, copy in Bernard Flexner Papers, Mudd Library.

6. Abraham Flexner to Anne Flexner, 21 April, 4 May 1929, Abraham Flexner Papers; Abraham Flexner to Bernard Flexner, 5 February 1929, Bernard Flexner Papers, Mudd Library.

7. Abraham Flexner to Anne Flexner, 25 May 1929, n.d. [1930], Abraham Flexner Papers.

8. Frank Aydelotte to Philip Kerr, 23 May 1927, Philip Kerr to Frank Aydelotte, [July 1927], Rhodes Lecture Archives, Rhodes House, Oxford University.

9. Philip Kerr to Abraham Flexner, 30 January 1928, list of Rhodes Trust lecturers, Rhodes Lecture Archives.

10. A. Flexner, *I Remember,* 347.

11. Anne Flexner to Mary Flexner, 28 April 1928, Bernard Flexner Papers, Mudd Library.

12. Abraham Flexner, "Bulletin" to family, 20 May 1928, Anne Flexner to Mary Flexner, 28 April 1928, Bernard Flexner Papers, Mudd Library; secretary of Rhodes Trust to Abraham Flexner, 30 January 1928, Rhodes House, Oxford University.

13. A. Flexner, *I Remember,* 347; A. Flexner, "Bulletin," 20 May 1928.

14. E. A. Lowe to Abraham Flexner, 5 May 1928, copy attached to "Bulletin"; H.A.L. Fisher to Abraham Flexner, 19 May 1928; A. Flexner, "Bulletin" to family, 20 May 1928.

15. Random notes in Rhodes Memorial Trust Lectures file, Rhodes House.

16. "Bulletins" to family, 20 May, 29 May, 8 June 1928, Bernard Flexner Papers, Mudd Library; Abraham Flexner to Simon Flexner, 11 June 1928, Simon Flexner Papers.

17. See, e.g., *New York Times*, 26 May 1928; *New York Post*, 26 May 1928; *Louisville Times*, 25 May 1928.

18. *New York World*, 26 May 1928; *New York Herald-Tribune*, 26 May 1928; *Louisville Times*, 25 May 1928; *New York Post*, 26 May 1928.

19. *New York World*, 26 May 1928; Abraham Flexner to Anne Flexner, 21 April 1929, Abraham Flexner Papers; Abraham Flexner to Bernard Flexner, 24 January, 12 February 1929, Bernard Flexner Papers, Mudd Library; Abraham Flexner to Anne Flexner, 21 April 1929, Abraham Flexner Papers.

20. Carl W. Ackerman, *George Eastman* (Boston: Houghton Mifflin, 1930), 476.

21. Abraham Flexner to George Eastman, 28 July 1928, George Eastman Papers, George Eastman House, Rochester, N.Y.

22. George Eastman to Frank Aydelotte, 11 June 1929, Frank Aydelotte Papers, Swarthmore College; List of Eastman Professors at the University of Oxford, George Eastman Papers.

23. Abraham Flexner, *The Burden of Humanism* (Oxford: Clarendon Press, 1928), 5–25.

24. A. Flexner, *I Remember*, 355; Abraham Flexner to Anne Flexner, 30 April 1929, Abraham Flexner Papers.

25. Abraham Flexner to Bernard Flexner, 12 February 1929, Bernard Flexner Papers, Mudd Library; *Hamburger Nachrichten*, 8 March 1929; Abraham Flexner to John D. Rockefeller Jr., 27 March 1929, Office of the Messrs. Rockefeller General Files, Rockefeller Archive Center, Sleepy Hollow, N.Y.

26. Abraham Flexner to Anne Flexner, 16 March 1929, clipping from *Paris Herald*, n.d., Abraham Flexner Papers.

27. John D. Rockefeller to Abraham Flexner, 2 May 1929, Office of the Messrs. Rockefeller General Files; Simon Flexner to Abraham Flexner, 8 April 1929, Simon Flexner Papers.

28. Abraham Flexner to Bernard Flexner, 5 February 1929, Bernard Flexner Papers, Mudd Library; Abraham Flexner to Anne Flexner, 13 April 1929, Abraham Flexner Papers.

29. Abraham Flexner to Thomas Jones, 13 September 1930, Thomas Jones Papers, National Library of Wales, Aberystwyth, Wales; Abraham Flexner to Anne Flexner, 21 April 1921, Abraham Flexner Papers.

30. Abraham Flexner, "Memorandum re German Universities," [1929], Office of the Messrs. Rockefeller General Files; Alanson Houghton to Abraham Flexner, 27 December 1929, copy in Julius Rosenwald Papers, Regenstein Library, University of Chicago; John D. Rockefeller to Abraham Flexner, 9 December 1929, Office of the Messrs. Rockefeller General Files.

31. Abraham Flexner to John D. Rockefeller, 27 May 1929, Office of the Messrs. Rockefeller General Files.

32. Abraham Flexner to Julius Rosenwald, 19 April, 25 April 1930, Julius Rosenwald Papers; Abraham Flexner to Frank Aydelotte, 2 July 1929, Frank Aydelotte Papers.

33. Richard Pearce diary, "Luncheon Conference Midday Club, September 15, 1928: Mr. Arnett, Mr. Flexner, Dr. Pearce," General Education Board Files, Rockefeller Archive Center, Sleepy Hollow, N.Y.; Trevor Arnett diary, "Interviews: Saturday, September 15, 1928: Doctor Abraham Flexner, Doctor R. M. Pearce (Midday Club)" and "Interviews: Mr. Abraham Flexner, with Trevor Arnett, March 4, 1932," Rockefeller Archive Center.

34. Lewis Weed to Abraham Flexner, 18 December 1930, Lewis Weed Papers, Alan M. Chesney Archives, Johns Hopkins University. The survey is described in a letter to David Edsall, 18 December 1929, David Edsall Papers, Countway Library, Harvard University School of Medicine, Boston.

35. Abraham Flexner to Franklin McLean, 1 April 1930, Franklin McLean Papers, Regenstein Library; Abraham Flexner to A. N. Richards, 6 November 1930, College of Physicians, Philadelphia.

36. Abraham Flexner to Milton Winternitz, 19 November 1930, Yale Medical School Archives, Yale University Library; Abraham Flexner to Rush Rhees, 2 January 1931, Edward G. Miner Library, University of Rochester School of Medicine; Abraham Flexner to G. Canby Robinson, 19 February 1931, Chancellor's Office files, Heard Library, Vanderbilt University.

37. Abraham Flexner to Clyde Furst, 26 August 1929, Abraham Flexner Papers.

38. *New York Times,* 18 September, 20 September 1928; *Jewish Daily Bulletin,* 19 September 1928.

39. Clifford L. Muse Jr., "An Educational Stepchild: Howard University during the New Deal, 1933–45" (Ph.D. diss., Howard University, 1989), 64–65; Minutes, semi-annual meeting, board of trustees, 28 October 1930, 12 April 1932, and special meeting, board of trustees, 14 March 1932, Moorland-Spingarn Research Center, Howard University, Washington, D.C.; Abraham Flexner to George Foster Peabody, 21 October 1932, Abraham Flexner Papers.

40. A. Flexner, *I Remember,* 355; A. Scott Berg, *Lindbergh: A Biography* (New York: G. P. Putnam's Sons, 1998), 234–39, 355–56; Charles Lindbergh to Abraham Flexner, 13 June 1933, Abraham Flexner to Charles Lindbergh, 15 June 1933, Abraham Flexner Papers.

41. Abraham Flexner to Thomas Jones, 6 February, 28 August 1930, Thomas Jones Papers, National Library of Wales, Aberystwyth, Wales; Abraham Flexner to Julius Rosenwald, 18 July 1930, Julius Rosenwald Papers; Abraham Flexner to Paul H. Hanus, 1 November 1930, Abraham Flexner Papers; Henry S. Pritchett to Abraham Flexner, 8 April 1930, Henry S. Pritchett Papers, Library of Congress.

42. A. Flexner, *I Remember,* 355.

43. Clark Kerr, *The Uses of the University* (Cambridge: Harvard University Press, 1964).

44. Abraham Flexner, "Symposium on the Outlook for Higher Education in the United States: Address by Abraham Flexner," *Proceedings of the American Philosophical Society* 69 (1930):264–68; Clark Kerr, "Remembering Flexner," introduction to *Universities: American, English, German* (New York: Oxford University Press, 1967), xvi.

45. Kerr, "Remembering Flexner," viii, xvi.

46. Abraham Flexner, "Aristocratic and Democratic Education," *Atlantic Monthly* 58 (1911):390; Abraham Flexner, *Universities: American, English, German* (New York: Oxford University Press, 1930), 134.

47. A. Flexner, *Universities*, 63.

48. Ibid., 202–8.

49. Ibid., 23.

50. Abraham Flexner, "Medical Education, 1909–1924," *Educational Record*, April 1924, 10.

51. L. D. Coffman, "Flexner and the State University," *Journal of Higher Education* 2 (1931):383; *New York Times*, 20 November, 7 December 1930.

52. *New York Evening Post*, 20 November 1930; *Louisville Herald-Press*, 20 December 1930.

53. Abraham Flexner to Anson Phelps Stokes, 10 June 1931, Abraham Flexner Papers; A. Flexner, *Universities*, 99–100, 133–34, 212.

54. A. Flexner, *Universities*, 59, 91; Abraham Flexner to Lewis Weed, 28 September 1931, Lewis Weed Papers.

55. A. Flexner, *Universities*, 112–22, 164–65; Abraham Flexner, "Failings of Our Graduate Schools," *Atlantic Monthly* 149 (1932):447; Abraham Flexner to Anson Phelps Stokes, 18 June 1931, Abraham Flexner Papers.

56. W. H. Cowley, "The University and the Individual," *Journal of Higher Education* 2 (1931):393; Robert Shafer, "University and College," *Bookman* 73 (1931):227; Albert Bushnell Hart, "A New Attack on American Universities," *Current History* 33 (1931): 728–31; Albert Guerard, "The American Way," *New York Herald-Tribune Books*, 7 December 1930, 1; Charles A. Beard to Abraham Flexner, 20 November 1930, Abraham Flexner Papers.

57. John Henry McCracken, "Flexner and the Woman's College," *Journal of Higher Education* 2 (1931):369; L. D. Coffman, "Flexner and the State University," *Journal of Higher Education* 2 (1931):381–82; Editorial, *Saturday Review of Literature*, 29 November 1930.

58. *International Journal of Ethics* 42 (1931–32):331–32.

59. Abraham Flexner to John Dewey, 29 March, 2 April 1932, Rare Book and Manuscript Library, Butler Library, Columbia University. For Flexner's comments on Dewey's "obscurity," see Abraham Flexner to Simon Flexner, 9 September 1930, Simon Flexner Papers. Neither the Dewey archives at Southern Illinois University, the Flexner Papers in the Library of Congress, nor the Dewey materials at Columbia seem to contain the Dewey letter.

60. A. Flexner, *Universities*, 217–18.

61. Abraham Flexner, "Louis Bamberger and Mrs. Felix Fuld," *American Jewish Historical Society Quarterly* 37 (1947):455–57; E. M. Bluestone, "Abraham Flexner (in Memoriam)," *Jewish Forum*, December 1959, 197–98; E. M. Bluestone to Abraham Flexner, 2 October 1956, Archives, Institute for Advanced Study, Princeton, N.J.; Beatrice M. Stern, "A History of the Institute for Advanced Study, 1930–1950," 3, unpublished manuscript, Archives, Institute for Advanced Study. This is a very valuable manuscript, originally commissioned by Director J. Robert Oppenheimer but never published, that contains interviews and reminiscences from the 1950s of persons no longer alive. I am grateful to Ms. Stern's sister, Flora Dean of Santa Rosa, Calif., for permission to use and quote from the manuscript.

62. Abraham Flexner to Sam Dorfman, 3 January 1944, Abraham Flexner Papers.

63. Abraham Flexner to Julius Rosenwald, 10 May 1930, Julius Rosenwald Papers.

64. Ibid.; *New York Times,* 22 October 1930; *New Republic* 66 (1931):60; Abraham Flexner to Frank Aydelotte, Frank Aydelotte Papers.

65. *New Yorker,* 22 November 1930, 29–32.

CHAPTER II: A LAST HURRAH

1. Abraham Flexner to Simon Flexner, 21 April 1932, Simon Flexner Papers, American Philosophical Society (several of the clauses in the letter have been transposed); Abraham Flexner to Frank Aydelotte, 15 October 1930, Frank Aydelotte Papers, Swarthmore College.

2. Abraham Flexner to Louis D. Brandeis, 22 March 1932, Abraham Flexner Papers; Abraham Flexner to Simon Flexner, 21 April 1932, Simon Flexner Papers.

3. Abraham Flexner to Simon Flexner, 21 April 1932, Simon Flexner Papers.

4. Abraham Flexner to Anne, Jean, and Eleanor Flexner, 11 July 1930, Archive, Institute for Advanced Study, Princeton, N.J.

5. Louis Bamberger to Abraham Flexner, 5 May 1930, Archive, Institute for Advanced Study; Abraham Flexner to Julius Rosenwald, 10 May 1930, Julius Rosenwald Papers, Regenstein Library, University of Chicago.

6. Abraham Flexner, "A Proposal to Establish an American University," [November 1922], 1, Abraham Flexner Papers; Abraham Flexner to Julius Rosenwald, 18 July 1930, Julius Rosenwald Papers.

7. A. Flexner, "A Proposal to Establish an American University," 9; Abraham Flexner to Thomas Jones, 7 January 1932, Thomas Jones Papers, National Library of Wales, Aberystwyth, Wales.

8. Ron Chernow, *Titan: The Life of John D. Rockefeller Sr.* (New York: Random House, 1998), 477.

9. Louis Bamberger and Mrs. Felix Fuld to trustees, 6 June 1930, Archive, Institute for Advanced Study.

10. Quoted in Laura S. Porter, "From Intellectual Sanctuary to Social Responsibility: The Founding of the Institute for Advanced Study, 1930–1933" (Ph.D. diss., Princeton University, 1988), 406. For a good discussion of the social significance of the Princeton site, see 160–68.

11. Abraham Flexner to Bernard and Mary Flexner, 24 June 1931, Abraham Flexner Papers.

12. Beatrice M. Stern, "A History of the Institute for Advanced Study, 1930–1950," MS., 53–54, Archive, Institute for Advanced Study; Porter, "Founding of the Institute for Advanced Study," 123–29. These are both excellent sources on the early history of the institute.

13. Abraham Flexner, *Universities: American, English, German* (New York: Oxford University Press, 1930), 213, 217.

14. Institute for Advanced Study, *Bulletin No. 1: Organization and Purpose* (New York: Institute for Advanced Study, December 1930), 9–11.

15. Simon Flexner to Abraham Flexner, 21 September 1931, Archive, Institute for Advanced Study; Simon Flexner to Abraham Flexner, 2 May 1932, Simon Flexner Papers.

16. Felix Frankfurter to Bernard Flexner, 5 March, 4 November 1931, Bernard Flexner Papers, Mudd Library, Princeton, N.J.; Abraham Flexner to Bernard and Mary Flexner, 24 June 1931, Abraham Flexner Papers.

17. Abraham Flexner to Jean Flexner, 5 April 1931, Abraham Flexner Papers. Letters and notes of his European trip are in the Institute for Advanced Study archive.

18. Abraham Flexner to Simon Flexner, 21 April 1931, Abraham Flexner Papers.

19. Arnold Toynbee to Abraham Flexner, 26 February 1931, Graham Wallas to Abraham Flexner, 8 December 1930, Abraham Flexner Papers.

20. Abraham Flexner to Eleanor Flexner, 22 June 1931, Abraham Flexner Papers; Joseph Schumpeter to Abraham Flexner, 31 May 1931, Archive, Institute for Advanced Study. Emphasis in original.

21. Minutes, board of trustees, Institute for Advanced Study, 8 October 1934, Archive, Institute for Advanced Study.

22. Abraham Flexner to Florence Sabin, 27 February 1935, Florence Sabin Papers, American Philosophical Society.

23. Abraham Flexner to Charles A. Beard, 23 December 1930, Charles A. Beard to Abraham Flexner, 25 December 1930, 15 August 1931, Charles A. Beard Papers, DePauw University, Greencastle, Ind.

24. Charles A. Beard to Abraham Flexner, 22 July 1931, Charles A. Beard Papers.

25. Abraham Flexner to Charles A. Beard, 27 July 1931, Charles A. Beard Papers.

26. Abraham Flexner to Charles A. Beard, 11 August 1931, Charles A. Beard Papers.

27. Charles A. Beard to Abraham Flexner, 15 August 1931, Charles A. Beard Papers.

28. Charles A. Beard to Abraham Flexner, 29 August 1931, Charles A. Beard Papers.

29. Charles A. Beard to Abraham Flexner, 15 August 1931, Charles A. Beard Papers.

30. Charles A. Beard, "Outline of Foundation Document," 29 August 1931, Charles A. Beard Papers.

31. Abraham Flexner to Jacob Flexner, 16 February 1932, Abraham Flexner Papers; "Confidential Memorandum to the Trustees, 28 March 1932," Archive, Institute for Advanced Study.

32. Abraham Flexner to Jean Flexner [Lewinson], 3 February 1932, Abraham Flexner Papers; A. Flexner, *I Remember,* 382.

33. Albert Einstein to Abraham Flexner, 8 June 1932, Albert Einstein Papers, Hebrew University, Jerusalem; A. Flexner, *I Remember,* 384.

34. Loren B. Feffer, "Oswald Veblen and the Capitalization of American Mathematics," *Isis* 89 (1998):489.

35. Stern, "History," 127–28.

36. George D. Birkhoff to Abraham Flexner, 17 March 1931, Archive, Institute for Advanced Study.

37. Oswald Veblen to Abraham Flexner, 19 June 1931, Abraham Flexner to George D. Birkhoff, 29 February 1932, George D. Birkhoff to Abraham Flexner, 7 March 1932, 20 March 1932, Archive, Institute for Advanced Study.

38. Abraham Flexner, "Memorandum Regarding Professor Weyl," 20 August 1932, Archive, Institute for Advanced Study.

39. Abraham Flexner to Oswald Veblen, 2 June 1932, Archive, Institute for Advanced Study.

40. *New York Times,* 11 October 1932; Charles A. Beard to Abraham Flexner, 12 October 1932, Charles A. Beard Papers.

41. Louis Bamberger to Abraham Flexner, 26 August 1932, Archive, Institute for Advanced Study; Felix Frankfurter to Abraham Flexner, 5 November 1932, copy in Bernard Flexner Papers, Mudd Library, Princeton University.

42. Abraham Flexner to Dean Luther P. Eisenhart, 12 November 1932, Archive, Institute for Advanced Study; Stern, "History," 151.

43. Abraham Flexner to Frank Aydelotte, 16 January 1933, Archive, Institute for Advanced Study.

44. Abraham Flexner to Oswald Veblen, 17 March, 27 March 1933, Oswald Veblen Papers, Library of Congress; Stern, "History," 156.

45. Abraham Flexner to Dean Eisenhart, 4 July 1934, Archive, Institute for Advanced Study.

46. *Princeton Alumni Weekly,* 15 February 1935.

47. Oswald Veblen to Frank Aydelotte, 4 August 1973; Minutes, board of trustees, 29 January 1934, 9, Archive, Institute for Advanced Study.

48. Abraham Flexner to Oswald Veblen, 14 September 1934, Oswald Veblen Papers, Library of Congress; Abraham Flexner to Oswald Veblen, 31 July 1933, Archive, Institute for Advanced Study.

49. Abraham Flexner to Oswald Veblen, 25 October 1934, Abraham Flexner Papers; 28 January 1935, Archive, Institute for Advanced Study.

50. Stern, "History," 167–68; Elsa Einstein to Mrs. Oswald Veblen, 21 September 1933, Oswald Veblen Papers.

51. Abraham Flexner to Simon Flexner, 25 September 1933, Simon Flexner Papers; Abraham Flexner to Felix Warburg, 28 September 1933, Felix Warburg to Abraham Flexner, 29 September 1933, Abraham Flexner to Felix Warburg, 2 October 1933, Felix Warburg Papers, American Jewish Archive, Hebrew Union College, Cincinnati.

52. Abraham Flexner to Julian W. Mack, 11 October 1933, Archive, Institute for Advanced Study, emphasis in original; Abraham Flexner to Albert Einstein, 13 October 1933, Albert Einstein Papers.

53. Albert Einstein to Abraham Flexner, 26 March 1933, Albert Einstein Papers.

54. Abraham Flexner to Simon Flexner, 18 October 1933, Simon Flexner Papers; Abraham Flexner to Elsa Einstein, 31 October 1933, Albert Einstein Papers.

55. This account is in a letter from Bernard Flexner to Felix Frankfurter, 6 November 1933, Bernard Flexner Papers, Mudd Library; Marvin McIntyre to Abraham Flexner, 4 November 1933, Archive, Institute for Advanced Study.

56. Abraham Flexner to Albert Einstein, 13 November 1933, Abraham Flexner to Elsa Einstein, 14 November, 15 November 1933, Albert Einstein Papers.

57. Albert Einstein to Abraham Flexner, 30 November 1933; Albert Einstein to members of the Board of Trustees, n.d. [December 1933], Albert Einstein Papers, cited in Porter, "Founding of the Institute for Advanced Study," 419–22. The archivist at the Hebrew University in Jerusalem was unable to find the memorandum in the Einstein Papers.

58. Abraham Flexner to Louis Bamberger, 11 December 1933, Archive, Institute for Advanced Study.

59. Abraham Flexner to Herbert Maass, 19 February 1934, Archive, Institute for Advanced Study.

60. Abraham Flexner to Simon Flexner, 28 May 1934, Simon Flexner Papers.

61. Stern, "History," 176.

62. Abraham Flexner to Florence Sabin, 29 September 1933, Florence Sabin Papers.

63. Minutes, Board of Trustees, 29 January 1934, Archive, Institute for Advanced Study; Abraham Flexner to Raymond B. Fosdick, 5 October 1933, copy in Bernard Flexner Papers, Mudd Library; Abraham Flexner to William Henry Welch, 16 March 1934, William Henry Welch Papers, Alan M. Chesney Archives, Johns Hopkins University.

64. Abraham Flexner to Caroline Fuld, 6 March 1934, Archive, Institute for Advanced Study.

65. The best account of these differences is in Stern, "History," esp. 305–12.

66. Ibid., 66, 99.

67. Draft of Oswald Veblen memo to Abraham Flexner, June 1931, Oswald Veblen Papers.

68. Abraham Flexner to Percy Straus, 22 October 1931, Archive, Institute for Advanced Study.

69. Abraham Flexner to Simon Flexner, 17 March 1931, 4 March 1932, Simon Flexner Papers; Abraham Flexner to Jacob Flexner, 24 March 1932, Abraham Flexner Papers.

70. Abraham Flexner, "The University in American Life," *Atlantic Monthly* 149 (1932): 620–27; Abraham Flexner, "Failings of Our Graduate Schools, "*Atlantic Monthly* 149 (1932):441–52.

71. Abraham Flexner, "Private Fortunes and the Public Future," *Atlantic Monthly* 156 (1935):215–24.

72. *New York Times,* 20 April 1933; Frances Blanshard, *Frank Aydelotte of Swarthmore* (Middletown, Conn.: Wesleyan University Press, 1970), 221; Abraham Flexner to Henry S. Pritchett, 25 October 1935, Carnegie Foundation Files, Butler Library, Columbia University; Anson Phelps Stokes to Abraham Flexner, 29 June 1931, Abraham Flexner Papers; Abraham Flexner–Franklin McLean correspondence, Franklin C. McLean Papers, Regenstein Library, University of Chicago.

73. Jacob Billikopf to Abraham Flexner, 13 April 1932, copy in Bernard Flexner Papers, American Jewish Archives, Hebrew Union College, Cincinnati.

74. Edwin Embree to Abraham Flexner, 28 September 1933, cited in Clifford L. Muse Jr., "An Educational Stepchild: Howard University during the New Deal, 1933–45" (Ph.D. diss., Howard University, 1989), 327; Harold Ickes, *The Secret Diary of Harold Ickes: The First Thousand Days, 1933–1936* (New York: Simon and Schuster, 1953), 47.

75. Kenneth R. Manning, *Black Apollo of Science: The Life of Ernest Everett Just* (New York: Oxford University Press, 1983), 269.

76. Minutes, Board of Trustees, Howard University, 10 June, 13 October 1934, Howard University Archives, Washington, D.C.; Rayford W. Logan, *Howard University: The First Hundred Years, 1867–1967* (New York: New York University Press, 1969), 297.

77. Minutes, Board of Trustees, Howard University, 18 March 1935, Howard University Archives, Washington, D.C.

78. A critical but full account of Flexner's role at Howard is in Muse, "An Educational Stepchild," 317–31; Abraham Flexner to Paul H. Hanus, 4 March 1935, Abraham Flexner Papers.

79. Minutes, Board of Trustees, 8 October 1934, Archive, Institute for Advanced Study.

80. Abraham Flexner to Eleanor Flexner, 21 May 1933, Abraham Flexner Papers.

CHAPTER 12: FINAL BATTLES

1. Jean Flexner Lewinson, "A Family Memoir, 1899–1989," 64, MS. in author's possession.

2. Eleanor Flexner to Thomas Jones, 27 December 1935, 11 November 1937, Thomas Jones Papers, National Library of Wales, Aberystwyth, Wales; Eleanor Flexner, *American Playwrights, 1918–1938: The Theatre Retreats from Reality* (New York: Simon & Schuster, 1938), ix.

3. Stephen Duggan and Betty Drury, *The Rescue of Science and Learning: The Story of the Emergency Committee in Aid of Displaced Foreign Scholars* (New York: Macmillan, 1948), 6–7, 19, 64, 78–79, 200–204. The committee's name was changed from "German" to "Foreign" scholars in 1938.

4. Obituary of Caroline Flexner, *New York Times,* 21 January 1958.

5. Abraham Flexner to Thomas Jones, 12 May 1933, Thomas Jones Papers.

6. Abraham Flexner to John von Neumann, 6 May 1933, John von Neumann Papers, Library of Congress; Abraham Flexner to Thomas Jones, 4 August 1934, Thomas Jones Papers.

7. Laura S. Porter, "From Intellectual Sanctuary to Social Responsibility: The Founding of the Institute for Advanced Study, 1930–1933" (Ph.D. diss., Princeton University, 1988), 434.

8. Abraham Flexner to Jacob Billikopf, 15 January 1935, Simon Flexner to Jacob Billikopf, 26 April 1939, Jacob Billikopf Papers, American Jewish Archives, Hebrew Union College, Cincinnati; Abraham Flexner to Lewis Weed, 21 August, 27 November 1933, Lewis Weed Papers, Alan M. Chesney Archives, Johns Hopkins University.

9. Abraham Flexner to Frank Aydelotte, 10 November 1938, Abraham Flexner to George Birkhoff, 12 September 1938, Abraham Flexner, "National Conference of Jews and Christians [sic]," 28 November 1938, MS., Abraham Flexner Papers, Library of Congress.

10. University College of Wales, *Thomas Jones, C.H., M.A., LL.D., 1870–1955* (Aberystwyth, Wales: University College of Wales, 1955), 1.

11. Abraham Flexner to Thomas Jones, 23 March 1933, 25 May 1936, Thomas Jones Papers.

12. Abraham Flexner to Thomas Jones, 30 July 1936, 19 August 1938, Thomas Jones Papers.

13. Abraham Flexner to Thomas Jones, 5 November 1936, 21 March 1938, Thomas Jones Papers.

14. Abraham Flexner to Thomas Jones, 25 September 1938, Thomas Jones Papers.

15. Abraham Flexner to Thomas Jones, 18 October, 2 November 1932, 6 April, 26 April 1933, 19 February 1934, 29 March 1935, Thomas Jones Papers.

16. Abraham Flexner to Thomas Jones, 2 October 1935, 25 May 1936, Thomas Jones Papers; Abraham Flexner to Henry S. Pritchett, 25 March 1937, Carnegie Foundation Files, Rare Book and Manuscript Library, Butler Library, Columbia University.

17. Abraham Flexner to Thomas Jones, 8 March 1938, Thomas Jones Papers.

18. Abraham Flexner to E.L. Woodward, 31 May 1945, Abraham Flexner Papers.

19. Abraham Flexner to Thomas Jones, 25 May 1936, Thomas Jones Papers.

20. Abraham Flexner to Thomas Jones, 25 April 1939, Thomas Jones Papers; Beatrice M. Stern, "A History of the Institute for Advanced Study, 1930–1950," 379, unpublished manuscript, Archives, Institute for Advanced Study, Princeton, N.J.

21. Porter, "Founding of the Institute for Advanced Study," 370–71.

22. Oswald Veblen and Winfield Riefler to Abraham Flexner, 9 October 1936, in John von Neumann Papers.

23. Abraham Flexner to Thomas Jones, 11 November 1937, Thomas Jones Papers.

24. Felix Frankfurter, untitled remarks to board of trustees, 3 November 1934, copy in Florence Sabin Papers, American Philosophical Society.

25. Stern, "History," 197–217.

26. Abraham Flexner to Warden, All Souls College, 18 January 1935, Archive, Institute for Advanced Study.

27. Stern, "History," 330–33.

28. Felix Frankfurter to Winfield Riefler, 16 January 1935, Archive, Institute for Advanced Study.

29. Abraham Flexner to Felix Frankfurter, 19 January 1935, Archive, Institute for Advanced Study.

30. Lewis Weed to Felix Frankfurter, 29 January 1935, Archive, Institute for Advanced Study; Felix Frankfurter to Oswald Veblen, 6 January 1935, Oswald Veblen Papers, Library of Congress; Frank Aydelotte to Felix Frankfurter, 18 February 1935, Archive, Institute for Advanced Study.

31. Frank Aydelotte to Abraham Flexner, 19 March 1935, Archive, Institute for Advanced Study. Aydelotte was chairman of the board committee on nominations. Here Aydelotte explains to Flexner his conversation with Frankfurter advising him of the committee's unanimous position against his renomination.

32. Stern, "History," 224.

33. Ibid., 233–37.

34. Abraham Flexner to Oswald Veblen, 2 March 1935, Archive, Institute for Advanced Study. The first part of the quotation is transposed from the original.

35. Minutes, board of trustees, 21 April 1934, Archive, Institute for Advanced Study.

36. Flexner and Meritt were lifelong friends. Their correspondence is in the Benjamin D. Meritt Papers at the American Philosophical Society, Philadelphia, and an oral memoir, which credits Flexner with important influence on the Agora project, by Lucy S. Meritt, is in the archives of the University of Texas, Austin. For Panofsky, see Abraham Flexner to Simon Flexner, 12 March 1935, Simon Flexner Papers, American Philosophical Society.

37. Minutes, board of trustees, 22 April 1935, 3–8, Archive, Institute for Advanced Study.

38. Louis Bamberger to Abraham Flexner, 29 October 1935, Archive, Institute for Advanced Study.

39. Stern, "History," 278–82.

40. Ibid., 289.

41. Abraham Flexner to Simon Flexner, 5 August 1937, Simon Flexner Papers.

42. Abraham Flexner to Oswald Veblen, 7 November, 4 December 1936, Oswald Veblen Papers.

43. Minutes, board of trustees, 11 October 1937, Archive, Institute for Advanced Study.

44. Bertrand Russell to Abraham Flexner, 28 December 1936, Archive, Institute for Advanced Study; Abraham Flexner to Simon Flexner, 6 June 1936, Simon Flexner Papers; Herbert Maass to Abraham Flexner, 18 August 1937, Archive, Institute for Advanced Study.

45. Abraham Flexner to Simon Flexner, 3 December, 16 December 1935, Simon Flexner Papers; Abraham Flexner to Sir Thomas Lewis, 2 May 1935, Library, Wellcome Institute for the History of Medicine, London.

46. Abraham Flexner to Frank Aydelotte, 17 October 1937, Archive, Institute for Advanced Study.

47. Abraham Flexner to Henry S. Pritchett, 26 September, 10 October 1935, Henry S. Pritchett Papers, Library of Congress; Abraham Flexner to Hortense Flexner (Jacob's daughter), 8 December 1937, Abraham Flexner Papers.

48. Abraham Flexner to Simon Flexner, 12 June 1936, Simon Flexner Papers; Raymond B. Fosdick to Abraham Flexner, 12 May 1937, Abraham Flexner Papers. Fosdick wrote, "The material which you prepared last summer will be of the greatest assistance."

49. Abraham Flexner to Raymond B. Fosdick, 16 July 1936, Rockefeller Foundation Files, Rockefeller Archive Center, Sleepy Hollow, N.Y.

50. Abraham Flexner, "The Prepared Mind," *School and Society* 45 (1937):865–72.

51. Abraham Flexner, "The Usefulness of Useless Knowledge," *Harper's Magazine* 179 (1939):544–72.

52. Abraham Flexner to Oswald Veblen, 29 January 1938; minutes, budget committee, board of trustees, 7 April 1930, 2, Archive, Institute for Advanced Study.

53. Minutes, board of trustees, 18 April 1938; Abraham Flexner to Louis Bamberger, 4 April 1938; Herbert Maass to Abraham Flexner, 14 June 1938, Archive, Institute for Advanced Study.

54. Stern, "History," 444–45, fn. 43.

55. Ibid., 388–89.

56. Abraham Flexner to Louis Bamberger, 16 July 1938, Archive, Institute for Advanced Study.

57. "Salaries and Pensions: General Policies," 5 November 1938, Archive, Institute for Advanced Study.

58. Abraham Flexner to Oswald Veblen, 1 July 1938, Oswald Veblen Papers.

59. Minutes, board of trustees, 23 January 1939, Archive, Institute for Advanced Study.

60. Minutes, School of Mathematics, 3 February 1939, Archive, Institute for Advanced Study.

61. Interview with James Alexander by Beatrice Stern, cited in Stern, "History," 409.

62. Abraham Flexner to Frank Aydelotte, 15 January 1939, Archive, Institute for Advanced Study; Stern, "History," 382; Frank Aydelotte to Abraham Flexner, [1939], Archive, Institute for Advanced Study.

63. Abraham Flexner to Alanson Houghton, 22 March 1939; Albert Einstein, Hetty Goldman, and Marston Morse to Flexner, 30 March 1939, Archive, Institute for Advanced

Study; Frances Blanshard, ed., *Frank Aydelotte of Swarthmore* (Middletown, Conn.: Wesleyan University Press, 1970), 317.

64. Edward Earle to Frank Aydelotte, 25 June 1939, Edward Meade Earle Papers, Mudd Library, Princeton University; Stern, "History," 421–22. Stern's judgment on this and other matters is based in part on extensive interviews conducted in the 1950s with all the principals involved.

65. Edward Earle to Abraham Flexner, 9 June 1939, Edward Meade Earle Papers; Stern, "History," 423.

66. Edward Earle to Abraham Flexner, 11 August 1931, Archive, Institute for Advanced Study.

67. Edward Earle to Oswald Veblen, 28 June, 13 July, 22 July 1939, Oswald Veblen Papers; Oswald Veblen to Frank Aydelotte, 17 July 1939, Archive, Institute for Advanced Study.

68. Abraham Flexner to Thomas Jones, 8 July 1939, Thomas Jones Papers.

69. Abraham Flexner to Bernard Flexner, 22 July 1939, Abraham Flexner Papers; Abraham Flexner to Simon Flexner, 7 August 1939, Simon Flexner to Abraham Flexner, 23 July 1939, Simon Flexner Papers.

70. Oswald Veblen to Abraham Flexner, 12 August 1939, Oswald Veblen Papers; Edward Earle to Abraham Flexner, 18 October 1939, Archive, Institute for Advanced Study.

71. Erwin Panofsky to Abraham Flexner, 15 October 1939, Hermann Weyl to Abraham Flexner, 16 October 1939, copies of both in Simon Flexner Papers.

72. Oswald Veblen to Albert Einstein, 18 August 1939, Oswald Veblen Papers; Edward Earle to Herbert Maass, 18 June 1939, Edward Meade Earle Papers.

73. Abraham Flexner to Frank Aydelotte, 28 August 1939, Archive, Institute for Advanced Study.

74. Edward Earle to Oswald Veblen, 4 September 1939, Edward Meade Earle Papers.

75. Abraham Flexner to Alanson Houghton, 26 September 1939, Louis Bamberger to Alanson Houghton, 2 October 1939, Archive, Institute for Advanced Study.

76. Minutes, board of trustees, 9 October 1939, Archive, Institute for Advanced Study.

77. "Resolutions Adopted by Board of Trustees and Faculty," [January 1940], Archive, Institute for Advanced Study.

78. *New York Times,* 17 October 1939.

79. "Berlin's Institute for Advanced Study Gives Scholars a Respite from Daily Grind," *Chronicle of Higher Education,* 14 August 1998, A39–40.

80. Abraham Flexner to Thomas Jones, 8 July 1939, Thomas Jones Papers; Simon Flexner to Abraham Flexner, [October 1939], Simon Flexner Papers.

81. Abraham Flexner to Bernard Flexner, 18 February 1940, copy in Simon Flexner Papers.

82. Abraham Flexner to Simon Flexner, 27 November 1939, Simon Flexner Papers.

CHAPTER 13: "I BURN THAT I MAY BE OF USE"

1. *New York Herald-Tribune,* 3 June 1939; Meharry Medical College Endowment Campaign file, Edward L. Tanner Papers, Archives, Meharry Medical College, Nashville.

2. Abraham Flexner to Simon Flexner, 5 November 1935, Simon Flexner Papers, American Philosophical Society.

3. A. Flexner, *I Remember,* 98.

4. Ibid., 405.

5. Simon Flexner to Abraham Flexner, 29 September 1940, Simon Flexner Papers.

6. *New York Times,* 6 October 1940, 4.

7. *Saturday Review of Literature* 22 (1940):41; *Living Age* 104 (1940):154; *Books,* 13 October 1940, 4; *Current Biography,* 1941, 289.

8. Abraham Flexner to Allan Nevins, 1 August 1940, Abraham Flexner Papers.

9. Abraham Flexner, *Henry S. Pritchett: A Biography* (New York: Columbia University Press, 1943), 198; Abraham Flexner, *An Autobiography: A Revision, Brought Up-to-Date, of the Author's* I Remember (New York: Simon & Schuster, 1960), 265.

10. Abraham Flexner to Thomas Jones, 21 April 1944, Thomas Jones Papers, National Library of Wales, Aberystwyth, Wales.

11. Abraham Flexner, *Daniel Coit Gilman: Creator of the American Type of University* (New York: Harcourt, Brace, 1946), 52, 141.

12. A. Flexner, *I Remember,* 52; Abraham Flexner to Florence Sabin, 22 March 1943, Florence Sabin Papers, American Philosophical Society.

13. Abraham Flexner to Thomas Jones, 7 June, 23 August 1940, Thomas Jones Papers.

14. Abraham Flexner to Thomas Jones, 6 November 1939, 6 August, 22 September 1941, Thomas Jones Papers.

15. Abraham Flexner to Thomas Jones, 9 September 1940, 18 February 1941, Thomas Jones Papers.

16. Abraham Flexner to Thomas Jones, 21 December 1940, Thomas Jones Papers.

17. Ibid.

18. Abraham Flexner to Thomas Jones, 1 May 1941, Thomas Jones Papers.

19. Abraham Flexner to Thomas Jones, 12 February, 2 April 1942, Thomas Jones Papers.

20. Abraham Flexner to Thomas Jones, 27 April 1943, Thomas Jones Papers.

21. Abraham Flexner to Benjamin Meritt, 6 May, 8 November, 12 November 1943, Benjamin D. Meritt Papers, American Philosophical Society.

22. Abraham Flexner to Thomas Jones, 27 April 1943, Thomas Jones Papers.

23. Minutes, Board of Directors, Palestine Economic Corporation, 8 May 1945, Abraham Flexner Papers; Abraham Flexner to Esther Bailey, 6 May 1946, Abraham Flexner Papers.

24. Abraham Flexner to Emma Murray Strong, 12 May 1950, Abraham Flexner to Esther Crawford, 19 January 1945, Abraham Flexner Papers; Abraham Flexner to Thomas Jones, 11 March 1947, Thomas Jones Papers.

25. Abraham Flexner to Thomas Jones, 17 June 1947, Thomas Jones Papers; Abraham Flexner to Allan Nevins, 30 August 1953, Allan Nevins Papers, Rare Book and Manuscript Library, Butler Library, Columbia University; Abraham Flexner to Thomas Jones, 11 May 1948, Thomas Jones Papers.

26. Abraham Flexner to Thomas Jones, 19 October 1948, 13 September 1951, Thomas Jones Papers.

27. Allan Nevins, "Introduction," in A. Flexner, *Autobiography,* ix, 279–80.

28. Abraham Flexner to Thomas Jones, 19 May 1949, Thomas Jones Papers; A. Flexner, *Autobiography,* 280–81; Abraham Flexner to Allan Nevins, 15 December 1951, Allan Nevins Papers.

29. A. Flexner, *Autobiography,* 281–85; John Flexner, interview by author, Vanderbilt University, 3 November 1997.

30. Harry Rosenberg, interview by author, Chicago, 22 July 1997. Rosenberg, a Chicago attorney, is the grandson of Abraham's younger sister Gertrude.

31. Abraham Flexner to Thomas Jones, 29 November 1954, Thomas Jones Papers.

32. A. Flexner, *Autobiography,* 275–76.

33. Abraham Flexner, *Funds and Foundations: Their Policies Past and Present* (New York: Harper, 1952), 88.

34. Ibid., 97, 133.

35. Abraham Flexner to Thomas Jones, 19 June 1952, Thomas Jones Papers; Abraham Flexner to Alan T. Waterman, 25 April 1952, Alan T. Waterman to Abraham Flexner, 30 July 1952, Abraham Flexner Papers.

36. Milton Winternitz to Abraham Flexner, 28 June 1952 (I am indebted to Steven Wheatley for making available a copy of his notes on this letter); Alan Gregg to Abraham Flexner, 15 August 1953, Abraham Flexner Papers.

37. Abraham Flexner to Thomas Jones, 14 December 1949, 19 June 1952, Thomas Jones Papers.

38. Abraham Flexner to Thomas Jones, 27 October, 10 December 1952, Thomas Jones Papers.

39. "A Foundation for Humanistic and Related Studies," 2 February 1953, MS., Abraham Flexner Papers; Abraham Flexner to George Sarton, 28 October 1952, George Sarton Papers, Houghton Library, Harvard University.

40. Abraham Flexner to Allan Nevins, 14 February 1957, Allan Nevins Papers.

41. Paul Mellon, *Reflections in a Silver Spoon: A Memoir* (New York: William Morrow, 1992), 347, 408–9.

42. Abraham Flexner to Samuel Leidesdorf, 29 October 1951, Abraham Flexner Papers.

43. John von Neumann to Abraham Flexner, 16 October 1944. Von Neumann thanks him for "all you say about our book" and promises to consult with the other readers Flexner suggested "in the order mentioned"; Benjamin Meritt to Abraham Flexner, 3 October 1949, Benjamin D. Meritt Papers.

44. E.M. Bluestone, "Abraham Flexner," *Jewish Forum,* December 1959, 198; Allan Nevins to Abraham Flexner, 3 July 1948, Abraham Flexner Papers; Abraham Flexner to Allan Nevins, 11 July 1949, Allan Nevins Papers.

45. Allan Nevins, oral memoir, 287–88, Oral History Project, Butler Library, Columbia University.

46. Detlev W. Bronk to Abraham Flexner, 21 April 1949, 16 March 1950, Abraham Flexner Papers. The Welch address can be found in the *Supplement to the Bulletin of the Johns Hopkins Hospital* 87 (1950):39–54.

47. Abraham Flexner to Thomas Jones, 28 October 1948, 23 May, 6 June 1949, Thomas Jones Papers.

48. Abraham Flexner to Thomas Jones, 20 April 1950, Jean Flexner to Thomas Jones, 30 August 1948, Thomas Jones Papers.

49. Abraham Flexner to Thomas Jones, 10 April 1952, 20 July 1954, Thomas Jones Papers; Abraham Flexner to Allan Nevins, 16 July 1953, 5 August 1955, 26 August 1956, Allan Nevins Papers.

50. Bernard Berenson to Abraham Flexner, 20 June 1954, Abraham Flexner Papers; Abraham Flexner to Thomas Jones, 20 April 1950, Thomas Jones Papers.

51. Abraham Flexner to Gilbert Highet, 5 August 1950, Gilbert Highet Papers, Rare Book and Manuscript Library, Butler Library.

52. Abraham Flexner to Thomas Jones, 1 February 1955, Thomas Jones Papers.

53. Abraham Flexner to Mrs. Peter Atherton, 8 January 1955, 22 May 1956, Abraham Flexner Papers.

54. Notes of Beatrice Stern, 23 October 1955, Archive, Institute for Advanced Study.

55. "Abraham Flexner: A Tribute," program of the National Fund for Medical Education," [1956], Abraham Flexner Papers.

56. *New York Times Magazine,* 11 November 1956, 50; *New York Times,* 13 November 1956.

57. Jean Flexner Lewinson, "A Family Memoir, 1899–1989," 83–84, MS. in author's possession.

58. Abraham Flexner to Cornelia Atherton, 8 January 1958, Abraham Flexner Papers; Lewinson, "Family Memoir," 84.

59. John W. Gardner, "Abraham Flexner, Pioneer in Educational Reform," *Science* 131 (1960):594–95; Clipping from *Washington Post,* [September 1959], Rockefeller Archive Center; *New York Times,* 22 September 1959; *Cleveland Plain Dealer,* 22 September 1959; *Oswego Palladium Times,* 23 September 1959; *Lancet,* 10 October 1959.

60. Abraham Flexner, *Medical Education in Europe,* Bulletin no. 6 (New York: Carnegie Foundation for the Achievement of Teaching, 1912) 299, 302; Ronald L. Numbers, *Almost Persuaded: American Physicians and Compulsory Health Insurance* (Baltimore: Johns Hopkins University Press, 1978), 68; Arthur J. Viseltear, "Compulsory Health Insurance and the Definition of Public Health," in *Compulsory Health Insurance: The Continuing American Debate,* ed. Ronald L. Numbers (Westport, Conn.: Greenwood Press, 1982), 36.

61. Diane Ravitch, *Left Back: A Century of Failed School Reforms* (New York: Simon & Schuster, 2000), 451.

A Note on Sources

The archival materials for a life of Abraham Flexner are spread widely across the United States and abroad. Flexner himself was not an avid collector, and there are gaps in his own papers. His letters to his wife, Anne, have been preserved, apparently by her, but little remains of her correspondence with him. He was much more interested in saving papers illustrating his official actions than those reflecting his own private views.

Fortunately, several of his correspondents preserved hundreds of his personal letters, and these are the best source of his views on passing events. The largest collections of these letters are in his brother Simon's papers and in his correspondence with his good friend the Welsh political figure Thomas Jones. Other personal letters are in the papers of Flexner's brother Bernard, Harvard president Charles W. Eliot, Chicago philanthropist Julius Rosenwald, historian Allan Nevins, and others.

The records of his work at the Carnegie Foundation for the Advancement of Teaching (1908–12) were preserved at the Carnegie Corporation until about 1990, when they were transferred to the Butler Library of Columbia University. At that time some of these important records were misplaced, and despite the best efforts of President Lee Shulman of the Carnegie Foundation for the Advancement of Teaching and officials at Columbia University, the records have not been located. Fortunately, I have had the assistance of Steven Wheatley and Kenneth Lindmerer, who used the materials before the transfer.

Flexner's years at the General Education Board (1912–28) are carefully documented at the very efficient Rockefeller Archive Center in Sleepy Hollow, N.Y. Not only are full records of his activities and correspondence at the board preserved, but Flexner materials are found in the files of the Office of the Messrs. Rockefeller and the Rockefeller Foundation, personal diaries of officials, and other collections.

His service as founding director of the Institute for Advanced Study (1930–39) is well covered in the archives of this institute. Especially helpful is a manuscript by Beatrice M. Stern, "A History of the Institute for Advanced Study, 1930–1950," commissioned by director J. Robert Oppenheimer in the 1950s but never published. She was able to interview almost all of the important figures of the Flexner period.

I was fortunate to be able to interview Flexner's daughter Jean, who was alert and helpful at age 97. She provided me with a family memoir, some personal letters and photographs, and even her parents' marriage certificate. Several other members of the family also offered assistance, especially Miriam Maderer, Flexner's niece, Harry Rosenberg of Chicago, who has accumulated a great deal of information about the family, and Professor John Flexner of the Vanderbilt University School of Medicine, who has brought together an Abraham Flexner Collection at the university.

353

LOCATION OF ARCHIVES

Aberystwyth (Wales)
   Thomas Jones Papers
Baltimore
   Johns Hopkins University, Alan M. Chesney Archives
      John J. Abel Papers
      Lewellys Barker Papers
      Thomas Cullen Papers
      William H. Halsted Papers
      Lewis Weed Papers
      William Henry Welch Papers
   Johns Hopkins University, Ferdinand Hamburger Archives
      File of Abraham Flexner, 1884–86
Boston
   Francis A. Countway Library
      Henry Christian Papers
      Deans' Office Papers
      David Edsall Papers
      Frederick Gates Papers
Cambridge
   Harvard University Archives
      Charles W. Eliot Papers
      A. Lawrence Lowell Papers
   Arthur and Elizabeth Schlesinger Library
      Eleanor Flexner Papers
Chicago
   American Medical Association Archives
      American Medical Association Proceedings, 1904–19
      Council on Medical Education, Minutes, 1907–17
      Council on Medical Education, Reports, 1904–12
   University of Chicago, Joseph Regenstein Library
      William Rainey Harper Papers
      Henry Pratt Judson Papers
      Franklin C. McLean Papers
      Presidents' Papers, 1898–1925
      Julius Rosenwald Papers
   Rush Medical Center, Archives and Records
      Arthur Dean Bevan Papers
Cincinnati
   Hebrew Union College, American Jewish Archives
      Jacob Billikopf Papers
      Bernard Flexner Papers, 1930–44
      Morris Jastrow Papers
      Nearprint File

> Adolphe Moses
> Abraham Flexner
> Felix Warburg Papers

Cleveland
> Case Western Reserve University
> > Charles Thwing Papers

Jerusalem
> Hebrew University, Jewish National and University Library
> > Albert Einstein Papers

London
> Wellcome Institute for the History of Medicine
> > Lord Haldane Papers
> > Thomas Lewis Papers
> > Sir William McCormick Papers

Louisville
> Filson Club
> > Barry Bingham Papers
> > Jewish Community Center Records
> Louisville Free Public Library
> > Scrapbooks on Louisville Schools
> > Works Progress Administration, Kentucky Writers Project, "Biographical and Critical Materials Pertaining to Kentucky Authors," mimeographed, 1941
> University of Louisville, Ekstrom Library
> > Brandeis Papers
> > Hortense Flexner King Papers
> University of Louisville, Kornhauser Health Sciences Library
> > Morris Flexner Papers

Montreal
> William Osler Papers (File on "Whole-time Clinical Professors")

Nashville
> Meharry Medical College
> > Deans' Office Papers
> > Edward L. Burner Papers
> Vanderbilt University, Eskind Medical Library
> > Abraham Flexner Collection
> Vanderbilt University, Heard Library
> > James H. Kirkland Papers

New York
> Columbia University, Butler Library, Rare Book and Manuscript Library
> > Minutes of Meetings of the Trustees, Carnegie Foundation for the Advancement of Teaching, and of the Executive Committee, 1909–15 (some files are missing)
> > Allan Nevins Papers
> Columbia University, Oral History Research Office
> > Abraham Flexner
> > Alan Gregg

William Henry Harvey
Allan Nevins
Flora Rhind
Oxford
Rhodes House
Trustee Archives
Philadelphia
American Philosophical Society
Rufus Cole Papers
Simon Flexner Papers
Benjamin D. Meritt Papers
Florence Sabin Papers
College of Physicians
Miscellaneous Flexner Letters
Swarthmore College Archives
Frank Aydelotte Papers
Princeton
Institute for Advanced Study
General File, 1930–39
Princeton University, Seeley G. Mudd Manuscript Library
Edward Meade Earle Papers
Bernard Flexner Papers
Raymond B. Fosdick Papers
Rochester
George Eastman House
George Eastman Papers
University of Rochester, Edward G. Miner Library
George H. Whipple Papers
University of Rochester, Rush Rhees Library
Rush Rhees Papers
St. Louis
Washington University, Bernard Becker Medical Library
Deans' Office Files
Marjorie Fox Grisham Papers
Phillip A. Shaffer Papers
Sleepy Hollow, N.Y.
Rockefeller Archive Center
Frederick T. Gates Papers
General Education Board Files
International Education Board Files
Office of the Messrs. Rockefeller General Files
Rockefeller Foundation Files
Washington, D.C.
Howard University, Moorland-Spingarn Research Center
Minutes, Board of Trustees, 1930–35

Presidents' Office Papers
Library of Congress, Manuscript Division
  Bollingen Foundation Papers
  Abraham Flexner Papers
  John von Neumann Papers
  Henry S. Pritchett Papers
  Oswald Veblen Papers
National Library of Medicine
  Alan Gregg Papers and Oral Memoir
  A. Baird Hastings Oral Memoir

DISSERTATIONS AND THESES

Cangi, Ellen C. "Principles before Practice: The Reform of Medical Education before and after the Flexner Report." Ph.D. diss., University of Cincinnati, 1983.

Carson, William H., Jr. "Medical Education Reform in America, 1868–1928: A Study of Abraham Flexner and His Direct Effect on the Reform of Medical Education for Blacks." Honors thesis, Harvard University, 1980.

Flicker, Bernard. "Abraham Flexner's Educational Thought and Its Critical Appraisal." Ph.D. diss., New York University, 1963.

Macleish, Marlene Y. "Medical Education in Black Colleges and Universities in the United States of America: An Analysis of the Emergence of Black Medical Schools." Ed.D. diss., Harvard University, 1978.

Movrich, Ronald F. "Before the Gates of Excellence: Abraham Flexner and Education, 1866–1918." Ph.D. diss., University of California, Berkeley, 1981.

Muse, Clifford L. "An Educational Stepchild: Howard University during the New Deal, 1933–1945." Ph.D. diss., Howard University, 1989.

Porter, Laura S. "From Intellectual Sanctuary to Social Responsibility: The Founding of the Institute for Advanced Study, 1930–1933." Ph.D. diss., Princeton University, 1988.

Steele, Ruth W. "Origin and History of the Medical Department of Washington University, 1891–1914." M.A. thesis, Washington University, 1944.

Yee, John D. "The Worship of Excellence: A Biography of Abraham Flexner." Honors thesis, Harvard University, 1986.

SECONDARY LITERATURE

The published materials used in this study are found in the endnotes.

The Published Writings of Abraham Flexner

Abraham Flexner: An Autobiography: A Revision, Brought Up-to-Date, of the Author's I Remember. Introduction by Allan Nevins. New York: Simon and Schuster, 1960.

"Adjusting the College to American Life." *Science* 29 (1909):361–72.

"Adventures in Money-Raising." *Harper's Magazine* 8 (1940):249–58.

The American College: A Criticism. New York: Century, 1908. Reprinted by Arno Press and the *New York Times,* 1969.

"Aristocratic and Democratic Education." *Atlantic Monthly* 108 (1911):386–95.

"Battleships and Higher Education." *New York Times,* 25 December 1927.

The Burden of Humanism. The Taylorian Lecture 1928. Oxford: Clarendon Press, 1928.

"Civilization Must Fling Down the Gauntlet." *Journal of Social Hygiene* 22 (1936): 419–20.

"College Entrance Examinations." *Popular Science Monthly* 63 (1903):53–60.

"The College President." *Association of American Colleges Bulletin* 26 (1940):587–89.

Daniel Coit Gilman: Creator of the American Type of University. New York: Harcourt, Brace, 1946.

Do Americans Really Value Education? The Inglis Lecture 1927. Cambridge: Harvard University Press, 1927.

"Education and Mental Discipline." *Atlantic Monthly* 119 (1917):452–64.

"The English Side of Medical Education." *Atlantic Monthly* 116 (1915):529–39.

"Failings of Our Graduate Schools." *Atlantic Monthly* 149 (1932):441–52.

"Fewer and Better Doctors: A Plan for the Reconstruction of American Medical Education." *American Review of Reviews* 42 (1910):203–10.

"A Freshman at Nineteen." *Educational Review* 18 (1899):353–62.

Funds and Foundations: Their Policies Past and Present. New York: Harper, 1952.

(With Frank P. Bachman) *The Gary Schools.* New York: General Education Board, 1918.

"Gates of Excellence." *Journal of Adult Education* 4 (1932):5–7.

The General Education Board: An Account of Its Activities, 1902–1914. New York: General Education Board, 1915.

"The German Side of Medical Education." *Atlantic Monthly* 112 (1913):654–62.

Henry S. Pritchett: A Biography. New York: Columbia University Press, 1943.

I Remember: The Autobiography of Abraham Flexner. New York: Simon and Schuster, 1940.

Is Social Work a Profession? New York: New York School of Philanthropy, 1915. Also in *Proceedings of the National Conference of Charities and Corrections* 42 (1915):576–90.

"A Layman's View of Osteopathy." *JAMA* 62 (1914):1831–33.

"Louis Bamberger and Mrs. Felix Fuld." *American Jewish Historical Society Quarterly* 37 (1947):455–57.

"Matthew Arnold's Poetry from an Ethical Stand-Point." *International Journal of Ethics* 5 (1895):206–18.

"Medical Colleges: The Duty of the State to Suppress Bad Ones and to Support Good Ones." *World's Work* 21 (1911):14238–42.

Medical Education: A Comparative Study. New York: Macmillan, 1925.

"Medical Education, 1909–1924." *Educational Record,* April 1924, 3–19.

"Medical Education in America." *Atlantic Monthly* 105 (1910):797–804.

Medical Education in Europe. Bulletin no. 6. New York: Carnegie Foundation for the Advancement of Teaching, 1912.

Medical Education in the United States and Canada. Bulletin no. 4. New York: Carnegie Foundation for the Advancement of Teaching, 1910.

"Medical Education in the United States and Canada." *Science* 32 (1910):41–50.

A Modern College and a Modern School. Garden City, N.Y.: Doubleday, 1923.

A Modern School. New York: General Education Board, 1916.

"A Modern School." *American Review of Reviews* 53 (1916):465–74.

"Modern University." *Atlantic Monthly* 136 (1925):530–41.

"Most Adult Education Is Mere Training," *School Topics* 14 (1922):3.

The *Nation.* Letters and Short Communications. 43 (1888):149, 249–50, 312–13, 395, 476; 49 (1899):410; 50 (1890):412–13; 51 (1891):11, 292–93; 56 (1893):158; 57 (1895):171–72.

"Parents and Schools." *Atlantic Monthly* 118 (1916):25–33.

"The Plethora of Doctors." *Atlantic Monthly* 106 (1910):20–25.

"The Preparatory School." *Atlantic Monthly* 94 (1904):368–77.

"The Prepared Mind." *School and Society* 45 (1937):865–72.

"Private Fortunes and the Public Future." *Atlantic Monthly* 156 (1935):215–24.

"The Problem of College Pedagogy." *Atlantic Monthly* 103 (1909):839–44.

Prostitution in Europe. New York: Century, 1914.

Public Education in Delaware. New York: General Education Board, 1919.

Public Education in Maryland. 2nd ed. New York: General Education Board, 1916.

"Purpose in the American College." *School and Society* 22 (1925):729–36.

"The Religious Training of Children." *International Journal of Ethics* 7 (1897):314–28.

"Symposium on the Outlook for Higher Education in the United States: Address by Abraham Flexner." *Proceedings of the American Philosophical Society* 69 (1930):257–69.

"The Ultimate Importance of the Kindergarten Idea." *Kindergarten* 3 (1889):199–201.

"The University in American Life." *Atlantic Monthly* 149 (1932):620–27.

"University Patents." *Science* 77 (1933):325.

Universities: American, English, German. New York: Oxford University Press, 1930.

"Upbuilding American Education: The National Work of the General Education Board," *Independent,* 9 August 1915, 188–91.

"The Usefulness of 'Useless' Knowledge." *Harper's Magazine* 179 (1939):544–72.

"William Henry Welch." *Bulletin of the History of Medicine* 87 (suppl.) (1950):39–54.

Acknowledgments

My debts for this book begin with Alan Raucher, a colleague in history, who persuaded me to undertake it rather than other projects I had in mind. Sherwin Nuland was the first to read parts of the manuscript and to encourage me to see Flexner as a more human, sympathetic figure. From my agent, Donald Lamm, I received numerous excellent suggestions for improving the manuscript.

Invaluable financial help, which enabled me to visit scores of archives and libraries and to travel abroad in search of Flexner materials, came from a multiyear grant from the National Library of Medicine. Additional help came from the research assistance program at Wayne State University and from the Director's Discretionary Fund at the Rockefeller Archive Center.

It would be impossible to list the many archivists and librarians whose assistance made this book possible. To each of them I send my heartfelt thanks.

A number of colleagues were kind enough to read the manuscript and to offer critical suggestions. I am deeply appreciative of their efforts. In alphabetical order, they are John Burnham, Daniel Fox, Roger Geiger, Hugh Hawkins, Kenneth Ludmerer, Eliot Shore, and Darwin Stapleton. I appreciate, too, the helpful suggestions of the reviewer for the Johns Hopkins University Press.

Of all those who read the manuscript, none read more carefully, suggested more changes, or raised more questions than Jacqueline Wehmueller, executive editor at the Johns Hopkins University Press.

Members of the Flexner family were uniformly helpful in providing information, documents, and photographs. Jean Flexner, one of Abraham's daughters, gave me a wonderful day shortly before her death. Harry Rosenberg, a grand-nephew, was a rich source of information about the Flexner family and provided some photographs. Abraham Flexner's niece, Miriam Maderer, answered dozens of questions and drew on her memories of "Uncle Abe." Finally, Dr. John Flexner, a grandson of Abraham's oldest brother, introduced me to the collection of Abraham Flexner materials that he has assembled at Vanderbilt University.

In the city of Louisville, Leo Loeb and Dr. Saleem Seyal, both students of Abraham Flexner's life, have shared information and undertaken important tasks on my behalf.

I was blessed to have two able research assistants, Mark J. McCreary of Wayne State University and Farshad Marvasti of Arizona State University. Their labors made easier the tasks of finding and organizing printed materials.

The typing of the manuscript was begun by my longtime friend and assistant, Annette Riley, who tragically succumbed to cancer about halfway through the manuscript. It was ably completed by Alison Landor.

Finally, this book would never have seen the light of day without the encouragement, love, and devotion of my remarkable wife, Sylvia.

Index

Aberhalden, Emil, 182
Abraham, Caroline (aunt), 3, 5, 6, 11
Adams, Herbert Baxter, 23
Adams, W.G.S., 242
Adenauer, Konrad, 221
Adler, Cyrus, 21
African Americans: conditions in
    Louisville, 9; education of, xv–xvi,
    117–19, 192; medical education of, 71,
    87, 162, 188–93; Rosenwald fellow-
    ships, 190–91; slow pace of change
    for, 119
Agora project, 201
Albany Medical College, 147
Alexander, James W., 250, 253, 283
All Souls College, Oxford, as model, 242,
    244
All Soul's Eve (drama), 175
American College, The (Flexner), xiv, 61,
    63–66
American Medical Association (AMA):
    and Bevan, xvii; Council on Medical
    Education, 73–75, 76, 106, 184, 188,
    189; and Flexner report, 67, 68; Flex-
    ner's attitude toward, 77; intimidation
    by, 188; medical school admission
    requirements, 151; southern medical
    school standards, 150; in survey of
    medicine, 224
American School of Classical Studies, 201
ancient Greek civilization, 200–201
anti-foreign sentiment, 266
antilynching laws, 9
anti-Semitism: and Flexner, 10–11, 141,
    221, 284, 295; at Princeton, 239, 255,

268, 283; against refugees, 265; rising
    in U.S., 283
archaeology, 200–201, 274
Arnett, Trevor, 173, 209, 210, 222, 240
Art of Teaching, The (Highet), 303–4
Atherton, John, 49
Austrian medical education, 97, 184
Aydelotte, Frank, 198; on anti-Semitism,
    283; on education, 195; and Flexner,
    240, 285; at Institute for Advanced
    Study, 239, 268–69, 283, 285–86, 287;
    at Lake Ahmic, 176; and Oxford:
    —American Studies program at, 219;
    —lectures, 215, 217; in salary contro-
    versy, 271; and teacher loyalty oath,
    277; and Veblen, 301–2

Bachman, Frank P., 123–24, 125, 129
Bailey, Esther S., 142, 296, 297, 298–99
Balfour Declaration, 179
Baltimore, 22–23, 25
Bamberger, Louis, 237; and Aydelotte,
    285; dislike of controversy, 275;
    financial problems of, 240; and
    Flexner, 239, 250, 262; in Institute for
    Advanced Study, management, 238,
    257–58, 269, 286; no-hire agreement
    with Princeton, 251; philanthropy
    of, 233–34, 257, 273, 275, 280, 281;
    reluctance to commit more money,
    270, 282; skepticism about economics
    studies, 269
Barker, Lewellys, 102, 105, 147
Barnes Hospital, 148
Barrett, John, 299

Barzun, Jacques, xiv

Baylor University, 161–62

Beard, Charles A., xvii, 232, 242, 244–46, 258, 279, 281

Beard, Mary, 244

Beit, Otto, 216

Benison, Saul, 32

Berchtesgaden, 91

Berenson, Bernard, 303

Berlin, 59–61

Bernard, Claude, 200

Bevan, Arthur Dean: on Canadian medical schools, 77; on contemporary medical instruction, 73; and Flexner, xvii, 150–51, 156, 236, 290; and full-time principle, 106, 157–58

Beveridge, William, xvi, 242

Billikopf, Jacob, 261

Billings, Frank, 71–72, 157

Billroth, Theodor, 76, 200

Birkhoff, George D., 248, 266

Blaine, James B., 30

Bluestone, E.M., 234

Boas, Franz, 11

Bohr, Niels, 181, 266

Booth, Edwin, 25

Borden, Robert, 215

Born, Max, 182

Bourne, Randolph, 126, 129

Bowers, Claude, 298

Boyd, William R., 168, 169, 299

Bragg, Braxton, 6

Brandeis, Louis D., 15, 179, 236, 244

Breasted, James H., 200

Brigham Hospital, 152–53, 154

Broadus, John A., 15

Brödel, Max, 176

Brookings, Robert, xvii, 80, 147–48, 149, 177, 202, 214, 240

Brookings Institution, 202, 219

Brookings School, 177

Bryce, James, 31

Bryn Mawr College, 35, 176–77, 278–79

Bureau of Social Hygiene, 107, 112

Burton, Ernest D., 197

Butler, Nicholas Murray: and Columbia reorganization, 158; and Flexner, xvii, 65, 66, 67, 156, 159, 230, 236, 302; on Flexner report, 69

Butlin, Henry, 92–93

Buttrick, Wallace, 116; and archaeological proposal, 200; and Chicago medical school, 156; departure of, 173, 174, 181; and Flexner, 113, 114, 122, 123, 140, 172, 180, 291; and Flexner report, 69; and full-time principle, 152, 155; and Gary plan, 127, 128; and Iowa City school project, 169; and Rochester school, 166; southern schools tour, 117; and teaching in America, 131; and Vanderbilt, 163

Caldwell, Otis W., 134

California Institute of Technology (Caltech), 246–47, 256

California Medical College, 79

Calkins, Mary, 58

Cambridge, Massachusetts, 56

Cambridge University, 176–77

Campbell, Oscar, 297

Campbell, W.A., 274

Campobello Island, 62

Canadian medical schools, 77

Capps, Edward C., 198, 239

Carman, Harry, 298

Carnegie, Andrew, xvii, 73, 88, 113, 163

Carnegie Foundation for the Advancement of Teaching: assignments from, 81; and Cincinnati, 165; evolution of leadership, 173; and Flexner, 63, 66–68, 113; grants from, 144; and new medical standards, 73; philanthropy of, 87; Presbyterian Hospital grant, 158; responsible for high standards in education, 116; tax-supported school policy, 169; and Vanderbilt, 164

Carothers, R.H., 16

Carrel, Alexis, 96, 225, 239

Century of Struggle (E. Flexner), 307
Chamberlain, Neville, 267
Chapman, Carleton B., 89
character education, 195
Christian, Henry, 151, 153
Churchill, Winston, 201, 216
Civil War, 6, 8–9
classics studies: difficulty of learning, 37; and Flexner, 21–22, 28–29; as outmoded, 38, 133; replacement by modern language studies, 133; for women, 119
Clay, Henry, 242, 280–81
Clemenceau, Georges, 215
Cleveland, Grover, 15, 30
clinical teaching: and commercial incentives, 103, 145; criticism of, 101; in England, 93–94; in Flexner plan, 94; full-time plan (*see* full-time teaching principle); in Germany, 97; and Harvard Medical School, 151–56; at Johns Hopkins, 101–3, 104–6; and profit motive, 103
Cobb, Stanley, 193
Coffman, L.D., 232
Cohen, Abraham, 62
Cohen, Wilbur, xvi
Cohn, Alfred, 214, 240
college admissions standards, 38, 71–72, 85–86, 195
college libraries survey, 122
College of Eclectic Medicine and Surgery, Georgia, 79
Columbia University: Flexner as mature student, 297–98; grants to, 146; humanities at, 199; modern medical school creation at, 156, 158–59; oral history archive, 302; Teachers College, 134
Colwell, Nathan P., 75, 77, 189
commercial impulse, in medicine, 103
Commonwealth Fund, 146
Communism, 183, 261, 264
Compton, Arthur, 219
Conant, James, 276

Cook County Hospital, 79–80
Cornell University, 165, 171
Councilman, William T., 75, 152
Council on Medical Education, AMA, 73–75, 76, 106, 184, 188, 189
Courant, Richard, 266
Crawford, Anne, xvi, 49, 51–52. *See also* Flexner, Anne (wife)
Crawford, William H., 49
Cremin, Lawrence, xviii
Croce, Benedetto, 215
Cubberly, Ellwood P., 127
Cullen, Thomas, 176
curriculum: in college-controlled secondary schools, 64, 138–39; in Germany, 97; lack of imagination in, 115; need for change in America, 99; rigid, 42–43, 61, 188; science in, 73, 131; standardization of, 188
Cushing, Harvey, 80–81, 104, 148, 151, 153, 154

Dabney, Charles W., xv, 80, 164–65
Darwin, Charles, 10, 13
Dembitz, Louis N., 15
democracy, 185, 195, 295
Dewey, John: Beard on, 245; on education, 61; and Flexner, xvii, 41–42, 232–33; on Gary school plan, 126; at Johns Hopkins, 23; Laboratory School of, xii, 41; and Wirt, 125
Dock, George, 148
Dramatists Guild, 120, 175
Dulles, John Foster, 303
Durac, Paul, 263

Earle, Edward Meade, 244, 270, 271–72, 282, 284–85, 286, 289, 290
Eastman, George, xiii, xvii, 166, 167, 190, 214, 218–19
Eaton, Harlow W., 16
eclectic medicine, 71
economic depression, 43–44, 45, 264, 268, 278, 282
economics studies, 244, 245–46, 252

Edsall, David: and Flexner, 206; and full-
time principle, 153, 160; at Harvard,
151, 154, 160, 171; matching gifts
request of, 223; and medical education
survey, 224; on Rosenwald fellowship
committee, 190; at Washington
University, 81, 148
education: of African Americans, xv–xvi,
9, 117–19, 192; classroom discipline, 28,
39–40; college as indiscriminate study,
64; criticism of —in American universities, xv; —in Oxford lectures, 217–18;
—in *The American College,* 63–66;
Dewey Laboratory School, xii, 41;
disciplinary theory of learning, 138;
equality for women, 119–20; father as
disciplinarian, 7; German university
ideal, 21, 60–61; government role in,
260; higher education direction and
purpose, 194, 195–96; individually
tailored, 187; inductive teaching, 186;
intellectual inquiry *vs.* job training,
228; kindergarten concept, 29–30;
learning theories, 41; Lincoln School
influences, xii, 135; literature of, 29,
57; meritocratic learning, 115, 229; pace
of learning, 38; private aid to tax-
supported schools, 168, 169, 170;
progressive education movement, 42,
135, 229; public attitudes toward,
195; secondary schools, 194–95; segregated schools, 125; as social process,
41; southern states surveys, 123–25;
specialization of, 278; teacher qualifications, 29, 132; teaching effectiveness
study, 131; theory *vs.* learning, 227. *See
also* medical education
education reform: active teaching
methods, 38; Eliot and, 38, 58; Flexner
on, 114–15; independent of politics,
42; questions of, xi–xii; science in
curriculum, 73, 131
Ehrlich, Paul, 266
Einstein, Albert: arrival in U.S., 253;
at Caltech, 246; for faculty self-

governance, 283; and Flexner, xi, xvii,
247, 249–50, 253–54, 255–56, 257, 284,
285, 289, 290; inscribed photo of, 298;
at Institute for Advanced Study, 248,
251; —absence at opening of, 252; —as
his choice, 276; Oxford lectureship
offered to, 215; as political symbol, 254–
55; on Princeton, 239; salary of, 281
Einstein, Elsa, 253, 254
Eischseler, Marie, 297, 298–99, 306
Eisenhart, Luther, 250, 251
Eisenhower, Dwight D., 302, 303, 305
elective system, 81
Eliot, Charles W.: and Flexner, 38–39, 51,
61, 67, 123, 277, 279; on Flexner
report, 88, 89; and full-time principle,
146, 151, 153–54, 155; and Gary school
plan, 127; as Harvard president, 58; on
Lincoln School, 135; on medical
schools, 73; retirement as Rockefeller
board member, 173; and teaching in
America, 131–32
Ely, Richard T., 23
Embree, Edwin, 173–74, 222, 261
Emory University, 161, 162
England: education in, 59, 63; medical
education in, 92–96, 184, 185; Oxford
life, 216
Erlanger, Joseph, 148
Europe: First World War, 115–16, 137, 179,
182, 183, 244; influences on Institute
for Advanced Study, 241–43; medical
education study, 184–88, 292; politics
in, 183; prostitution report, 107–12;
refugees from Nazism, 248, 264–66,
276; Second World War, 229, 268,
294–96
European medical report, 91–92; Austria,
97; English medicine, 92–96; France,
96–97; Germany, 97–98; reactions to,
99–100; success of, 98; writing of, 99
European universities, 63

Faculté de Médicine, 96
Farrand, Max, 244

Fascism, 183, 264, 267

Fermi, Enrico, 181, 266

Fine, Benjamin, 306

Finney, J.M.T., 104

First World War, 115–16, 137, 179, 182, 183, 244

Fisher, H.A.L., 217, 242

Fiske, Harrison Gray, 52

Fiske, Minnie Maddern, 52–53

Flexner, Abraham, 42–43, 64, 65, 115, 137, 139, 183, 227, 229, 279, 295; activism, 3, 225; articles on education, 29–31, 41, 138, 146, 259–60, 276–77, 292; autobiography, 290–92; awards and tributes to, 305–9; birth, xvi, 8; childhood, 9, 11–14, 14–15; children's births, xvi, 52, 62; death, 307; engagement to marry, 48–50; financial responsibilities, 34–36, 44, 46, 48, 51, 122; health, 141–42, 180, 288, 289, 305; higher education, 18, 21–22, 24, 54, 55–58, 298; honorary degrees, 220, 302, 305; influence of Royce, 57; Jewish heritage, xvi, 2, 10–11, 221, 254; and Louisville, 27, 54, 55; love letters, 121; marital discord, 175, 209; marriage, xvi, 51–52; and music, 298; and opera, 298; parents, 1–8, 11–12, 13, 18, 27, 33; physical appearance, 18–19, 48, 180; politics, 236–37, 302–3; primary education, 7, 14, 16–17; prosperity, 43–44; on racial issues, 224–25, 295; on radio and television, 299; reading preferences, 14–15, 16, 221, 277, 298; removal from General Education Board, 209, 210–12, 213; retirement from Institute of Advanced Study, xi, 284, 285–87; salaries of, 38, 113, 117, 210; separations from wife, 62, 90, 107–8, 111, 263; study abroad, 58–61; as teacher, 27–29, 31, 39–40; traits, 25–26, 44, 75, 81, 89, 140–41, 180–81, 208; vacations, 82, 91, 176, 218, 263, 298–99, 306; at work in youth, 15

Flexner, Anne (wife): death, 304–5; health, 120–21, 289; marital discord, 175, 209; mental deterioration, 296–97; as playwright, 52–54, 62, 120, 175; separations from husband, 62, 90, 107–8, 111, 263; social graces, 57–58, 59, 257; success of, 175–76, 291; support for husband, 215; at Tyringham Valley house, 82

Flexner, Bernard (brother): birth, 6; bookstore business of, 35; consultation with Flexner, 210, 240, 241, 246, 285; death, 296; in economic depression, 43–44; and Einstein, 253; establishment of Abraham Flexner Lectureship, 164; on Flexner's departure from General Education Board, 218; helped by brother Jacob, 18; law career of, 46, 164; as paterfamilias, 122; refugee placement, 264–65; at work in youth, 12, 27; as Zionist, 179

Flexner, Caroline (niece), 265

Flexner, Eleanor (daughter), 177; abroad, 91; birth, 62; *Century of Struggle*, 307; closeness to father, 52, 120; education, 177–78; family discord, 175; liberal views of, 277; in Lincoln School, 136; in New York, 263; political activism, 264; separation from father, 90, 107–8; at Tyringham Valley house, 82; visits to mother, 296–97

Flexner, Esther Abraham (mother), 1–3, 4–7, 27, 33

Flexner, Gertrude (sister), 8, 35, 37, 40, 46

Flexner, Henry (brother), 6, 12, 18, 27, 46, 122

Flexner, Isadore (brother), 6, 12, 18, 27, 43, 46, 263

Flexner, Jacob (brother): birth, 6; bluster of, 46; college education, 45–46; death, 263; drugstore business of, 27, 32, 33; in economic depression, 43–44, 45; and Flexner, 33, 34, 240; health, 122; help to brothers, 17–18, 35; medical career of, 46, 51; as paterfamilias, 13–14; as teacher, 40; at work in youth, 12

Flexner, James Thomas (nephew), 5, 44, 136

Flexner, Jean (daughter): abroad, 60; birth, 52; at Cambridge University, 119–20; closeness to father, 52, 306; and family crisis, 209; marriage, 209–10; as McCarthy investigation subject, 303; political activism, 177, 264; separation from father, 62, 90, 107–8; and sister, 62–63; at Tyringham Valley house, 82; visits to mother, 296–97; in Washington, 263

Flexner, Mary (sister), 8, 35, 37, 40, 44, 296

Flexner, Morris (father), 1–8, 11–12, 13, 18

Flexner, Simon (brother), 178–79; birth, 6; closeness to Flexner, 178–79, 296; consultation with Flexner, 210, 240–41, 246, 252, 285; death, 296; and doctor title confusion, 124; as Eastman professor, 219; in economic depression, 44; and European medical report, 99; in family conferences, 121–22; and Flexner report, 69, 76, 81, 82; on Flexner's autobiography, 291; on Flexner's departure from General Education Board, 218; guidance from, 54, 55, 63; and Johns Hopkins report, 101, 105; medical education, 32–34; and prostitution report, 107; and refugee placement, 265; retirement, 263; at Rockefeller Institute for Medical Research, 51, 58, 73, 100, 148, 173, 178, 238; support from, 220; traits, 14, 46; as Welch assistant, 44–45; at work in youth, 12, 18, 27

Flexner, Washington (brother), 8, 12, 26, 35, 43–44, 122, 265

Flexner family, success of, 1, 51, 178–79, 279

Flexner report, xiii–xiv, xv; acknowledged but unread, 292; and Canadian medical schools, 77; codification of medical education essentials, 83; initial reports, 75; in medical education reform, 85–87; methodology of, 76–77, 78–79; phases of, 74; publication of, 78; reactions to, 69–70, 87–89; repercussions from, 72; travel involved, 77–78; and Washington University, 80–81; writing of, 81–83

Flexner School: family members as teachers, 35, 36, 40, 44; Flexner's learning from, 55, 83; inception, 36–38; learning strategies, 39–40; sale of, 54–55

Fogg Museum of Art, 199

Fosdick, Harry Emerson, 140

Fosdick, Raymond: and conflict among Rockefeller boards, 203, 204, 208, 209; and Flexner, 139, 140, 141, 174, 178, 222, 240; on Iowa grant debate, 169; and peace proposal, 201–2; as Rockefeller Foundation president, 277–78

Fox, Daniel, 180

Frankfurter, Felix: and Bernard Flexner, 179, 241; as Eastman professor, 219; and Flexner, 246, 250, 290; on disinterested scholar, 242; on Institute for Advanced Study board, xvii, 269–71, 272, 281; and law schools, 172

Franklin, Fabian, 23, 293–94

Franks, Oliver, 302

French medical education, 96, 184–85, 186

Friedenwald, Harry, 25

Friedenwald, Julius, 25, 239

Froebel, Friedrich, 29

Fuld, Caroline, 233–34, 237, 257, 280

full-time teaching principle, 159; abandoned, 206; conflict over, 172–73; and Flexner, 145–46, 159–60, 171, 207; as General Education Board policy, 159; and Harvard Medical School, 154–55, 160; at Johns Hopkins, 105–6, 147; and Meharry Medical College, 222; as model, 159; opposition to, 150–51, 157–58, 207; public reaction to, 207; at Rochester, 167; as suppression of part-time departments, 155; and

University of Chicago, 206; and Vanderbilt, 206, 222; at Washington University, 147–48, 149; weakening of programs, 223–24; at Yale, 147–48, 150
Funds and Foundations (Flexner), 299–300

Gardner, John, 299, 305–6, 307
Garfield, James, 15
Gary plan, 125–26; controversy over, 127–29; discussion of, 126; New York City demonstration, 126–29; praise for, 130
Gasser, Herbert, 193
Gates, Frederick T., 116; on African American education, 118; and clinical medicine, 100–102; departure of, 172; and Flexner, xvii, 107, 112–13, 114, 122, 123, 140, 178, 207, 290, 291, 306; and Flexner report, 69; and full-time plan, 145, 146; and Harper, 156; and Iowa City school project, 169, 170; and Johns Hopkins report, 103–4, 105–6; and philanthropy, 116; praise for *A Modern School*, 138; proposals to, 143; retirement of, 117; and Rochester school, 166; and tax-supported school policy, 168; and teaching in America, 132; and University of Chicago medical school, 156; withdrawal from board affairs, 173
Gaynor, William Jay, 107
General Education Board: activities of, 116–17, 122–23; and archaeology, 200; attacks on, 206–7; and Cincinnati, 165; education for African Americans, 117–18; evolution of leadership, 174; as favoring science and medicine over humanities, 198; Flexner at: —arrival, 106, 113, 114; —departure from, 209, 210–12, 213; —value of, 116–17; fragmentation of, 203; and full-time teaching policy, 159; and Harvard Medical School, 152–53, 154–55; and humanities, 201; and Iowa, 168, 169; and medical education: —national system of, 161, 172; —reform grants,

146, 148–49; and Meharry Medical College, 189–90; mission of, 116; modern school project, 130–31, 132–34; plans for, 208; Presbyterian Hospital grant, 158; reorganization of, 204; revision of contracts, 206; and Rochester, 168; Rose as president, 181; and Rush Medical School, 157; termination of programs, 210; and southern high schools, 150–51; undergraduate programs deemphasis, 197; and Vanderbilt, 163, 164; work ending, 181–82, 203; written history, 117, 123. *See also* Rockefeller Foundation
German education, 21, 58–61, 73, 87
German-Jewish immigrants, 1–2
German medical education, 97–98, 184–85, 186
Germany, 58–61, 91, 182, 221, 249
Gildersleeve, Basil, 23, 273
Gilman, Daniel Coit: and Flexner, 23–24, 27, 35, 277, 279, 289, 291, 293–94; plans for Johns Hopkins, 21; succeeded by Remsen at Johns Hopkins, 67; vision of education, 61, 236, 294; wisdom of, 252
Godkin, E.A., 15
Gödl, Kurt, 266
Goldman, Hetty, 274, 283
Goodnow, Frank J., 197
graduate programs, 65–66, 122, 195–96, 240, 259
Great Depression, 264, 268, 278
Greene, Jerome, 151, 152
Gregg, Alan, 141, 172, 205, 206, 207, 300
Groton School survey, 139–40
Guerard, Albert, 232

Haber, Fritz, 182
Haldane, Richard, 93, 94, 95, 216
Hale, Ellery, 246–47
Halévy, Elie, 215
Hall, G. Stanley, 24
Halsted, William S., 102, 142, 147
Hampton Institute, 118

Hardin, John, 285
Harding, Warren, 183
Harkness, Edward, 158, 159, 190
Harper, William Rainey, 156
Harrison, Benjamin, 30
Hart, Albert Bushnell, 231–32
Harvard, 54, 55–58, 139, 199, 206, 222–23, 231
Harvard Medical School, 151–56, 160
Harvey, A. McGehee, 160
Haskins, Caryl, 301
Hawkins, Hugh, 23
Heady, Morrison, 15
Hegan, Alice, 53
Heidelberg, 61
Herbart, Johann Friedrich, 29
Herzfield, Ernst, 274
Hess, Alfred, 91
Heuer, George, 165
Highet, Gilbert, 86, 303–4
Hill, Bert Hodge, 201
Hind, Florence, 180
His, Wilhelm, 187
Hitler, Adolf, 221, 251, 254, 266–67, 268
Hoffman, Paul, 299
Holmes, Oliver Wendell, 244
homeopathic colleges, 71
homework, 39
honors, 305–6
Hoover, Herbert, 266–67, 305
Hotel Adams suite, 297
Houghton, Alanson, 182, 221, 239, 286, 287
Howard University: absorption of trainees, 191; and AMA standards, 150, 188–91; bookkeeping questions, 261–62; difficulty retaining white teachers, 190; Flexner as board member, 260–62; Flexner's appraisal of, 71; needs of, 222; support of, 87, 162
Howland, Charles P., 136
Howland, John, 147, 148
Hubble, Edwin, 215
Hull, Cordell, 253, 295
humanities, 133, 197–200, 219–20, 228–29, 243–44, 252, 273–74, 300–301

Hurt, Ashley B., 16
Hutchins, Robert Maynard, 231
Huxley, T.H., 10, 13, 41
Hylan, John F., 128

Ickes, Harold, 261, 262
immigrants, 1–2, 3–4
individual teaching, importance of, 39, 187
inductive teaching, 186
Institute for Advanced Study: academic politics, 279, 282, 288; Aydelotte on board, 198; faculty: —life/staffing, 240–41, 247–52, 257, 273–74; —self-government, 245, 248, 275–76, 283, 284–85, 288; finances, 239–40, 257, 262, 270–71, 272, 273–74, 280–81; first year of operation, 256; and Flexner: —focus on, xviii, —as founder, 1, 36, 187, 212; —retirement of, xi, 284, 285–87; —successor, 268–69, 283, 285–86, 287; Frankfurter forced off board, xvii; management of, 238, 257–59, 288; negotiations to create, 234–35; opening, 252–53; as place of undirected learning, 279; planning, 237–38, 241–47, 251–52; as postdoctoral institution, 252; power struggles/tensions, 270–71, 272–73, 275; and the press, 249–50; Princeton location, 238–39; recruitment of American scholars, 251; refugee placement in, 265; salaries, 246, 259, 270–71, 275, 281; School of Economics and Politics, 269–72, 273, 280–81, 282, 284; School of Humanistic Studies, 273–74; School of Mathematics, 241, 245–46, 247–48, 249–50, 251, 275, 280, 282–83; similar endeavors, 287; success of, 276; trustees, 239, 269–70, 284
Insull, Samuel, 179
International Education Board, 181, 201, 203
International Health Board, 173, 181, 203–4, 208

Introduction to the Study of Experimental Medicine (Bernard), 200
I Remember (Flexner), 290–92

James, William, 57
Jameson, J. Franklin, 23, 244
Janeway, Theodore C., 147, 160
Jefferson Medical College, 34
Jessup, Walter, 168–69
Jewish medical college, proposal for Newark, 233–34
Jews: in American intellectual life, 11; at Bryn Mawr College, 35; in Europe after First World War, 179; homeland for, in Palestine, 179; in Institute for Advanced Study, 239; marrying outside faith, 51; and Nazi Germany 249; —refugees from, 265; —sympathy for cause of, 254
Johns Hopkins University, 20–21; brother Simon's education at, 33–34; emphasis on graduate over undergraduate programs, 196–97; in Flexner report, 79, 101–6; Flexner's choice of, 18; and full-time principle, 105–6, 147; under Gilman, 23–24; grants to, 146, 149; group system, 22; high standards of, 73; as humanistic environment for physicians, 199; Institute of the History of Medicine, 222; as model, 156, 157; pathology studies, 32–33, 34; recruitment efforts, 98; reforms begun at, 97; School of Medicine, 88; student housing, 21
Johnson, Mordecai W., 261
Johnston, Virginius D., 261, 262
Jones, Thomas: death, 304; and Flexner, 176, 216, 221, 225, 240, 242, 298, 299, 302; and Nazism, 266, 267
Jordan, David Starr, 67
Judson, Harry Pratt, 156–57
Just, Ernest E., 191, 261

Kaiser Wilhelm Institute, 182
Kansas Medical College, 79

Kelly, Howard, 176
Kennan, George, 298, 303
Kennedy, Joseph P., 267
Kentucky bluegrass region, 6
Kerr, Clark, 226, 227
Kerr, Philip, 217
Keynes, John Maynard, xvi, 176, 268
Kirby, Morris, 27, 28
Kirkland, James H., 80, 162–64, 176
Ku Klux Klan, 8

laboratory movement, 83–84
La Guardia, Fiorello, 264
laissez-faire economy, 260, 268
Lake Ahmic resort, 162, 176, 218, 263, 297, 299, 306
Lambert, Samuel, 158
Laski, Harold, 17, 264
Laue, Max von, 266
Laura Spelman Rockefeller Memorial Fund, 173, 201, 203, 204, 208
Lawrenceburg, Kentucky, 6, 7
Lehmann, Herbert H., 179, 239, 265
Leidesdorf, Samuel D., 234, 284
Levene, Phoebus, 225
Lewinson, Jean. *See* Flexner, Jean (daughter)
Lewinson, Paul, 209–10, 297
Lewis, Thomas, 277
Lincoln School, 134–35; anti-amalgamation campaign, 290; criticism of, 136–37; Flexner's association with, xviii; influences from, xii, 135; lessons applied to, 36; students, 135–36, 177
Lindbergh, Anne Morrow, 277
Lindbergh, Charles, 225, 294
Lloyd George, David, 267
Loeb, Jacques, 11
Louisville: African American conditions in, 9; Author's Club, 53; bicycling, 50; German-Jewish immigrants in, 1–2; Jewish community in, 4–5, 19; library, 15; Male High School, 16–17, 23, 27–28; separation of Jews and gentiles in, 8
Louvre, 222

Lowe, E.A., 217, 274, 289
Lowell, A. Lawrence, xvii, 98–99, 138, 139,
    152–53, 154, 224, 236
Lowes, John Livingston, 219, 239
Ludmerer, Kenneth, xviii, 72, 83

Maass, Herbert H., 234, 276, 284, 286
MacInnes, Helen, 303
Mack, Julian W., 253
Madariago, Salvador de, 303
Mall, Franklin: and European medical
    report, 99, 259; and Flexner, 76, 91–92,
    291; and Flexner report, 76, 81, 82; and
    Johns Hopkins report, 101, 102, 103
"Man's Woman, A" (Anne Flexner), 52–53
Marriage Game, The (drama), 120
Marshall, Louis, 179
Marx, Karl, 177
Maryland education survey, 123–25
Mason, A.E.W., 52
Massachusetts General Hospital, 153–54,
    223
mathematics studies, 21–22, 38, 42–43, 64,
    135, 136
Maxwell, William H., 127
McCarthy, Joseph, 303
McCormick, William, 93, 95
McCracken, John Henry, 232
McIntyre, Marvin, 254
McLean, Franklin, 223
medical education: admission require-
    ments, 71–72, 85–86; for African
    Americans, 71, 87, 162, 188–93; classical
    studies as preparation, 99; clinical
    professor hiring standards, 84;
    comparative study of, 184–88, 292;
    costs of, 85–86; English physician
    training, 92–96; hands-on training,
    83–84; major Western systems of,
    185–86; on modern basis, 160–61;
    national system of, 160–61; number of
    schools, 70; premedical student
    preparation, 72–73; profit motive in,
    72, 85, 96, 103, 155–56; progress in U.S.,
    185; reconstruction process, 79–80;

southern schools, 161–65; standards for,
    74–75; surveys of, 224; typical school
    conditions, 70–71, 73–74; for women,
    71, 87, 119. See also education
Medical Education: A Comparative Study
    (Flexner), 185
medical education reform: beginnings of,
    70, 71; Flexner on, 43, 85–87; at Johns
    Hopkins, 97, 103–6; through philan-
    thropy, 144–45, 160, 170–72; special
    program for, 142–43; at University
    of Cincinnati, 164–65; at Vanderbilt,
    162–64
medical fellowships, 139, 190–91, 193, 194
Medical Sciences in the German University,
    The (Billroth), 76, 200
Mees, C. Leo, 16
Meharry Medical College: absorption of
    trainees, 191; and AMA standards, 150,
    188–91; difficulty retaining white
    teachers, 190; fellowships for graduates,
    192; Flexner's appraisal of, 71; and full-
    time plan, 222; fund raising for, 290;
    Mullowney as president, 189; needs of,
    222; support of, 87, 162, 219
Mellon, Paul, 299, 300–301
Memphis College of Physicians and
    Surgeons, 79
Menuhin, Yehudi, 221
Meritt, Benjamin, 273, 288–89, 295, 299,
    302
Metchnikoff, Elie, 97
Millikan, Robert, 215, 246–47, 256
Mitchel, John Purroy, 126, 127–28, 129
Mitchell, Wesley, 219
Mitrany, David, 270, 272, 282
Modern School, A (Flexner), 134, 137
"modern school" project, 130–31, 132–34
Morey, Charles R., 243, 273, 274
Morgan, Hugh, 193
Morgan, J.P., xvii
Morgan, John Hunt, 247
Morgan, Thomas Hunt, 246–47
Morris, Charles D'Urban, 22
Morris, Henry, 94

Morse, Marston, 262–63, 283
Moses, Adolph G., 15
Mrs. Wiggs of the Cabbage Patch (drama),
    53–54, 58, 120, 175
Müller, Friedrich von, 91–92, 182
Mullowney, John J., 189–90, 192
Münsterberg, Hugo, 54, 56, 57, 58, 75
Murray, Gilbert, 137, 216
Mussolini, Benito, 183, 267

Nazis: appeasement of, 267; bounty on
    Einstein, 253; Flexner on, 265, 266–67;
    refugees from, 248, 264–66, 276; rise
    of, 266–67
Nevins, Allan, 176, 292–93, 298–303,
    306–7
Nevins, Mary, 299
New Deal, 264, 268
Newman, George, 184
New York City, 58, 62, 106–7, 126–29
New York Hospital, 171
Noether, Emily, 266

O'Brien, John, 254
occupational training, 195, 227, 228
Ochs, Adolph, 11
Opie, Eugene L., 148
Oppenheimer, J. Robert, 181, 302
Oriental Institute, 200, 274
Orthodox Judaism, 2, 10
Osler, William, 93, 100, 104, 113, 164
osteopathic schools, 71
Oxford University: All Souls College, 242,
    244; American Studies professorship,
    167, 219; Flexner as lecturer at, 211–12,
    214–18; Taylorian lecture, 218, 219

Page, Walter Hines, 23
Panofsky, Erwin, 273, 286, 289
Paris, 96
Pasteur Institute, 96–97
Pauli, Wolfgang, 266
Paulsen, Friedrich, 59–60
Peabody, Endicott, 139–40
Peabody, Francis, 206

peace, promoting, 201–2
Pearce, Richard M., 173, 181–82, 206, 222
Pearl Harbor, 229, 295
Perkins, Frances, 267
Pershing, John J., 112
Pestalozzi, Johann Heinrich, 29
pharmacy schools survey, 122
philanthropy: best use of, 116; of Eastman,
    166; Flexner on, 260, 299; for human-
    istic studies, 300–301; for medical
    education, 73; private aid to tax-
    supported schools, 168, 169, 170;
    prominent organizations, 173; of
    Rockefeller organizations, 100; special
    projects donations, 278. *See also*
    individual foundations
Pirquet, Clemens von, 98
politics: after Civil War, 8; education
    reform independent of, 42; Einstein
    used as symbol, 254–55; electoral
    reform, 30; in Europe, 183; study of, 252
Poll, Heinrich, 182, 184, 220, 266
Pound, Roscoe, 172
prejudice, 24. *See also* anti-Semitism
Presbyterian Hospital, 158–59
Princeton, New Jersey: and anti-Semitism,
    238, 255, 283; location of Institute for
    Advanced Study at, 238–39, 274
Princeton, 268, 282; recruitment from,
    250, 251
Pritchett, Eva, 293
Pritchett, Henry S.: agreement with *The*
    American College, 63; and European
    medical report, 92, 99; and Flexner,
    66–68, 75–76, 113, 122, 187–88, 194,
    207, 226, 277, 291, 293, 305–6; and
    Flexner report, 69, 73–74, 79, 80, 82,
    87–89, 98; and full-time principle,
    159–60; and Iowa City school project,
    169; and Johns Hopkins report, 102; as
    mediator, 151; and philanthropy, 116,
    144, 164, 165; and prostitution report,
    107, 110; and Rochester school,
    167–68; and Washington University,
    81; withdrawal from activity, 173

Progressive Education Association, 126–27, 135

progressive education movement, 42, 83, 135, 229

prostitution report, 106–7; conclusions, 108–9, 111–12; in Europe, 107–12; informants, 109–10

psychology, 24, 29, 60

Public Works Administration, 261–63

Quinland, William S., 190–91

Rappleye, Willard, 224

Reform Judaism, 9–10

Remsen, Ira, 23, 67, 104

Rhees, Rush, 166, 167, 223–24

Rhodes Trust, 219

Richards, Alfred N., 223

Riefler, Winfield, 270–71, 272, 281, 286, 289

Rise of American Civilization (Beard & Beard), 244

Rivers, Tom, 225

Robinson, G. Canby, 164, 206, 224

Robinson, James Harvey, 133, 245

Rockefeller, John D.: biography of, 292; and Flexner, xvii, 291; and Harper, 156; and Lincoln School, xii; philanthropy of, 73, 143, 144, 160–61, 165

Rockefeller, John D., Jr.: assignments from, 100; and Chicago medical school, 156; and conflict among Rockefeller boards, 203, 204; and Flexner, xvii, 112, 114, 122, 123, 178, 181, 210, 213, 220, 291; and Gary plan, 126, 127, 128–29; and medical education in New York, 158; proposals to, 201–2, 221–22; and prostitution report, 106–7, 110; and teaching in America, 131–32; withdrawal from activity, 173

Rockefeller, Nelson, 201–2

Rockefeller Foundation: creating university medical center in London, 95; English grants, 185; Flexner's influence, 146; Fosdick as president,

277–78; grants from, 144; and Iowa, 168; medical teaching fellowships, 193; Presbyterian Hospital grant, 158; and Rush Medical School, 157; Vincent as president, 123. *See also* General Education Board

Rockefeller Institute for Medical Research, 73, 148, 173, 238

Rockefeller organizations: anti-Flexner sentiment, 205–8; confused boundaries among, 202–3; reorganization of, 203–5, 208–9, 210

Roosevelt, Eleanor, 267

Roosevelt, Franklin D., xvii, 254, 264, 266–67, 268, 294–95, 298

Roosevelt, Theodore, 16, 53

Rose, Wickliffe: and Flexner, 181–82, 197, 218; as General Education Board head, 174; peace quest, 201–2; retirement of, 209; in Rockefeller organization, 173, 208

Rosenwald, Julius: fellowships of, 190–92; and Flexner, xvii, 214, 225, 240; Flexner's proposals to, 156–57, 200, 222; and refugee placement, 265

Rousseau, Jean-Jacques, 29

Royal Commission on University Education in London, 92, 93, 94–95

Royce, Josiah, 23, 54, 56–57

Ruml, Beardsley, 203, 204

Rush Medical School, 156, 157, 231

Rusk, Dean, 299, 300, 306

Russell, Bertrand, 276

Russia, 183

Sabin, Florence, 239

salaries, 100, 124, 228, 246, 259, 270–71, 275, 281

Sarton, George, 244, 301

Schrödinger, Erwin, 251, 263

Schumpeter, Joseph, 243

science: in Austrian medicine, 97; in curriculum, 73, 131; and medical training, 93–94, 95–96, 100; union with medicine, 83–84

Second World War, 229, 268, 294–96
Semple, Ellen, 15
Semple, Patty, 15
seniority: in English hospitals, 93–94; *vs.* merit at Harvard, 98
sex education, lacking in Europe, 109
Shafer, Robert, 231
Shaffer, Philip A., 148
Sigerist, Henry, 223, 277, 295
Simmel, George, 60
Simon, John, 221
Smuts, Jan, 215
social class system, in England, 96
Socialism, 183, 303
Southwestern Homeopathic Medical College, 75–76
Soviet Union, 261, 303
Spencer, Herbert, 10
Staley, Frank S., 203
Starling, Ernst, 184
Starr, Louis, 298
Stern, Beatrice, 275
Stevenson, Adlai, 303
Stewart, Walter, 269, 280–81, 286, 289
stock market collapse, 240
Stokes, Anson Phelps, 80, 207
Story, William E., 22
Straus, Percy, 259, 273
Strickland, William, 176
student governments, Flexner on, 227
Stumpf, Karl, 60
Sutton, Carrie J., 191
Swarthmore College, 178, 198, 232, 260

Tammany Hall, 106–7, 127–28, 129
Tawney, R.H., 177
teachers: clinical training, 191–93; in Flexner ancestry, 2–3; shortage in humanities, 199; white, at Meharry Medical College, 190
Terry, Robert J., 148
Thayer, William, 104, 154
theater, 48–49, 52–54, 57–58, 120, 175, 298
Thomas, M. Carey, 95, 119, 277
Thwing, Charles, 171

Toscanini, Arturo, 298
Toynbee, Arnold, 242
Tulane University, 161, 162, 222
Turner, Frederick Jackson, 23
Tuskegee Institute, 118
Tyringham Valley house, 82, 99

undergraduate programs, 65–66, 196–97
Union Gospel Mission, 35
Universities: American, English, German (Flexner), 227–30, 233; basis in Oxford lectures, 217; as boost to Flexner's reputation, 233; debate over, 227, 230–32; Dewey review, 232–33; planning stage, 220; praise for, 244; publication, 230; on term "university," 240; writing of, 225–27
University in Exile, 265
University of Chicago: and archaeology, 200; emphasis on graduate over undergraduate programs, 196–97; and full-time plan, 206; grants to, 146; modern medical school creation at, 156–58; physician training at, 230–31
University of Cincinnati, 164–65
University of Colorado, 171
University of Georgia, 161, 162
University of Iowa, 165, 168–71
University of Louisville, 17, 33
University of Maine, 79
University of Michigan, 199
University of Oregon, 171
University of Pennsylvania, 171
University of Rochester, xiii, 165–68, 206, 223–24
University of Tennessee, Memphis, 161
University of Texas, Galveston, 161–62
Untermeyer, Samuel, 254
Upjohn, Everard, 298

Vanderbilt University: Flexner's advice to, 80; and full-time plan, 206, 222; grants to, 146, 163; medical school restructuring, 162–64
Vaughan, Victor, 190

Veblen, Oswald: on anti-Semitic climate at Princeton, 283; and Aydelotte, 302; and Flexner, 250–51, 252, 262–63, 275, 285, 289, 290; at Institute for Advanced Study, 247–48, 257, 258, 269, 272–73, 282, 284, 285–86; and refugee placement, 265; and salary issues, 271; 281; and Weyl, 249

Veblen, Thorstein, 248

venereal disease, 109, 112

Versailles Treaty, 183, 266

Vincent, George E.: for administrative reform, 203–4, 208; and Flexner, 137, 240; on full-time teaching, 207; and Germany after First World War, 182; and Iowa grant, 169; in Rockefeller Foundation, 123

vocationalism, Flexner warns of, 278

von Neumann, John, 251, 253, 288–89, 299, 302

Wallas, Graham, 177, 242

Warburg, Felix M., 179, 253

Warburg, Paul, 244

Warren, Robert B., 280–81, 289

Washington University: Flexner's advice to, 80–81; and full-time principle, 147–48, 149; grants to, 146, 149; reorganization of, 148

Wasson, Gordon, 301

Waterman, Alan, 300

Watterson, Henry, 53

Webb, Sidney, 177

Weed, Lewis, 187, 199, 223, 239, 271

Weiskotten, H.G., 305

Welch, William Henry: centennial birth celebration, 302; clinical situation in Baltimore, 100–102; and Flexner, 278, 279, 291, 306; on Flexner report, 88; grants to, 147; Institute for the History of Medicine at Johns Hopkins, 222; and Johns Hopkins report, 103, 104–5; retirement of, 199, 223; on Rosenwald fellowship committee, 190; as Simon Flexner's professor, 32–34, 76; on St. Louis reforms, 149

West, Andrew F., 137

Western Reserve School of Medicine, 171, 192

Weyl, Hermann, 249, 250–51, 252, 281, 286, 289

Wheatley, Steven, xviii, 116, 155, 208, 213

Whipple, George H., xiii, 167

Wilbur, Ray Lyman, 172, 224

Williams, J. Whitridge, 147

Wilson, Woodrow, 23, 118–19, 121, 183

Winternitz, Milton C., 147, 149–50, 206, 223, 300

Wirt, William A., 125–26, 129, 130

Wise, Isaac M., 10

Wise, Stephen S., 254

women: equality in education, 119–20; medical education for, 71, 87, 119; in Rosenwald fellowship, 191

women's suffrage, 121

Woodward, E.L., 176, 216, 242–43, 299

Yale, 146, 147–48, 149–50, 199, 231

Zimbalist, Efrem, 176, 299

Zinsser, Hans, 206–7, 224, 292

Zionism, 179